The Image of God, Personhood and the Embryo

The Image of God, Personhood and the Embryo

Calum MacKellar

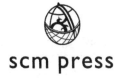

scm press

First published in 2017 by SCM Press
Editorial office
3rd Floor, Invicta House,
108–114 Golden Lane,
London EC1Y 0TG

SCM Press is an imprint of Hymns Ancient & Modern Ltd
(a registered charity)

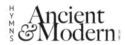

Hymns Ancient & Modern® is a registered trademark
13A Hellesdon Park Road, Norwich,
Norfolk, NR6 5DR, UK

www.scmpress.co.uk

British Library Cataloguing in Publication data

A catalogue record for this book is available
from the British Library

978 0 334 05521 1

Typeset by Regent Typesetting
Printed and bound in Great Britain by
CPI Group (UK) Ltd, Croydon

Contents

Preface

I was encouraged to write this book because a specific and detailed examination of how the image of God may be reflected in the embryo seemed to be missing from the accumulated heritage of Christian study.

A lot had already been written, over the past decades, concerning the moral status of the human embryo. Even more had been published, over the past centuries, concerning the image of God in humankind. Surprisingly, however, the combination of these two great themes had not resulted in any significant volume of literature. This is interesting since, from a Christian perspective, any discussion relating to the moral status of the human embryo cannot be dissociated or separated from a consideration of how the image of God may be reflected in this embryo. For example, the Church of England ethicist Brendan McCarthy writes:

> This concept of the dignity and status of humans being fundamentally determined by the image of God is an important one in our attempt to evaluate the human embryo. If it can be demonstrated that the image is to be found in the human embryo, then any destruction of it or experimentation on it ought to be opposed.[1]

My hope, therefore, is that this study will be a useful tool for readers wanting to know more about a topic that has challenged both society and the Christian Church.

Indeed, it may be suggested that, because of the discomfort associated with any appropriate discussions relating to the moral status of embryos, this subject matter may have been put aside or even avoided. It has become somewhat taboo, including in local church situations, and may unfortunately only seldom be addressed.

This may have happened in order to show appropriate compassion and sensitivity towards those affected by the very difficult experiences of infertility, miscarriage and abortion with all the very deep suffering generally associated with such occurrences.

But this may also mean that many parishioners are being singularly deprived of any guidance about how to consider and regard the human embryo. The situation may have been compounded by pastors themselves feeling (1) often unqualified from a theological and scientific perspective to address such a subject or (2) unprepared to speak to their congregations on a deeply moral issue out of an understandable fear of causing deep upset to, or even alienating, some church members. Regrettably, this silence may, at the same time, have led many Christians to resemble the Israelites in the time of the Judges when 'everyone did as they saw fit' (Judg. 17.6).

The American theologian and bioethicist John Kilner argues that the silence and inaction of most churches in this arena is distressing.[2] Similarly, the American politician and Christian leader Charles Colson (1931–2012) and the Scottish-American theologian Nigel Cameron are concerned that churches are 'sleeping through another moral catastrophe … [for which] our churches are ill-prepared'.[3] Living a life in a context of love and self-sacrifice to God, thereby expressing a form of praise to God, has often been relegated to the responsibility of other generations.

I also wrote this book because I had become particularly aware of the dearth of theological material relating to the destructive embryonic research procedures currently being developed. These had indeed been considered by the 30-member Church and Society Council of the Church of Scotland during its 2005–6 discussions on the matter. I had been a member of this council from 2005 to 2013 having been an elder of this church since 1998.

The Protestant Church of Scotland is one of a very few Reformed and Presbyterian national churches in the world, and the Church and Society Council was responsible for preparing all the reports concerning societal issues, including those on biomedical ethics, for this church's General Assembly. This is the sovereign and highest court of the Church of Scotland which, since 1560, has usually met for one week every year to guide and govern its members.

When the General Assembly of 2006 agreed to debate the moral consequences of destructive embryological research from a theological perspective, I became increasingly concerned that it seemed to be doing so without any thorough or robust grounding. This was especially the case relating both to a theological understanding of the image of God and to current developments in embryology. Unfortunately, this shortage of appropriate resources became a real handicap at the time of the discussions.

The scarcity of appropriate material was only redressed somewhat when I became aware, some years later, of an excellent Master's degree thesis which sought to address the topic of the moral status of the human embryo from a Protestant theological perspective. This document, 'The incarnation and the status of the human embryo', had been written by the Rev. Andrew Rollinson who is a Baptist pastor and zoology graduate. It had been submitted in 1994 to the Religious Studies Department of the University of Newcastle upon Tyne in the UK, a town in which Andrew Rollinson was ministering at the time.

Concerned by the realization that this valuable manuscript might not be used by future readers, I eventually contacted Andrew Rollinson to ask whether he would agree to his thesis, and especially the sections relating to the incarnation and the image of God, being used in the preparation of a new book about how the image of God can be reflected in the embryo. To this he kindly agreed. As a result, it is impossible to express my indebtedness to the Rev. Andrew Rollinson for letting me use the original basis of his thesis in the preparation of this book.

In reading this work, it will become clear that the volume is distinctive from a number of other perspectives. First, the contents are considerably influenced by Scottish Protestant churches and theologians. This is especially the case with respect to the theology of the Very Rev. Prof. Dr Thomas F. Torrance (1913–2007), who was a minister of the Church of Scotland, Professor of Christian Dogmatics at the University of Edinburgh, Moderator of the General Assembly of the Church of Scotland from 1976 to 1977 and the 1978 Templeton Prize winner for progress in religion. Indeed, I would like to very much recognize, in this book, T. F. Torrance's past work in theological ethics.

Second, because it would be impossible to do justice to the manner in which the image of God can be reflected in the human embryo without studying the very rich arguments coming from other Christian denominations, such as the Roman Catholic and Orthodox Churches, this volume is intentionally ecumenical.

Third, the book does not represent a study on the image of God, as such, since many publications have already addressed this complex matter. Instead, it seeks to examine the manner in which the image of God may be considered and articulated in the specific case of the human embryo.

It is also essential for the volume to begin with a certain amount of careful preparation with respect to notions of personhood and human dignity. For example, when the important themes of being a person and the image of God are considered, the work will demonstrate that an intrinsic convergence of ideas takes place which plots a way forward in understanding the moral status of the human embryo.

Moreover, all too often this status has been reduced to being examined from just a human or worldly perspective, thereby limiting any appropriate understanding of the embryo's true nature. This is in contrast to seeking to appreciate the moral status of embryos from a more comprehensive theological (and Godly) perspective while recognizing that this may not always be achievable.

At the same time, the book does not only examine aspects of the image of God which are already well developed in theology, such as substantive, functional and relational aspects, but investigates relatively new angles, such as the way the incarnation and the creation of humankind by God are important for this image. In more specific terms, these last two themes may be more relevant to understanding the true value and worth of human embryos because they enable them to be seen as being created from God's love while also being destined to remain in this love for all eternity.

This means that an embryo's existence on earth, and the manner in which it is considered by human persons in society, is but a very short period in time compared to its overall existence in eternity.

Of course, this is the same for all human beings. The real meaning of humankind's creation can only be understood in fellowship with the eternal God and not just through the lens or context of human life on earth, including physical aspects such as size or functionality. What is far more important is the emphasis that human embryos exist before God as living wholes – whole persons whom he loves.

In preparing this book, I also sought to examine all the scientific, philosophical and theological arguments which became the basis, a number of decades ago, for many legislations in the UK and elsewhere. From this perspective it was interesting to note that, though many arguments had now moved on, old legislation had, unfortunately, remained unchanged.

This new study was written, therefore, to help the conversation in society move forward while being informed by the latest scientific developments including, for example, the 2008 discussions which occurred in the UK on the moral status of human–nonhuman interspecies chimeric and hybrid embryos. Because new dilemmas arose in these discussions in seeking to determine whether the image of God is even reflected in such living entities, fresh insights were studied which were later used to develop a better understanding of the moral status of completely human embryos.[4]

Inevitably, of course, some Christians will reach different conclusions from the ones presented in this book. But if the claims being made are correct and embryonic human lives can be considered as being made in the image of God, then the deliberate destruction of these countless embryos represents the deliberate destruction of those whom God loves very deeply.

Finally, I should indicate that a significant amount of embryological science will, initially, be presented in lay language in order to address and explain some of the arguments being made.

In the text itself, repetition of some of the information being presented may also take place in order to emphasize certain ideas while enabling readers to study certain chapters and follow the arguments without having to go back to earlier sections. Moreover, a large number of quotations are presented in order to do justice to the very careful wording of the authors being mentioned in addressing some of the complex and very precise theological arguments.

Calum MacKellar
Edinburgh 2017

Notes

1 Brendan McCarthy, 1997, *Fertility & Faith*, Leicester: InterVarsity Press, pp. 126–7.

2 John F. Kilner, 2015, *Dignity and Destiny: Humanity in the Image of God*, Grand Rapids: Eerdmans, p. 327.

3 Charles W. Colson and Nigel M. de S. Cameron (eds), 2004, *Human Dignity in the Biotech Century*, Downers Grove, IL: InterVarsity Press, pp. 20–1. For an interesting study about how Christian congregations seek to avoid addressing some of these issues, see Jennifer Baines, 'An Investigation into the Theological and Pastoral Issues Surrounding Abortion, and its Place in the Main Body of Christian Teaching and Ministry Today', MTh in Practical Theology Dissertation, Mattersey Hall in association with Bangor University, Wales.

4 Calum MacKellar and David A. Jones (eds), 2012, *Chimera's Children*, London: Continuum.

Acknowledgements

I am very grateful to the Rev. Andrew Rollinson for kindly letting me use, in the preparation of this book, his Master's thesis entitled 'The incarnation and the status of the human embryo', which was submitted in November 1994 to the Religious Studies Department of the University of Newcastle upon Tyne.

I would also like to thank Mrs Natalia Pelttari, Mrs Barbara MacKellar, the Rev. Iain MacKellar, the Rev. Prof. Dr Donald M. MacDonald and Dr David Prentice for all their help in preparing this book (though it should not necessarily be assumed that they would endorse all of its contents).

All biblical quotations are from the New International Version unless otherwise noted.

Introduction

Ever since the Christian Church came into being, ethical debates have taken place relating to the moral status of human beings, including embryos and foetuses, as well as to the manner in which they should be regarded. The very nature of human persons and how they should behave towards each other went to the very heart of these discussions.

In this context, it was natural for the early Christian thinkers to build on their Jewish roots in seeking to understand the uniqueness and special importance of humankind as arising from the reality that human beings were created in the image of God. Indeed, it is impossible to understand the moral status of human beings, either before or after birth, from a theological perspective without also examining this great and wonderful theme of the image of God.

As the influential Anglican theologian John Stott (1921–2011) wrote, 'The sanctity of human life arises from the value of God's image bearers (Genesis 9:6).'[1] Seeking to obtain a biblically accurate and theologically comprehensive perspective of this image, however, is no easy matter.

Different Understandings of the Image of God

Early church theologians and biblical scholars have always been inquisitive about what makes humanity so special in the eyes of God. Many volumes have been prepared discussing the importance and implications of the image of God in humanity. But the intermittent usage of the term 'image' in the Bible together with its origins and its development as a word with complex meanings makes any interpretation challenging. That human beings are created in the image and likeness of God is indeed only explicitly stated in three passages in the Old Testament: Genesis 1.26–28; 5.1–3; 9.6.

This has led to numerous interpretations about the manner in which human beings reflect the divine image.[2] In the Christian tradition these are generally complementary, expressing different angles, while also emphasizing the unique character of humanity. For example, the concept of the image of God has been understood to:[3]

- relate to human rationality and humankind's capacity to think, since these characteristics imitate the ultimate rationality of God;
- reflect aspects of freedom in a human person. The Syrian monk St John of Damascus (c. 675–749) wrote that, for a man, 'being after God's image signifies his capacity for understanding, and for making free decisions, and his mastery of himself';[4]
- emphasize the role of stewardship and humanity's responsibility to rule over creation in its care for the natural world;
- represent humankind's capacity to be moral and understand the concept of the existence of God;
- express the creative capacity of human beings which is the most important reflection of God the creator;
- articulate a unique status in all of creation reflecting a special kind of dignity ascribed to humanity;
- reflect the relational capacity of human beings since God is inherently relational;
- express a distinct calling in the world, which springs from a special relationship to God;
- inform human beings concerning something about God and how they can know God. It tells them that God, though completely different from his creation, communicates himself to his children in creative love, in a way that offers precious clues about who he is, including his transcendence, triune life, incarnation and intentions for human life.[5]

Of course, it is very likely that the image of God includes all these ideas and much more besides since it is a multifaceted concept. Accordingly, all these notions should be understood as being interrelated and supporting one another, instead of competing against each other, though some may be more relevant to the specific case of the human embryo than others. For example, aspects such as functional or rational characteristics, so often emphasized in the past as being necessary for the presence of the image of God, may not be so relevant to the embryo (or the adult with severe mental disability).

It is also important not simply to read into God's image whatever human traits contemporary culture values, including capacities such as reason, human virtues such as righteousness, or human functions such as rulership over creation.[6]

In contrast, the great themes of creation and incarnation and how they can be understood in the context of the image of God are far more robust in providing appropriate arguments in recognizing the status of the human embryo. It should also be noted that the themes of creation by God and of re-creation through the incarnation cannot be dissociated from each other. It is because God created, that he re-created. Similarly, there would be no incarnation without creation and no creation without the Son of God.

This book will not, therefore, have as its goal an exhaustive definition of the image of God in human beings before or after birth. This would be impossible to achieve since the very nature of the image of God reflects something in God who is outside humanity's complete understanding. Instead, this study will explore the way in which the central Christian doctrine of the image of God can inform a reflection on the moral status of the human embryo.

This will be achieved by first examining how the theology of the image of God and being a person has fundamentally shaped Christian anthropology. Further study will then be attempted to understand the image of God from five of the most relevant perspectives. These were chosen because they can either be seen as the most helpful in considering the image of God in embryos, namely from the angle of (1) the concept of creation and (2) the doctrine of the incarnation, or because they are the most common and have already been studied by scholars, as with (3) substantive, (4) relational and (5) functional perspectives.

In undertaking such a study, science and theology will also be considered as handmaids to each other. The divide which, historically, has often caused a breakdown in communication between the two disciplines will seek to be challenged while examining how this separation can be bridged. New accounts of scientific understanding relating to the human embryo will be studied while considering how this image of God can be understood. This is crucial in that the very definition of a person may be considered as any being who reflects this image. As will be explained in the different chapters, being a person and the image of God are theologically inseparable and will be discussed together in the different sections.

By examining the relevance of a central Christian doctrine for a present-day ethical dilemma, the book will also demonstrate that theological ethics has a key role in both setting a comprehensive agenda and prioritizing that agenda. It is hoped, therefore, that this volume will be a useful tool, foundation or sign-post in the complex and sensitive debates that arise.

This means that theological ethics still has a key role to play in modern society for all those who are convinced that a transcendent God is the ultimate reference point of all that exists. As the American theologian Reinhold Niebuhr (1892–1971) claimed: 'There are resources in the Christian Faith for an understanding of human nature which have been lost in modern culture.'[7]

This emphasizes the importance of taking seriously theological ethics to rediscover precepts and directions in the context of human behaviour such as in bioethics and especially the manner in which human embryos may be considered.

Notes

1 John Stott, 2006, *Through the Bible Through the Year*, Oxford: Lion Hudson, p. 18.

2 Colin Gunton, 1998, *The Triune Creator: A Historical and Systematic Study*, Grand Rapids: Eerdmans, p. 193.

3 Nathan MacDonald, 'The *Imago Dei* as Election: Reading Genesis 1:26–28 and Old Testament Scholarship with Karl Barth', *International Journal of Systematic Theology* 10:3 (2008), pp. 303–27; J. Richard Middleton, 2005, *The Liberating Image: The* Imago Dei *in Genesis 1*, Grand Rapids: Brazos; Colin E. Gunton, 1998, *The Triune Creator*.

4 Cited by Aquinas, *Summa Theologica*, 1a.93.5. In Gunton, *The Triune Creator*, p. 194.

5 Ian A. McFarland, 2005, *The Divine Image: Envisioning the Invisible God*, Minneapolis: Fortress Press.

6 John F. Kilner, 2015, *Dignity and Destiny: Humanity in the Image of God*, Grand Rapids: Eerdmans, pp. 18 and 49.

7 Reinhold Niebuhr, 1943, *The Nature and Destiny of Man*, London: Nisbet, Vol. I, Preface, p. vii.

I

The Moral Status of the Embryo

An extensive literature has developed concerning the moral status of the human embryo and this book will not be able even to begin providing an overview or summary of all the different positions and arguments.[1]

Ever since the embryo was perceived by philosophers and studied by scientists, debates have arisen concerning its moral status and the manner in which society should recognize its worth and value as well as any corresponding protection.

For example, both at the time when a number of countries were legalizing abortion and during the subsequent discussions relating to the possibility of undertaking research on embryos, fierce disputes in churches, parliaments and societies took place concerning how embryos should be considered. These usually included the question of whether it would be ethically acceptable to destroy human embryos with intent.

Once parliamentary decisions were eventually made, these debates usually became more subdued. But they continued, nonetheless, to remain on the back-burner since an ethical appreciation of the embryo in society cannot be conclusively decided through majority votes in assemblies.

It follows that, even though many commentators may be somewhat tired of all the different arguments and discussions over the decades, there is still room for new perspectives in the understanding of the moral status of the embryo – an understanding that may enable some members of society to appreciate better the different theological and scientific aspects of the debate.

At this stage it is important to first consider the very being of the embryo, what the embryo actually 'is', which must be examined from the complementary perspectives of science and theology before a society decides how it 'ought' to evaluate this being from a moral perspective. Indeed, it is only because an embryo can be recognized as a specific kind of being that it can (or ought to) be respected in a special moral manner.

But what kind of being, then, is the embryo? In this regard, it should be remembered that, from the restricted viewpoint of science, embryos (and for that matter any human being) are only collections of cells destined to become, with time, collections of dust or ashes. This means that the worth and value of an embryo cannot be demonstrated from a scientific perspective and any moral appreciation becomes impossible. It is only because of the manner in which God, the only true source of value, chooses to consider this being that it has any worth and deserves to be recognized with moral status. This is the real challenge for modern societies as they struggle to evaluate the embryo from a secular moral perspective.

Early Embryonic Developments

In investigating the history of the debate relating to the moral status of the embryo, it is necessary to begin by introducing some of the relevant scientific aspects. In this regard, it will be useful to understand both how an organism is actually characterized in science and why this is important in defining an embryo.

Defining an Organism

Before the actual process of bringing an embryo into existence is examined, it is important to first seek to comprehend why this embryo can be considered as a living organism and how this is defined. This is crucial since it is only because the embryo is an organism from a biological perspective that it can be considered as a 'whole' with all the philosophical and theological meaning that this entails.

As the word implies, an organism entails an organization of the participant, cooperative and interdependent elements in an overarching unity which forms a harmonious whole. This means that a living biological organism is an entity with an integrated, self-developing and self-maintaining organized communion which retains in both space and time a wholeness which precedes and produces its organic parts. Thus, a biological living organism is not merely a sum of biochemical reactions; it is, rather, a dynamic and ordered collection of interdependent, coherent functional cells and structures which coordinate all their integrated functions for the sake of, and from within, this whole organism.[2] This enables emergent properties to be expressed which are far more complex than their substituent intrinsic parts. In other words, a living organism must precede and be considered prior to its constitutive, organic and functional elements.

'Wholeness' in this sense represents the totality of the person; that nothing from within has been taken out and that nothing is missing from an inherent or intrinsic perspective. A 'wholeness' cannot be reduced to mere biology and it relates, as well, to the notion of individuality and 'oneness'.[3] Accordingly, an individual wholeness cannot be part of a greater whole.[4] Wholeness is also defined from the perspective of the observer and the individual whose wholeness is being considered (if he or she is self-aware).

This also means that some biological entities, such as human cadavers, cannot be considered as living organisms since they no longer function as integrated wholes even though some human cells in such entities may still be living.[5]

Already from the one-cell stage (24 hours after fertilization), the early human embryo shows all the properties of an organism. Moreover, when subsequent early cells are formed in the embryo, they all act as an integrated whole, and not separated parts of the whole, to form a multi-cellular entity of the same original organism. As such, the one-cell embryo can be accepted as the stage when the whole begins its life. It then retains, and continues in, its identity of living being, through all the stages of its development in time, as a whole living member of the species *Homo sapiens*.[6] It is a being that never loses its wholeness throughout its life.

From a scientific perspective, however, it will never be possible to determine the exact moment when this organism is brought into existence before the first one-cell embryo is formed. Science can only confirm that a one-cell embryo is already an organism and continues as an organism in its subsequent development.

What distinguishes an organism from a constituent cell is that all the parts of an organism function together in an interdependent and organized fashion in maintaining life as well as in the continued development of the organism as a whole. Individualized cells, on the other hand, do not demonstrate any higher level of properties for organization beyond the functions that they already express. A skin cell, for example, removed from a body and left to develop on its own in a laboratory, will divide and continue to live but will never be able to develop into the body from which it was removed.[7]

In addition, the development of early embryonic cells should not always be considered as the development of an embryo as such. Sometimes, embryonic cells can divide and differentiate into cancerous tumours such as teratomas which cannot be considered as organisms. Similarly, an egg from which its chromosomes are removed can sometimes begin to divide upon activation into a number of further cells. There seems to be an initial and intrinsic biological capacity for an egg to divide before coming to a stage in which it stops, but this again cannot be considered as an organism. Thus, a limited tendency for cells to organize themselves does not mean that an organism is present. As the American physician William Hurlbut explains: 'Incompletely constituted or severed from their source in which they are a natural coherent part, embryonic fragments may have a certain developmental momentum, but ultimately they become uncoordinated and disorganized growth.'[8]

This is what is so remarkable about the one-cell embryo. It is not just an individualized cell but an organism with all the intrinsic properties necessary to continue development as a whole. The organization of the one-cell embryo does not come from outside but originates from inside. A one-cell embryo is also defined as totipotent in that it can develop into all the different cells of a mature organism while, at the same time, organizing these cells into a functioning, integrated and ordered whole.[9]

According to these characteristics of an organism, scientists can reliably distinguish a multi-cellular organism, including an embryonic human being, from other amalgamations of cells which do not have the properties of an integrated whole. They can do this by carefully studying the composition and behaviour of the cells in question, as in the development of normal healthy embryos.

Normal Development of Embryos

Before considering how embryos are brought into existence through the fertilization of a human egg by a sperm cell, it may be useful, first of all, to examine how these cells are generated by the individuals concerned.

Egg and Sperm Cell Formation

The preliminary egg cells of a woman are formed during her own development as an embryo or foetus. In other words, the immature eggs develop with the woman's own foetal body and about two million of these are present in a newborn girl. Once puberty is reached, one of these preliminary eggs is then matured and released in the fallopian tubes of the woman in a monthly cycle. This means that of all the immature eggs available only about 400 mature during a woman's fertile life with the others eventually degenerating.

The formation of preliminary sperm cells in a man, in contrast, is very different since they do not exist in a newborn boy. It is only when the boy reaches puberty that he can then produce these reproductive cells which mature into functional sperm cells.

Generally, each mature sperm and egg cell contains 23 chromosomes (that is, they are haploid, from the Greek meaning 'single') which include most of the DNA inside these cells. Because of the manner in which each sperm and egg cell is produced, each one has a unique combination of different gene variations. In both the sperm and egg cells, the chromosomes are regrouped together in what is called the pronucleus (plural: pronuclei) which is surrounded by a nuclear membrane.

Fertilization and Development of the Embryo[10]

When a maturing egg of a woman is released, about every month, into her fallopian tubes it measures just about 0.1 mm in size and is surrounded by a trans-lucid membrane layer called the zona pellucida. If sperm cells are then discharged into the vagina, through a sexual relationship, they take 5 to 70 minutes to reach the egg in the fallopian tubes[11] where they can survive up to 2–3 days and fertilization becomes possible. If this happens, the following events will then occur.

The head of a sperm cell membrane binds to the zona pellucida in order to enter into the egg; this takes less than a few seconds to complete. As soon as this happens, biochemical changes take place (within the first 1–3 minutes) and the zona pellucida modifies its surface so that other sperm cells cannot get through.

Inside the fertilized egg the pronuclei of the sperm cell and of the egg are still separated and generally remain distinct and visible entities until 10 to 20 hours after fertilization; this is called the pronuclear stage. They have, by this time, duplicated their number of chromosomes in preparation for cell division in a coordinated pattern of development. Interestingly, the entire process of fertilization up to and including the pronuclear stage is believed to be reversible in humans.[12]

By approximately 20–24 hours, the two pronuclei of the egg and the sperm cell begin to come together in a gradual process and the nuclear membranes dissolve.[13] It is only at the end of this stage (called syngamy) that fertilization is considered to be complete and a one-cell embryo (called a zygote) is obtained. This one-cell embryo can no longer be compared to a fertilized egg or the sum total of a sperm and egg cell since, from a molecular perspective and its developmental behavioural pathway, it is totally new. In some countries, such as Germany, it is only when fertilization has been completed that it is recognized, in law, that a new human embryo, as such, has come into existence. It should be noted, however, that there is no actual fusion of the pronuclei at this zygotic stage in human beings to form a single clearly defined cell nucleus with 46 chromosomes since, at syngamy, the cell begins immediately to divide to form a two-cell embryo.

Significantly, the fertilization process taking place in the first 24 hours after fertilization is extremely important for the subsequent embryonic developmental stages. It is from the first moment when the sperm cell binds to the egg and during the subsequent 24 hours that the embryonic organism comes into existence, though scientists still disagree about when, precisely, this occurs.[14] However, it is generally accepted that the one-cell embryo which is obtained at the end of these 24 hours, just before cell division, is already an organism and behaves as such.[15]

After division of this one-cell (zygote) embryo, which is the end of the first cycle, a two-cell embryo is formed in which both cells now normally contain 46 chromosomes in their nucleus of which 23 come from the father and the other 23 from the mother. This means that it is only at this two-cell embryonic stage that paternal and maternal chromosomes are present together in the nucleus of each of the two cells.

Once the two-cell embryo is obtained, animal research suggests that each one of the cells of the two-cell embryo may already be slightly different in that they may be biased to develop into specific elements of the future animal body.[16]

But science shows that these early cells are relatively 'plastic' in that they can change their developmental direction without any negative consequences if they are disturbed for some reason. In addition, in normal development, all the cells from the two-cell stage onwards seem to divide and enter into distinct developmental pathways which are mutually coordinated in cell–cell interactions. By the four-cell stage of the developing embryo, there are already distinct molecular and developmental variations among the cells. At this point, if one of the cells is removed, the embryo may not always recover to normal growth, which means that the removed cell may have started to specialize in the coordinated matrix of development which is important for survival.

The subsequent normal development of the embryo in the fallopian tubes of the woman takes place with a division of the cells about every 12–36 hours without the embryo really growing in size, which means that the cells in the embryo become increasingly smaller. Unless a problem occurs, all these cells have exactly the same genetic composition. At about the eight-cell stage, the cells are seemingly arranged as a uniform structure and are only loosely associated with one another[17] though molecular differences between the cells exist.

Interestingly, it is believed that if one of these cells is removed from the eight-cell embryo it could, in appropriate circumstances, be able to develop on its own into a second embryo. Because of this, the cells are defined as totipotent, a property that is believed to be lost after the eight-cell stage in humans. Since this second embryo would have exactly the same genetic composition in its chromosomes as the first, it would be genetically identical to the first one. This is how certain forms of identical twins are believed to arise, though they are usually the result of a group of several cells detaching themselves together (not just by themselves) from an original eight-cell embryo or its earlier stages.[18]

After this point, the inner cells in the embryo are seen to divide relatively faster than the larger ones on the outside. Glue-like junctions (called desmosomes) and other strong attachments continue to be developed. These can be considered as highly specific permeable seals which form on the outer cells. Communication junctions also appear at this stage, enabling small elements to be exchanged which help to regulate the inter-actions between the embryonic cells.[19]

At the 16-cell stage the structure of the embryo (now called a morula, which is Latin for a mulberry, since it resembles such a berry) changes and some parts begin to flatten. At this point, a number of dynamic inter-actions develop between the cells, and in particular between the inner and outer cells. It is believed that when the inner cells reach a certain number the outer ones are prevented from dividing, making them spread around the more adhesive inner cells. If the number of inner cells is not sufficient for some reason, some of the cells on the outside can become inner cells until an appropriate balance is obtained. This suggests that it is the inner cells that control the fate of the cells on the outside of the embryo at a stage when their developmental potential has not yet been irreversibly fixed.[20]

Between about three and five days, when further divisions have taken place and the embryo (now called a blastocyst) reaches about the 120-cell stage, an internal fluid-filled cavity appears and two different parts are formed. The first part contains a large number of embryonic outer cells (which becomes what is called the trophectoderm). This develops pre-dominantly into extra-embryonic tissue such as protective and nutritive tissue including the placenta which enables an exchange of substance between the mother and the embryo. The second part of the embryo contains a small group of inner cells (called the inner cell mass) which eventually becomes the body of the baby itself.[21]

During this time, the embryo moves from the fallopian tubes into the uterus. At about the sixth or seventh day after fertilization, the embryo then begins to discard its zona pellucida in order to implant itself into the uterus of the mother.

Implantation is usually complete 14 days after fertilization. This 14-day stage is also when the primitive streak begins to appear from which the first rudiments of the nervous system are developed. In addition, it is the point in time when identical twins can no longer be obtained through an eventual division of the inner cell mass of the embryo.

In normal circumstances this embryo then becomes a foetus after eight weeks of gestation and is born after about 36 weeks of development.

It should be emphasized that it is now possible for scientists to fertilize an egg with a sperm cell outside the body by bringing together these reproductive cells in a glass (*in vitro*) or transparent dish through the help of a technician in a laboratory. This is called *in vitro* fertilization (IVF). The resulting embryo is then usually implanted into the woman's uterus on the second or third day after fertilization whereby, if all goes well, a normal pregnancy will develop. It is also possible, in some instances, to implant an embryo into the uterus of a woman on the fourth to seventh day after fertilization though the success rate is very much diminished.

The Moral Status of the Embryo – Historical Perspective

This section will seek to briefly summarize the manner in which the early Church sought to consider or regard the moral status of the human embryo or foetus. Such an examination has relevance not only to put present ethical discussions into their historical context but also to emphasize the reality that, already in the first centuries, the Christological and Trinitarian implications of the image of God were being carefully considered.

Trying to understand the manner in which the Church Fathers considered the moral status of the human embryo will, however, not always be easy. The American Religious Studies scholar Wayne Meeks, in his book, *The Moral World of the First Christians*, purposely sought to avoid questions such as 'What did the early Christians teach about abortion?' Among a number of reasons, he did this because 'the temptation is too great to subject the early Christians to our own agenda' and a real risk of oversimplification exists.[22]

The early Christians were called to live in a way that was very different from the reality of those around them. This meant that most Church Fathers were asked to address wider Christian ethical and moral questions such as those related to abortion and infanticide, which were very common in Greco–Roman society[23] and which they generally opposed.[24] This was reflected by the Didache, an important Christian document from the first Christian century, which states: 'You shall not kill the foetus by abortion, or destroy the infant already born.'

As a result, the moral status of the embryo and foetus, as such, was only indirectly considered by many of these early Christian scholars when discussing these practical moral questions[25] or when making theological inquiries into, for example, the origins of the soul. Moreover, at the time, no real distinction was made at the eight weeks stage after fertilization between an embryo and a foetus, such as now exists in modern biology.

Interestingly, the reasoning behind the prohibition on abortion for Christians varied,[26] and in order to understand the different theological reflections of the early Church on the topic it is necessary to note two important influences.

The first was the philosophical understanding that existed at the time relating to the status of early human embryos. A number of Church Fathers were indeed influenced by the Platonic suggestion that the body and the soul were to be considered in a dualistic manner.

The transcripts of *On the Generation of Animals*,[27] by the Greek philosopher Aristotle (384–322 BC), suggested that the early embryo went through a three-stage process. It first has a vegetative existence, animated by a nutritive soul, which develops into an animal-like embryo with a 'sensitive' soul, finally becoming a formed foetus with a rational animated soul. In Aristotelian philosophy, this final animation, from the Latin word *anima* (meaning 'soul'), occurs for the male embryo at about 40 days while the female embryo takes 90 days.[28] As a result, such a philosophical understanding of the development of the embryo was probably already present in the minds of the translators of the Hebrew Bible into Greek (the Septuagint), which then influenced patristic writings.

Another important influence, of course, was their Jewish heritage which considered abortion as contravening the will of God.

However, the exact moral status of the embryo or foetus remained ambiguous. This is especially exemplified by the different understandings of Exodus 21.22–25 and what should happen when a pregnant woman incurs an accidental injury caused by others. Interestingly, these different ways of understanding the text are also reflected in some of the English translations. For example, the English Standard Version translation of Exodus 21.22–25 (which is a good literal translation) reads:

> When men strive together and hit a pregnant woman, so that her children come out, but there is no harm, the one who hit her shall surely be fined, as the woman's husband shall impose on him, and he shall pay as the judges determine. But if there is harm, then you shall pay life for life, eye for eye, tooth for tooth, hand for hand, foot for foot, burn for burn, wound for wound, stripe for stripe.

This passage is difficult because it is unclear whether it is the foetus or the mother who is referred to as being harmed. Indeed, it can be understood in three different manners.[29] The first was influenced by Greek philosophy and the Septuagint translation of Exodus 21.22:

> And if two men are fighting and strike a pregnant woman and her infant departs not fully formed, he shall be forced to pay a fine: according to whatever the woman's husband shall lay upon him, he shall give with what is fitting. But if it is fully formed, he shall give life for life.[30]

This reflected a difference between a 'formed' and 'unformed' foetus in the context of an assault on a pregnant woman who received a mortal blow to her foetus. If the foetus was considered 'not yet formed' only a fine was demanded as a penalty. On the other hand, if the foetus was 'formed', which was understood to mean when the foetus could be recognized as having a human form, then the death penalty was demanded.[31]

As the Anglican Lord Bishop of Oxford, Richard Harries, stated in 2001 during the UK House of Lords discussion on the Church's tradition relating to the moral status of the human embryo:

> Abortion ... was always regarded as gravely sinful. But there was a distinction in the gravity of the offence depending on whether it occurred before or after the foetus was 'formed'. The distinction arose on the basis of the Septuagint translation of Exodus 21:22. That refers to a fight between two men, as a result of which a pregnant woman loses her child. If the child is in the early stages of embryonic development, then the penalty is a financial one. If it is in the later stages of pregnancy, then the penalty is death. The Greek word there literally means 'not yet so formed as to be a copy or portrayal of the human form'.[32]

But according to the former Chief Rabbi of the UK, Lord Immanuel Jakobovits (1921–99), the Septuagint translation of the Hebrew words 'if there be no accident', which, according to the earliest rabbinic scholars, are applied to the mother surviving the assault, seem to have been mistranslated as 'if it be without form'. This mistake in the Septuagint was then interpreted as exempting the attacker from the death penalty if the foetus was not yet formed with a human shape though he or she was liable to the capital punishment for any destruction of a foetus at any subsequent stage.[33]

In other words, there is no mention of the distinction between formed and unformed or stages of development, implied or otherwise. The mistake in the Septuagint was probably the result of a misunderstanding of the text or a simple mistranslation.[34] The British theologian Gordon Dunstan (1917–2004) explains that the Septuagint was the version of the Bible used most frequently by the early Christian Fathers. It was then followed by old Latin versions used in the disputes and discussions of the Western Christian Church.[35]

This means that even though abortion was always opposed, it was because of early Hellenistic Jewish influences that a significant difference was suggested between formed and unformed foetuses.

The second view used the Hebrew text of Exodus 21 to make a difference between the accidental abortion of the foetus, in which case a fine was paid, and the death of the pregnant mother, in which case the death penalty was demanded. This is reflected in the New American Standard 1977:

> And if men struggle with each other and strike a woman with child so that she has a miscarriage, yet there is no further injury, he shall surely be fined as the woman's husband may demand of him; and he shall pay

as the judges decide. But if there is any further injury, then you shall appoint as a penalty life for life.

Here the harm or the injury refers only to the woman since the foetus miscarried and died. This also means that the foetus was not considered to have the same moral status as an adult person. It is also the interpretation given by Josephus in the first century AD:

He that kicks a woman with child, so that the woman miscarry, let him pay a fine in money ... as having diminished the multitude by the destruction of what was in her womb ... but if she die of the stroke, let him also be put to death.[36]

It implies that some therapeutic abortions could be considered though intentional non-therapeutic abortions remained unacceptable. This remains the present perspective of conservative orthodox Jews for whom the full moral status of the foetus is not attained until birth.[37] Though any deliberate abortion remains a sin, it is not the sin of homicide.

There is, however, a third view which suggests that the foetus does have the same moral status as an adult person and that the harm mentioned in Exodus 21.22–25 applies to both the mother and the foetus.

The NIV translation of Exodus 21.22–23 may reflect this perspective:

If people are fighting and hit a pregnant woman and she gives birth prematurely but there is no serious injury, the offender must be fined whatever the woman's husband demands and the court allows. But if there is serious injury, you are to take life for life.

This would mean that when no serious harm is experienced by either the woman or the foetus, who is born prematurely because of the accident to the woman, there would be a fine. But if there is serious harm for either of them, then there should be 'life for life' and 'eye for eye'.[38]

Some who hold this third perspective also interpret Genesis 9.6 as saying: 'Whoever sheds human blood, ... [within other] humans shall their blood be shed', suggesting that 'human blood within other humans' is the foetus.

A good, though controversial, introduction of the manner in which the status of the embryo was considered by early Church writers can be obtained from Dunstan's very influential 1984 article 'The Moral Status of the Human Embryo: A Tradition Recalled'. In this paper he argued:

The claim to absolute protection for the human embryo "from the beginning" is a novelty in the Western, Christian and specifically

Roman Catholic moral traditions. It is virtually a creation of the later nineteenth century, a little over a century ago; and that is a novelty indeed as traditions go.[39]

Because of this, Dunstan sought to re-emphasize the position which supported the formed/unformed difference. But his proposal may be somewhat prejudiced since, as already indicated, other traditions can be considered and the relevance of Dunstan's evidence may not be as significant as he claims. This was emphasized by the British Catholic bioethicist David A. Jones who presented a more comprehensive history of the theological discussions relating to the moral status of the human embryo in his excellent (2004) book *The Soul of the Embryo*.[40]

Furthermore, Dunstan often gives the impression that the moral status of the embryo can simply be determined by studying Christian historic tradition. But though tradition is important, it cannot be considered as the basis for determining the moral status of an entity such as an early human embryo.

There are also omissions in Dunstan's references. For example, he seems to overlook the Church Father Clement of Alexandria (*c.* 150–215), who agrees with an anonymous Christian text of the mid second century that suggests that it is an angel who puts a soul into the womb of a woman at the stage of conception. This means that for Clement the earliest human embryo already has a soul.[41]

The second-century Greek apologist Athenagorus is also seen to support a similar perspective in his book *De Resurrectione*.[42] In it he states that there is a permanence of the unity between the body and the soul at resurrection. What was united when a person was created will continue to be united by God at the resurrection. In this way, Athenagorus is expressing his clear understanding that the unity between the body and the soul of a human being stretches back to his or her earliest existence, 'For human nature universally considered is constituted by an immortal soul and body which has been united with it at its creation.'[43]

The Latin Church Father Tertullian (*c.* 160–225), from Carthage (North Africa), gives further indications on this theme of human creation though some remain ambiguous. He argued that the clay body of Adam was ensouled when God breathed into it his breath of life. For subsequent human persons, however, he believed that the soul is derived from the parents by generation through conception (Traducianism). In Tertullian's *Apology*, written in 197, he defends Christianity against accusations of immorality:

> In our case, murder being once for all forbidden, we may not destroy even the foetus in the womb, while as yet the human being derives

blood from other parts of the body for its sustenance. To hinder a birth is merely a speedier man-killing; nor does it matter whether you take away a life that is born, nor destroy one that is coming to birth. That is a man which is going to be one; you have the fruit already in its seed.[44]

It is interesting that Dunstan, who mentions Tertullian as one of the writers who forms an exception to the Christian tradition he wants to emphasize, does not also quote his later work in *De Anima*. In a section in which Tertullian mentions the Septuagint version of Exodus 21.22–23 the Church Father states: 'The embryo therefore becomes a human being in the womb from the moment that its form is completed.'[45]

This seems to contradict his earlier account which suggested that an embryo should be protected as soon as it is created.[46]

In this respect, the American theologian Michael Gorman suggests that Tertullian did not quote Exodus 21.22 in order to question his understanding of the very high moral status of the early human embryo but to emphasize Moses' penalty for abortion. In other words, because a 'rudimentary man' was already in existence the embryo has already 'been entered into the book of fate'.[47]

A clearer and more unambiguous protective stance is given by the Greek Bishop of Caesarea (in modern Turkey), St Basil the Great (*c.* 329–79), who strongly rejected the difference between the formed and unformed status. He emphasized: 'A woman who deliberately destroys a foetus is answerable for murder. And any fine distinction as to its being completely formed or unformed is not admissible among us.'[48]

Unfortunately, when Dunstan mentions this statement he then seems to question its importance by quoting a contradictory statement from Basil's brother St Gregory (*c.* 330–95) who was the Greek Bishop of Nyssa (in modern Turkey). This is awkward because Gregory is actually not contradicting Basil, nor does Dunstan indicate that Basil's position has become an important tradition in Eastern Orthodoxy. The British theological commentator Gerald Bonner (1926–2013) actually maintains that Basil's perspective was the majority position of the Church Fathers.[49] In this he is supported by D. A. Jones, who states: 'Basil ... was wholly in conformity with the dominant tradition of church legislation in the first millennium ... which treated abortion as homicide without distinction as to the stage of development of the embryo.'[50]

With respect to Gregory, who has been characterized as one of the most versatile theologians of his century,[51] further insights relating to the commencement of life can be gathered. In fact, the Scottish theologian Thomas. F. Torrance (1913–2007) argued that he presented the most complete exposition of the beginning of human existence of any Church Father. Gregory developed his thinking in *De Anima et Resurrectione*, arguing that, because a human being is a unity of soul and body, then the beginning of his or her existence must also reflect this unity which continues to develop. Gregory comments: 'No intelligent man would suppose that the birth of souls occurs later or earlier than the formation of bodies. We must conclude that the soul and the body have a single beginning.'[52]

For Gregory, therefore, there cannot be any form of body–soul dualism in the embryo or the foetus. In this, he was generally in agreement with the position of most Greek Church Fathers that there is always a coexistence between the soul and the body and that they come into existence together.[53] Torrance further comments:

> This idea that the human being is already potentially complete in 'the human germ', as Gregory expressed it, is startlingly similar to the modern scientific finding that the human being is genetically complete in the embryo from the moment of its conception.[54]

Interestingly, however, Dunstan quotes a divergent perspective from Gregory's *Adversus Macedonianos*:

> For just as it would not be possible to style the unformed embryo a human being, but only a potential one – assuming that it is completed so as to come forth to human birth, while so long as it is in this unformed state it is something other than a human being – so our reason cannot recognise as a Christian one who has failed to receive, with regard to the entire mystery, the genuine form of our religion.[55]

It is interesting that Dunstan does not try to further develop this quotation in the context of Gregory's more extensive theological perspective and that Torrance does not take this passage into account in his own understanding of Gregory's views. There seems to be some unresolved ambiguity[56] concerning this quotation, in that it may not actually be referring to a differentiation within a pregnancy between the formed and unformed embryo but to a distinction between the born and unborn child.[57]

At this stage it is also important to emphasize that the Third Ecumenical Council of Ephesus (a council of Christian bishops convened in AD 431 by the Roman Emperor Theodosius II) condemned the teaching of Nestorius (c. 386–450), Patriarch of Constantinople, that the Virgin Mary may be called the Christotokos, 'Birth Giver of Christ', but not the Theotokos, 'Birth Giver of God'. This difference was rejected because her son, Jesus Christ, was one divine person with two natures (divine and human) intimately, hypostatically, united. 'Theotokos' is also sometimes translated as 'God-bearer', which means that the Virgin Mary was not just bearing a foetus with no value but was, instead, bearing the creator of the universe.

The solemn declaration of the Fourth Ecumenical Council of Chalcedon, in 451, also stated that 'for God the Word became flesh and was made man and from the moment of conception united himself to the temple he had taken from her'.[58] The early Church recognized thereby that, at least in the case of Jesus Christ, his immeasurable status and worth was already present at conception.

In this brief historical overview, it is also necessary to examine the position of one of the most influential Latin Christian theologians, the North African St Augustine, Bishop of Hippo (354–430), and the manner in which he understood the distinction between formed and unformed.

Augustine was apparently influenced by the Septuagint interpretation of Exodus 21.22 and did not, therefore, seem to consider the destruction of the unformed foetus as murder in his writings on this text. But D. A. Jones writes that a more correct quotation from Augustine relating to his commentary on Exodus should be:

> If what is brought forth is unformed but at this stage some sort of living, shapeless thing (since the great question of the soul is not to be rushed into rashly with a thoughtless opinion), then the law of homicide would not apply, for it could not be said that there was a living soul in that body, for it lacks all sense, if it be such as is not yet formed and therefore not yet endowed with its senses.[59]

Hence, there is a tension and even agnosticism in Augustine's account about the origins of the soul, since he remained open to the position that the soul was generated by the parents (implying its presence from conception) which may have arisen as a result of the mistakes in the Septuagint.[60] In *Enchiridion*,[61] Augustine suggests that foetuses which die before birth would be resurrected at the resurrection of the dead. Because of this, he was concerned about the stage at which the formed and unformed distinction should be characterized. Augustine's acceptance of the difference between the formed and unformed foetus became the basis of the *Canon Aliquando* which was included in the famous 'Concordance of Discordant Canons' put together in the twelfth century as a legal textbook.

Bonner, however, makes the point[62] that in the year 1234, Pope Gregory IX in the Western Church promulgated a canon where the distinction between formed and unformed could be considered as being abolished. But Dunstan does not present this part of the tradition of the Catholic Church.

When the Italian St Thomas Aquinas (1225–74), one of the principal philosophers and theologians of the medieval Church in the tradition of scholasticism, began to discuss his reflections in the Catholic Roman West, another perspective was presented. Aquinas was a scholar who was heavily influenced by pre-Christian Greek philosophy, and especially by the Aristotelian understanding of the development of a soul, while also following the Septuagint version of Exodus 21.22. Aquinas therefore came to accept a distinction between a formed and unformed foetus, though he did believe that ensoulment took place when the body was 'formed'.[63] As a result, he held the standard Catholic position of the time in stating that 'the intellectual soul is created by God at the end of human generation',[64] by which he meant about 40 days for male foetuses.

As developed later in this volume, Aquinas also believed that Christ's incarnation as a human person began at conception although he was never an embryo but was conceived as a fully formed foetus (though a very small one).[65] Human embryos, on the other hand, only became persons when a rational soul, which was created by God, was infused into the body at a later stage.[66]

Why this difference existed in Aquinas' mind was probably because of the dual origins of his thinking, and his attempt to reconcile Christian doctrines with Greek philosophy.

A few centuries after Aquinas, in 1588, Pope Sixtus V (1521–90) enacted legislation against abortion as well as contraception and sterilization. But this attempt at reform proved difficult to implement and his successor, Pope Gregory XIV (1535–91), was forced to compromise by restricting excommunication to those who directly aborted a 'formed' foetus while insisting that early abortion remained a grave sin.[67]

With the development of medicine and an understanding of human biology in the eighteenth and nineteenth centuries the number of abortions began to rise, which was considered by the Catholic Church as a moral threat. As a result, Pope Pius IX (1792–1878), in his Bull of 1869, declared the spiritual penalty of excommunicate all who procured abortion, without any distinction as to whether the foetus was formed, animate or inanimate. In this context, his extension of ecclesiastical sentences to abortions at all stages of pregnancy represents only a small change in the direction of the dominant legal and moral stance of the earlier tradition.[68]

This perspective is also reflected in the continued opposition to abortion by the Eastern Orthodox Church ever since the Great Schism of 1054 when communion was broken with the Catholic Church. Even now, the Eastern Orthodox Church returns to the position of the Oriental Fathers to substantiate its condemnation of abortion, at any stage, as a very grave offence. This has enabled, for instance, the Synod of Bishops of the Orthodox Church of America to state in 2001: 'Human life is sacred from its very beginning, since from conception it is ensouled existence. As such, it is "personal" existence, created in the image of God and endowed with a sanctity that destines it for eternal life.'[69]

Moreover, in many of the historical Protestant churches which separated themselves from the Catholic Church at the Reformation in the sixteenth century, such as the Church of Scotland (whose first General Assembly took place in 1560), abortion was always considered to be a very grave offence. This still remains the position of the Church of Scotland, the only exception being when the continued pregnancy involves a serious risk to the life or grave injury to the health of the pregnant woman.[70]

Actually, in the very same year of Pius IX's Bull, the Presbyterian Church in the USA stated in its General Assembly: 'This Assembly regards the destruction by parents of their own offspring, before birth, with abhorrence, as a crime against God and against nature ...'[71]

These positions also reflect the standpoints of a number of leading Protestants, including the French Reformer John Calvin (1509–64), who wrote that: 'For the fetus, though enclosed in the womb of its mother, is already a human being.'[72]

Later on, and until the end of the twentieth century, the moral status of the human embryo was still not generally examined as such but, similarly to the early Church Fathers, was being considered as a result of indirect discussions about the moral stance on abortion.

The Swiss Protestant theologian Karl Barth (1886–1968) wrote in 1961:

The unborn is from the very first a child. It is still developing and has no independent life. But it is a man [a human being] and not a thing, nor a mere part of the mother's body ... He who destroys germinating life kills a man and thus ventures a monstrous thing of decreeing concerning the life and death of a fellow man, whose life is given to him by God, and therefore, like his own, belongs to Him.[73]

And the German pastor and theologian Dietrich Bonhoeffer (1906–45) adds: 'Destruction of the embryo in the mother's womb is a violation of the right to life which God has bestowed on this nascent life ... And that is nothing but murder.'[74]

In this brief historical overview, a number of significant elements have emerged. In the first place, it is incorrect to suggest that early human embryos were only considered to deserve full protection in the Christian Church in comparatively modern times. This is especially the case if the position of the Catholic Church is carefully considered and if the doctrines of the Eastern Orthodox as well as the historical Protestant churches are taken into account.

As D. A. Jones and 23 other leading scholars from theology and ethics, representing these three important denominations, have stated:

> The great weight of the tradition, East and West, Orthodox, Catholic and Reformed, from the apostolic age until the twentieth century, is firmly against any sacrifice or destructive use of the early human embryo save, perhaps, 'at the dictate of strict and undeniable medical necessity';[75] that is, in the context of seeking to save the mother's life.[76]

Moreover, the historical Christian figures who believed that there was a difference between the formed and unformed foetus were often influenced either by a mistranslation in the Septuagint of Exodus 21.22–23 or by an Aristotelian pre-Christian philosophical understanding of the embryo. This means that, had the Church Fathers had access to modern translations and more extensive information about embryology, it is very unlikely that they would have considered the early human embryo as having a different moral status from that of any other person who has been born.

This survey has been important to set the scene concerning how Christian tradition has considered the human embryo. It is in this context that the current debate in both theology and embryology should be examined as well as the manner in which it is moulding modern thinking.

The Current Debate on the Moral Status of the Human Embryo

During the past few decades, a number of reproductive procedures have been developed which have raised new questions about the way human embryos should be used. These include the final destiny of 'spare embryos' resulting from *in vitro* fertilization procedures, the genetic screening of embryos, the cloning of embryos and embryos created for research.

But the original question of the moral status of the embryo continues to be one of the fundamental unresolved problems in many of these developments. It is also a question that cannot be dissociated from the worldviews of each and every person. This is especially the case in procedures which lead to the destruction of embryos. For example, for persons with a strong utilitarian perspective, issues relating to the moral status of human embryos are considered secondary in comparison to making sure healthy children are born. The English IVF pioneer and 2010 Nobel Prize winner for Physiology or Medicine, Robert Edwards

(1925–2013), is typical of many commentators when he argues: 'The most important ethical point is to avert the birth of a severely handicapped baby, and this to my mind far outweighs the ethical disadvantages of discarding a cleaving embryo or blastocyst.'[77]

In the same way, many feminist critiques of the new reproductive procedures do not consider the moral status of the early embryo as being paramount. The primary question is that of women's rights and autonomy as well as a rejection of male domination and paternalism. They argue that what 'external human fertilization' really means is that it is 'external-to-women' fertilization.

Many feminists insist that the discussion is limited and incorrect precisely because it is embryo-centric instead of being woman-centric. In other words, it is 'foetalist' instead of 'feminist'. The feminist author Patricia Spallone comments: 'The term "status of the human embryo" is about the power of men, of the state and of medicine and science over women.'[78]

But such critiques of the moral status of the early embryo are often based on presuppositions instead of a full knowledge and consideration of all the aspects, including the important question of when human embryos begin to matter morally.

A number of scientists working in human embryonic research do consider the embryo to have some kind of value. But it is often the extent of this worth and the basis on which a decision is made that gives rise to debate. Moreover, seeking to side-step the question is not very helpful. For example, the use of the term 'pre-embryo' for the first 14 days of an embryo's existence is inappropriate because it does not reflect scientific reality and is often used simply to avoid the real moral debate.[79]

In the end, the amount of respect given to the early human embryo is always dependent on the manner in which it is perceived from a moral context. But the influential UK Warnock Committee on embryological research in 1984 resisted this approach:

> Although the questions of when life or personhood begin appear to be questions of fact, susceptible to straightforward answers, we hold that the answers to such questions in fact are complex amalgams of factual and moral judgements. Instead of trying to answer these questions directly, we have therefore gone straight to the question of how it is right to treat the human embryo.[80]

The 1985 Anglican study *Personal Origins* disagreed with such a methodology since it recognized that the key question was indeed the moral nature of the early human embryo. This, moreover, could be examined only once the nature and the very being of the embryo had been defined.[81]

It is the difference between an essentially empirical perspective based on observation and a perspective that seeks to understand the nature of the very being of the human which is the most important divide in the debate.

A number of moral theologians were also opposed to destructive research on the human embryo for other reasons. For example, the British theologian Oliver O'Donovan maintained that it was impossible to know, for certain, how to consider the moral status of the early embryo since it is 'ambiguously human'. In other words, it is similar enough to a person who has been born to be of interest in human biological research but is also different enough for certain persons not to be troubled about its moral status. Indeed, it is because of this ambiguity that many forget their own embryonic origins as 'begotten' in the sense that, as embryos, they had a similar moral status to their parents.[82] O'Donovan also suggested that, as soon as parents or other persons begin to consider certain human beings as no longer having the same moral status as their own, they necessarily stop loving them in an appropriate manner. An early human embryo then becomes an object that can be used by society and not a fellow human person whom society can welcome as an equal.[83]

Another concern for O'Donovan, which reflects the earlier disquiet of the Protestant American ethicist Paul Ramsey (1913–88) in his book *Fabricated Man*, is the considerable risks associated with the production, manipulation and implantation of embryos.[84] For O'Donovan, it is this much broader issue of the manner in which society considers human embryos, rather than the more specific questions of the very nature of their being, that is of concern.

But, from a theological perspective, the question of the moral status of human embryos remains, and this can only be answered by examining the image of God.

Notes

1 Robert W. Evans, 2000, 'The Moral Status of Embryos', in J. F. Kilner, P. C. Cunningham and W. D. Hagar (eds), *The Reproduction Revolution*, Cambridge: Eerdmans, pp. 60–76.

2 Maureen L. Condic, 2011, 'Preimplantation Stages of Human Development: The Biological and Moral Status of Early Embryos', in Antoine Suarez and Joachim Huarte (eds), *Is This Cell a Human Being?*, Berlin-Heidelberg: Springer, p. 29; William B. Hurlbut, 2011, 'The Boundaries of Humanity: The Ethics of Human–Animal Chimeras in Cloning and Stem Cell Research', in Suarez and Huarte, *Is this Cell a Human Being?*, p. 161.

3 This is in contrast to the concept of 'Completeness' in the sense that nothing is missing from an external perspective. Something is complete when different parts are

brought together from an external viewpoint – such as a jigsaw puzzle or a complete musical orchestra.

4 Norman M. Ford, 1988, *When Did I Begin? Conception of the Human Individual in History, Philosophy and Science*, Cambridge: Cambridge University Press, p. xv.

5 Maureen L. Condic, 'When Does Human Life Begin? A Scientific Perspective', White Paper, *The Westchester Institute for Ethics & The Human Person* 1:1 (2008), http://www.westchesterinstitute.net/images/wi_whitepaper_life_print.pdf (accessed 21 December 2011), p. 6 (article 1–18).

6 Hurlbut, 'Boundaries of Humanity', p. 163.

7 Condic, 'Preimplantation Stages', p. 29.

8 Hurlbut, 'Boundaries of Humanity', pp. 166, 161.

9 Condic, When Does Human Life Begin?, p. 11.

10 The following presentation is a simplified version.

11 M. J. K. Harper, 1982, 'Sperm and Egg Transport', in C. R. Austin and R. V. Short (eds), *Germ Cells and Fertilization, Book 2, Reproduction in Mammals*, Cambridge: Cambridge University Press, pp. 109, 111 and 112.

12 In rabbits, the male pronucleus can be removed at the pronuclear stage and replaced by another male pronucleus in the fertilized egg which can then continue to develop. P. R. Koninckx and P. Schotsmans, 'Frozen embryos: too cold to touch? Spare embryos: symbols of respect for humanity and freezing in the pronuclear stage', *Human Reproduction*, 11:9 (1996), pp. 1841–2.

A procedure called Pronuclear Transfer actually uses the reversible nature of this stage to create a new human embryo. In this technique the two pronuclei of a fertilized human egg are transferred to another fertilized human egg, from which its own pronuclei have been removed, giving rise to a new embryo which can then be left to develop and grow.

13 H. Balakier, N. J. MacLusky and R. F Casper, 'Characterization of the first cell cycle in human zygotes: implications for cryopreservation', *Fertility and Sterility* 59 (1993), pp. 359–65.

14 In its ruling on 18 October 2011, the European Court of Justice gave a clear legal definition of the concept of 'human embryo', thus closing any loophole in the interpretation of the 'morality clause' (Article 6) of the 1998 EU Patent Directive (98/44/EU). Any human ovum must, as soon as it is fertilized, be regarded as a 'human embryo' if that fertilization is such as to commence the process of development of a human being. A non-fertilized human ovum into which the cell nucleus from a mature human cell has been transplanted (somatic cell nuclear transfer – SCNT), or a non-fertilized human ovum whose division and further development have been stimulated by parthenogenesis, must also be classified as a 'human embryo' (Court of Justice of the European Union, 2011a).

15 Condic, 'Preimplantation Stages', p. 30.

16 Most of the experiments undertaken in this area use mice as a model. But since their early embryonic development has been shown to be similar to that of nonhuman primates, it is assumed that embryonic development in mice can be considered as comparable to that of humans, though a lot less is known about early human development as such. For example, one of the cells in the two-cell embryo of a mouse tends to divide earlier than the other one and to be the precursor of the cells that become the embryo proper which develop into the baby. The other cell which divides later, however, generally tends to generate the extra-embryonic tissue including the placenta. See: Condic, 'Preimplantation Stages', p. 30.

17 Early cell division is not always uniform. Moreover, it is possible that some early cells in an embryo may stop dividing or even die without changing the development potential of the embryo as a whole. In other words, on the third day after fertilization, the embryo may often have between six and ten cells.

18 Condic, 'Preimplantation Stages', pp. 28 and 31.

19 M. A. H. Surani and S. C. Barton, 'Spatial Distribution of Blastomeres is Dependent on Cell Division Order and Interactions in Mouse Morulae', *Developmental Biology* 102 (1984), pp. 335–43; Anne McLaren, 1986, 'Prelude to Embryogenesis' in The Ciba Foundation, *Human Embryo Research: Yes or No?*, London: Tavistock Publications, p. 9.

20 Ford, *When Did I Begin?*, p. 148.

21 If the inner cell mass is separated in two this would give rise to another route of twin formation. It is when this separation is only partial that Siamese twins are created.

22 Wayne Meeks, 1987, *The Moral World of the First Christians*, London: SPCK, pp. 16, 17.

23 Aristotle argued that the size of a family should be determined by the state. If children were conceived in excess of the permitted number then abortion should occur 'before sensation and life develops in the embryo', Aristotle, *Politics* VII.xii.15 (1335B). But the Hippocratic Oath (third century BC) explicitly denounced abortion. Roman attitudes, following Stoic philosophy, were more liberal. Stoics viewed the foetus as being no more than a part of the mother's body.

24 A useful overview can be found in: Michael Gorman, 1982, *Abortion in the Early Church: Christian, Jewish and Pagan Attitudes in the Greco-Roman World*, Downer's Grove, IL: Paulist Press.

25 Jean Boboc, 2014, *La grande métamorphose: Éléments pour une théo-anthropologie orthodoxe*, Paris: Les Éditions du Cerf, p. 266.

26 G. Bonner states: 'One cannot simply argue that the Fathers saw the embryo as a human being from the moment of its conception and based their condemnation of its destruction upon that assumption; their theology was, in fact, more varied than their denunciation.' In G. Bonner, 1985, 'Abortion and Early Christian Thought', in C. H. Channer (ed.), *Abortion and the Sanctity of Human Life*, Exeter: Paternoster Press, p. 113.

27 Aristotle, *De Generatione Animalium*, in *Aristotle, De generatione animalium*, trans. and ed. D. M. Balme, Oxford: Clarendon Press, 1972, 731a, p. 25.

28 Aristotle, *History of Animals* 7.3, 583b 3–5.

29 In this passage the Hebrew word *yasa* is used, which is generally employed for the birth of a child, and not the word *shakal* which is normally associated with a miscarriage. See Gleason Archer, 1990, *Encyclopedia of Bible Difficulties*, Grand Rapids: Zondervan, pp. 246–9. The analysis of the Jewish attitude to abortion relies on V. Apowitzer, quoted in Gorman, *Abortion in the Early Church*; David A. Jones, 'Abortion', *Triple Helix* 45 (Summer 2009), pp. 16–18.

30 David A. Jones, 2004, *The Soul of the Embryo*, London: Continuum, p. 48.

31 Exodus 21.22 was interpreted as, 'If two men fight and they strike a woman who is pregnant and her child comes out while not yet fully formed, the one liable to punishment will be fined; whatever the woman's husband imposes will be fitting. But if it is fully formed, he will give life for life.'

32 Lords *Hansard*, 22 January 2001, Columns 35–7.

33 Immanuel Jakobovits suggests that the mistake in the Septuagint is based on a variant Samaritan reading or simply a mistranslation. Immanuel Jakobovits, 1988, 'The Status of the Embryo in the Jewish Tradition', in G. R. Dunstan and Mary J. Seller (eds),

The Status of the Human Embryo: Perspectives from Moral Tradition, Oxford: Oxford University Press, pp. 62–73.

34 Andrew R. Rollinson, 1994, 'The Incarnation and the Status of the Human Embryo', a thesis submitted for the degree of M.Litt. with the Religious Studies Department of Newcastle University, p. 122.

35 Gordon R. Dunstan, 'The moral status of the human embryo: a tradition recalled', *Journal of Medical Ethics* 1 (1984), pp. 38–44.

36 Josephus, *Antiquities of the Jews* 4.8.33.

37 Immanuel Jakobovits writes: 'All these [biblical] passages clearly exempt feticide from the laws of murder, and they therefore firmly refuse to establish full human status before birth.' Jakobovits, 'Status of the Embryo', p. 62.

38 Peter Barns, 2010, *Abortion*, Edinburgh: The Banner of Truth, p. 29.

39 Dunstan, 'Moral status', pp. 38–9. Dunstan notes that the significant change in Roman Catholic law came in 1869 in the Bull *Apostolicae Sedis* by Pope Pius IX. Here, excommunication is threatened to all who procure abortion whatever the age or formed/unformed status of the foetus. This was to combat the growing incidence of abortions. See https://www.theguardian.com/world/2016/nov/21/pope-francis-makes-priests-ability-to-absolve-abortion-permanent-church-forgiveness-sin.

40 Jones, *Soul of the Embryo*, pp. 72–4 and 245–6. See also David A. Jones, 'Aquinas as an Advocate of Abortion? The Appeal to "Delayed Animation" in Contemporary Christian Ethical Debates on the Human Embryo', *Studies in Christian Ethics* 26:1 (February 2013), pp. 97–124.

41 Clement of Alexandria, *Ecologue Propheticae*, Patrologia, Series Graeca, J. P. Migne, 9, 697.

42 Athenagorus, *Concerning the Resurrection of the Dead*. The authorship is disputed. *Legatio and De Resurrectione*, trans. by W. R. Shoedel, Oxford: Clarendon Press, 1972.

43 Athenagorus, *De Resurrectione* 15.2. This could, of course, be a reference to Adam's creation, but is more likely a reference to procreation.

44 Tertullian, *Apologia* 9:8, Ante-Nicene Christian Library, Vol. XI, p. 72.

45 Tertullian, *De Anima*, ch. 37, Ante-Nicene Christian Library, Vol. XV, p. 498.

46 Tertullian wrote: 'We indeed maintain that both [body and soul] are conceived and formed and perfected simultaneously, as well as born together; and that not a moment's interval occurs in their conception.' *De Anima* ch. 27. He also said that: 'For although we shall allow that there are two kinds of seed – that of the body and that of the soul – we still declare that they are inseparable, and therefore contemporaneous and simultaneous in origin.' *De Anima*, ch. 27.

47 Gorman, *Abortion in the Early Church*.

48 St Basil, *Ep.* 188, Canon 2. *Ad Amphilochium* II, Patrologia, Series Graeca, J. P. Migne, 32. Quoted in Dunstan, 'Moral status', p. 40.

49 Bonner, 'Abortion and Early Christian Thought', p. 98.

50 David A. Jones, 'The Human Embryo in Christian Tradition: a reconsideration', *Journal of Medical Ethics* 31 (2005), pp. 710–14 (p. 711).

51 Hans von Campenhausen, 1963, *The Fathers of the Greek Church*, London: Lutterworth Press, p. 109.

52 Gregory of Nyssa, *De Anima et Resurrectione*, Patrologia, Series Graeca, J. P. Migne, 46, 125–8.

53 Boboc, *La grande métamorphose*, p. 271.

54 Thomas F. Torrance, 1989, 'The Soul and Person in Theological Perspective in Religion, Reason and Self', in S. R. Sutherland and T. A. Roberts (eds), *Essays in Honour of Hywel D. Lewis*, Cardiff: University of Wales Press, p. 110.

55 Gregory of Nyssa, *Adversus Macedonianos*, in H. Walce and P. Schaff (eds), Library of Nicene and Post-Nicene Fathers, Series 2, Vol. V, 1893, 320. Quoted in Dunstan, 'Moral status', p. 40.

56 Rollinson, 'Incarnation and the Status of the Human Embryo', p. 126.

57 Jones, 'Human Embryo', pp. 710–14.

58 Epistle of St Cyril to John of Antioch, in Norman P. Tanner (ed.), *Decrees of Ecumenical Councils*, London: Sheed & Ward, 1990, p. 70.

59 St Augustine of Hippo, *Quaestionum in Hept*, I.II n. 80. Quoted in Jones, 'Human Embryo', p. 711.

60 Jones, 'Human Embryo', p. 711.

61 Augustine, *Enchiridian*, Patrologia, Series Latina, J. P. Migne, 40, 685.4.

62 Bonner, 'Abortion and Early Christian Thought', p. 110.

63 For example, Aquinas wrote: 'We simply admit that souls were not created before bodies but were created at the same time as the bodies into which they were infused'. *Summa Theologica* I, q. 118, a. 3, ad.3. In the writings of the early centuries, the issue of formed/unformed and un-ensouled/ensouled were two separate issues. As Brendan Soame points out, it was possible to hold at one and the same time that the soul was given at conception, but the foetus not formed till later. For Aquinas and most commentators, however, the two issues coincided. See: Brendan Soame, 1988, 'Roman Catholic Casuistry and the Moral Standing of the Human Embryo', in Dunstan and Seller, *The Status of the Human Embryo*, p. 76.

64 Aquinas, *Summa Theologica* I, q. 118, a. 2, ad.2.

65 Aquinas, *Summa Theologica* III, q. 34, a. 2, ad.3; Jones, ch. 9.

66 David. A. Jones, 'Thomas Aquinas, Augustine, and Aristotle on delayed animation', *The Thomist* 76:1 (2012), pp. 1–36.

67 Jones, 'Human Embryo', pp. 710–14.

68 Jones, 'Human Embryo', pp. 710–14.

69 Holy Synod of Bishops of the Orthodox Church of America, 'Embryonic Stem Cell Research in the Perspective of Orthodox Christianity' (2001), 2003, in B. Waters and R. Cole-Turner (eds), 2003, *God and the Embryo*, Washington, DC: Georgetown University Press, p. 172.

70 The Church of Scotland 1966 Deliverance of the General Assembly on the topic of abortion remains valid to this day. This states: 'the criteria for abortion should be that the continuance of the pregnancy would involve a serious risk to the life or grave injury to the health, whether physical or mental, of the pregnant woman'. There is, however, a moral tension in this stance as regards the status of human embryos since subsequent General Assemblies have accepted that they could be used in research.

The full protection of the embryo and foetus is also the position of the more 'orthodox' Free Church of Scotland which separated from the Church of Scotland in 1843: it states that 'we must treat [human embryos] with the respect due to all innocent human life, and they must have the full protection of the law ... No procedure should be carried out on an embryo which is not designed for the survival and benefit of that embryo', 1990 General Assembly Report of the Free Church of Scotland, p. 58.

It adds: 'We are equally opposed to abortion, except where the mother's life is in grave danger. Our position on these questions we believe to be based on the principles which have played the major part in shaping the morality and public laws of this nation', 1994 General Assembly Report of the Free Church of Scotland, pp. 45–6.

71 1869 Minutes of the General Assembly of the Presbyterian Church in the USA, pp. 937–8.

72 John Calvin, *Commentary in Exodus*, 21.22.

73 Karl Barth, 1961, *Church Dogmatics*, Edinburgh: T&T Clark, Vol. III.4, pp. 415–16.

74 Dietrich Bonhoeffer, 1995, *Ethics*, New York: Touchstone, p. 174.

75 Lambeth Conference 1958 report, 'The Family in Contemporary Society', in *What the Bishops Have Said about Marriage*, 1968, London: SPCK, p. 17.

76 David A. Jones et al., 2003, 'A Theologian's Brief on the Place of the Human Embryo within the Christian Tradition, and the Theological Principles for Evaluating its Moral Status', in Waters and Cole-Turner, *God and the Embryo*, p. 194.

77 R. Edwards, 1990, 'Ethics and Embryology: The Case for Experimentation', in Anthony Dyson and John Harris (eds), *Experiments on Embryos*, London: Routledge, p. 48.

78 Patricia Spallone asks: 'Why do embryo interests supersede women's interests, but the interests of medical science supersede embryo interests? Why are scientists allowed to argue for their authority to handle and manipulate embryos because of some greater "good", which they define, while a pregnant woman who might wish to have an abortion is denied self-determination over her own body and life? Why do scientists ignore this moral paradox as if it is reasonable and just?' Patricia Spallone, 1989, *Beyond Conception: The New Politics of Reproduction*, Granby, MA: Bergin & Garvey, p. 55.

79 Patricia Spallone states: 'The coining of the term "pre-embryo" was a political act. It was invented for the purpose of human embryo research.' Spallone, *Beyond Conception*, p. 53.

80 Warnock Report, 1984, London: Her Majesty's Stationery Office, paragraph 11.9.

81 Board for Social Responsibility for the Church of England, 1985, *Personal Origins; Report on Human Fertilisation and Embryology*, C10 Pub. This perspective was also seen as important by other commentators. See: Teresa Iglesias, 1990, *I. V. F. and Justice*, London: Linacre Centre for Health Care Ethics, p. 87.

82 'The laws of operation cease to be the laws of natural procreation, aided discreetly by technical assistance; they become the laws of production, which swallow up all that is natural into their own world of artifice.' Oliver O'Donovan, 1984, *Begotten or Made?*, Oxford: Clarendon Press, p. 73.

83 O'Donovan, *Begotten or Made?*, p. 65.

84 O'Donovan, *Begotten or Made?*, p. 81; cf. Paul Watson and David Attwood, 1991, *Researching Embryonic Values – a Debate*, Nottingham: Grove Ethical Studies, p. 83, also ch. 2 by David Attwood.

2

The Image of God

As already indicated, in order to appropriately understand the moral status of a living entity from a Christian perspective it is crucial to consider whether the image of God is reflected in this entity. But the concept of the image of God is deeply theological and will never be, by its very nature, fully understood since it represents something in God who cannot be defined.

Nonetheless, this does not mean that the concept of the image of God has no real meaning or that it cannot be understood to some degree when it is considered from different angles giving different insights into its nature.[1] Some of these may even be more convincing than others in affirming that all persons reflect this image of God. Still, it is important not to reduce the image of God to only one set of considerations. A better 'view' is certainly obtained in bringing all these different angles together, all at once, while not seeing them as competing, in any way, against each other.

The Image of God – Origins and Meaning

The creation narratives in Genesis cannot be understood without noting the crucial words of Genesis 1.26–27: 'Then God said, "Let us make mankind in our image, in our likeness ..." So God created mankind in his own image, in the image of God he created them; male and female he created them.'

In the light of this, if the term 'likeness' (*demūth* in Hebrew) is considered to be a parallelism of 'image' (*tselem* in Hebrew) then the phrase is repeated four times in these two verses. This expression is also used in Genesis 5.3 in referring to Adam having a son, Seth, 'in his own likeness' and in Genesis 9.6 in which murder is prohibited because 'in the image of God has God made mankind'.

Other than in Genesis the expression is used only rarely but its importance is far greater than its frequency.

If one of the principal ideas in Hebrew thought is the vastness that exists between human beings and God, then the description of humanity being 'in the image of God' must be significant. It has been presented by the French Protestant theologian Henri Blocher as 'the most concise summary of biblical anthropology', with the Scottish Protestant theologian David Cairns (1904–92) commenting: 'The subject of the image of God in man is really the great subject of the Christian doctrine of man.'[2]

In Genesis, two main accounts of creation are presented, in 1.1—2.3 and 2.4—3.24. Though these two accounts present different aspects of God's creation and do not completely coincide, it is likely that they were both accepted as complementary descriptions of the creation narrative. As such, they do not only witness to the history of God's creation but are theological in nature and a reflection of the way God is involved in his creation.

Because Genesis 2.4—3.24 is believed to have been an earlier account of creation by God, it will be examined first in the present study.

Genesis 2.4 – 3.24

In contrast to Genesis 1, the order of creation in Genesis 2.4—3.24 begins with man, continuing with plants and animals to finally end up with the woman who is man's companion. The man is also brought into existence from the dust and portrayed as having been created in a very different manner from the rest of creation. Moreover, man is complete only when the woman is created to be his partner so that they can exist in a harmonious relationship.

The way in which man is formed out of the earth is emphasized by a play on words since in Hebrew the word for 'man' (*adam*) sounds like, and may be related to, the Hebrew for 'ground' (*adamah*). Human beings are therefore part of the material – the earth – of this world. Man became a living soul, an animated being (*nephesh* in Hebrew) only when God breathed into his nostrils the breath of life (*ruah* in Hebrew).[3] This breath of life is portrayed as the source of all life (see Gen. 1—2). But the word for living being (*nephesh*) can reflect a number of meanings, including the unquenchable need that a living being experiences (Prov. 25.25; Ps. 42.1) and the aspect of desire (Prov. 16.26).

Finally, in this account, Adam is responsible for cultivating the earth with the help of God who sends the rivers to water this earth.

Genesis 1.1 – 2.3

In Genesis 1, God brings into existence entities and beings in an ascending order of nobility, concluding with human beings created in the image of God (1.26–27). Interestingly, in all these different stages of creation God simply commands the different elements or beings into existence.

It is only when creating human beings that God seems to deliberate or discuss within himself the creation of such beings with his image. This portrayal of God deliberating within himself underlines the reality that God is not simply going through another stage of creation but is actually doing something totally new. In other words, human beings made in the image of God are completely different from all the other animals and the rest of creation.

In Genesis 1.26–28, it is also indicated that humankind should rule over creation and has dominion over nature. Theologians disagree over the significance and meaning of this position or place of authority. Some believe that this dominion is simply a consequence of human beings having been created in the image of God and not a necessary feature of this image. As the German Protestant theologian Claus Westermann (1909–2000) asserts, 'according to the text, dominion over other creatures is not an explanation, but a consequence of creation in the image of God'.[4]

Most theologians agree, however, that the dominion of humankind over the earth is an important feature of the image of God. In the same way as God rules over all of creation (Gen. 1), human beings are appointed by God to rule over the earth as his representatives.[5]

It is in the Genesis 1 account that mention is made of man being created by God 'in our image, in our likeness' (Gen. 1.26–27). There is considerable discussion about the translation of this expression. As already indicated, the word 'image' is usually understood as a translation from the Hebrew *tselem* (*eikon* in Greek), and the word 'likeness' is generally accepted as a translation from the Hebrew *demūth* (*homoiosis* in Greek). But in the Hebrew there is no conjunction between the two terms. Thus, an appropriate translation of the expression is 'let us make man in our image, after our likeness'. This contrasts with both the Septuagint[6] and the Vulgate[7] which insert the word 'and' between the two terms, perhaps implying that 'image' and 'likeness' refer to two different characteristics. But most commentators accept that, though the words may have different origins, they essentially express similar concepts.

The Hebrew word for image, *tselem*, can be understood as expressing a concrete or even bodily concept since the word itself is derived from a root word meaning 'to carve' or 'to cut'.[8] This means that *tselem* may express the image in the sense of a carving or representation of a likeness of a person in, for example, a sculpture. As the American bioethicists Ben Mitchell et al. explain:

As a human child was considered the *tselem* of a parent (Gen. 5), and the *tselem* in ancient Near East could refer to a statue reminding people of a king's presence, human beings were created to have a special, personal relationship with God that includes their being God's representative in the world. Accordingly, the Bible speaks of people not only as being in the image of God but also as being the image of God.[9]

In other words, human beings are created by God on this earth in his image in such a fashion that they represent God's sovereign emblem.[10]

The Hebrew word for likeness, *demūth*, on the other hand, tends to be understood as qualifying a more abstract concept while also including the notion of comparison. In Hebrew, *demūth* has its origin in the root word for 'to be like'.[11] Its use could, therefore, be understood in Genesis 1 as expressing 'an image which is like us'.[12]

Nevertheless, it should be emphasized that the two words *tselem* and *demūth* essentially mean the same thing in Hebrew, with the expression 'after our likeness' only being a different way of saying 'in our image'. In the whole of the Bible, including in Genesis, the two words seem to be used almost synonymously and interchangeably.[13]

Though it is in Genesis that the 'creation ordinances' are presented which characterize the original principles that apply to all human beings,[14] the 'image of God' expression is only infrequently used in the New Testament to portray humanity, as in James 3.9. In addition, it is used a number of times to depict the unique dignity and divine Sonship of the incarnate Word of God.

In Colossians 1.15, Christ is described as 'the image [*eikon*] of the invisible God'; in Hebrews 1.3, 'the exact representation [character] of … [God's] being'; and in 2 Corinthians 4.4, 'the glory of Christ, who is the image of God'.[15] A further use of the expression is to portray the purpose and final outcome of salvation, as in Colossians 3.10 when the new identity of Christians is portrayed which is 'being renewed in knowledge in the image of its Creator'. In this sense, of course, human beings are not the original. But they do reflect an image of God who is the real origin of this image.

The New Testament also covers the concept of the image of God more fully, especially in passages addressing the restoration of the image which has been hidden by sin in the redemptive work of Christ.

The Image of God from a Historic Perspective

The Patristic and Medieval Periods

The concept of the image of God in the history of theology has been complex, with a number of important debates taking place throughout the centuries.[16] The following very brief survey will begin with St Irenaeus of Lyon (now in central France).

St Irenaeus (c. 130–c. 200)

St Irenaeus was born in Asia Minor (now Turkey), became Bishop of Lyon in 177 and was one of the earliest Christian theologians to discuss in detail the concept of the image of God. Though disagreement exists, it is generally believed that Irenaeus made a distinction in Genesis 1.26 between 'image' and 'likeness'.[17] In other words, God created humankind in the beginning in his image (*tselem*) and likeness (*demūth*) but, through the Fall, the likeness to God in all human beings (humankind's original righteousness and supernatural graces that make it godlike) was lost, though the image of God (the natural qualities of humankind, such as its rational and free nature, that make it resemble God) remained.[18] Because of the incarnation of the Son of God in Jesus Christ, it is thought that Irenaeus believed that the likeness to God (lost at the Fall, regainable by redemption) is being restored in Christians by making them one with God the Father.[19] Irenaeus writes:

> And then, again, this Word was manifest when the Word of God was made man, assimilating himself to man and man to himself, that by means of his resemblance to the Son, man might become precious to the Father. For in the times long past, it was said that man was created after the image of God, but it was not yet shown; for the Word was as yet invisible, after whose image man was created. Wherefore also he did easily lose the similitude. When, however, the Word of God became flesh, he confirmed both these: for he both showed forth the image truly, since he became himself what was his image; and he re-established the similitude after a sure manner, by assimilating man to the invisible Father through means of the visible Word.[20]

Although the position, associated with Irenaeus, that the likeness was lost through the Fall but the image remained is now generally considered inappropriate, it was useful from the perspective of making a clear argument. In his writings and preaching, Irenaeus was active in opposing Gnostic beliefs. These suggested that the creator of the universe was not considered to be the true God and that the human body in particular, and the created cosmos more generally, were somewhat suspicious. Many scholars believe that, by stating that the 'likeness' was lost through sin though the 'image' was retained, Irenaeus was seeking to insist that humankind maintained its dignity as God's special creation.

Even though Irenaeus is thought to have misinterpreted the Bible verses, his work was significant. This was because he was one of the first Christian thinkers to appropriately clarify the distinction between human beings' nature as God's creatures, which they retain even in their sin, and their destiny through Christ's redemption. As Cairns says, 'By drawing attention to [this] cleavage, Irenaeus has done a service to theology.'[21]

Irenaeus also suggested that non-Christians had only two components in their being, namely a body and a soul, whereas Christians were composed of a body, a soul and a spirit. In this regard, the spirit in a believer is awakened or activated by the indwelling of the Holy Spirit which enables him or her to experience moral transformation and begin to know and follow the divine will. For Irenaeus, it is thus in this spirit, which was lost by humankind through the Fall but now indwells all Christians, that it may be possible to recognize the likeness to God.[22]

Tertullian (c. 160–c. 225)

As with the position ascribed to Irenaeus, the Carthaginian Tertullian also believed that God created human beings in his image which could never be lost or destroyed, but that the likeness of God can be lost through sin.[23] In this, he was apparently misled in believing that the two concepts reflected different meanings.

Epiphanius (c. 310–403)

Epiphanius, who was Bishop of Salamis in Cyprus, was troubled that many in his time were seeking to specifically define the image of God, which he believed was impossible. He wrote:

> For some of them say that the image of God which Adam had previously received was lost when he sinned. Others surmise that the body which the Son of God was destined to take of Mary was the image of the Creator. Some identify this image with the soul, others with sensation, others with virtue. These make it baptism, those assert that it is in virtue of God's image that man exercises universal sway ... But we, dearly beloved, believe the words of the Lord, and know that God's image remains in all men, and we leave it to Him to know in what respect man is created in His image.[24]

Epiphanius also argued that it is the whole, and not just a part, of a human being that reflects the image of a whole God.[25]

St Gregory of Nyssa (c. 330–395)

St Gregory of Nyssa believed that the nature of human beings is impossible to define since God is unfathomable and his image in human beings is also unfathomable.[26] In a very direct and humble manner, therefore, Gregory was prepared to accept that he would never be able to fully understand the image of God and that any prospect of seeking to do so would eventually end in failure.

St Augustine (354–430)

In contrast to earlier Christian writers, St Augustine did not make a distinction between image and likeness but emphasized a more personal, psychological and existential account of the image of God. He wrote:

> There is no doubt that man was made to the image of God that created him, not according to the body, not according to any part of the soul, but according to the rational mind wherein the knowledge of God can exist.[27]

Augustine also suggested a sort of trinitarian structure to this image expressed either in the tripartite structure of what he termed the human soul (spirit, self-consciousness, love) or in the three aspects of psyche (memory, intelligence, will). For Augustine, moreover, though this image of God in human beings could be obscured or defaced, it could never be lost and enables human persons to open up to God in invocation, knowledge and love.[28]

St Thomas Aquinas (1225–74)

St Thomas Aquinas' views on the image of God are drawn from his most important book, *Summa Theologica* (Summary of Theology), in which he states that he did not believe in a distinction between image and likeness while recognizing that these two words could be used in different ways.[29] Aquinas also accepted that the image of God is present in all human beings (even after the Fall) and could be described in terms of a certain theoretical capacity or endowment that all human beings possess, rather than the ability to actively express this endowment.[30] For Aquinas, this image is also generally associated with humanity's intellectual capacity or ability to reason.[31]

Human beings reflect the image of God because they are, like God, rational in nature. In this, Aquinas seems to have been influenced by Greek philosophy which emphasizes the special nature of human beings through their intellect.[32] This enabled human beings to have a natural ability to know and come into a relationship of love with God. Aquinas admits, however, that this natural capacity should be considered in humanity as a whole, and may not be equally expressed in every person.[33]

The Reformation

With its emphasis on the Bible, the Protestant Reformation sought to return to the initial meaning of the original texts by interpreting the nature of humanity. But the distinction, suggested by Irenaeus, between human beings' nature as God's creatures, which they retain even in their sin, and their destiny through Christ's redemption, was one that many Protestant theologians sought to maintain in some form.

The German Reformer Martin Luther (1483–1546) sought to express this point in proposing that there was a 'public' and 'private' image. The public image was considered to be universal to all humankind while the private image was the special reflection of Christians.

Interestingly, Luther also suggested that fallen humanity retained a 'relic' (a remnant reflection) of the original image of God. Maybe this was because he recognized the importance of seeking to maintain a difference between a 'given' for all humanity and a 'potential' for those who are redeemed in Christ.

Similarly, Calvin, building his reflection on Luther's earlier work, considered that there were two elements to humankind's dignity. The first was based on humankind's presence before God, the originator of the image, while the second was based on the divine purpose for human beings. Calvin also emphasized that humankind's dignity cannot be the basis for any inappropriate pride since it is a gift given through grace to humanity by God.[34]

In this regard, Calvin believed that the Bible showed that the image of God was found primarily in the soul of the human being: 'For although God's glory shines forth in the outer man, yet there is no doubt that the proper seat of his [God's] image is in the soul.' But he qualified this by stating that, 'although the primary seat of the divine image was in the mind and heart, or in the soul and its powers, yet there was no part of man, not even the body itself, in which some sparks did not glow'.[35] For Calvin, therefore, there is something that always remains of immense value in a human being even in the greatest of miseries or wretchedness. This something is the image of God. He summarized this idea by explaining:

> We are not to consider that men merit of themselves but to look upon the image of God in all men, to which we owe honor and love ... Therefore, whatever man you meet who needs your aid, you have no reason to refuse to help him ... Say, 'he is contemptible and worthless'; but the Lord shows him to be one to whom he has deigned to give the beauty of his image ... Say that he does not deserve even your least effort for his

sake; but the image of God, which recommends him to you, is worthy of your giving yourself and all your possessions.[36]

In this, Calvin follows Luther in not shying away from using the notion of a 'relic' that retains the image of God in sinners to emphasize the importance of continuing to respect them as persons with a special worth and dignity.[37]

He also believed that God created humankind after his image so that his truth might shine forth in his children. Since he portrayed God as a creative, dynamic being, it was natural for Calvin to understand humankind as being created in God's image in that persons could dynamically reflect this image. Human persons are in the image of God insofar as they reflect back God's glory to him in thankfulness.[38] The picture of a mirror is the governing one in Calvin's mind.[39]

God never intended that human persons should negate the grace that he had bestowed on them. Doing so would have completely hidden his image. Instead, Calvin's position seems to suggest that as God comes nearer to a person who responds to his presence, then the image grows in this person and shines forth all the more.

In contrast to a number of Church Fathers and other medieval theologians, Calvin also argued that there was no real difference between the likeness and the image of God.[40] This was taken up by other Protestant writers who suggested that, if a distinction between 'image' and 'likeness' was emphasized, while at the same time focusing on the spiritual development of the Christian into the likeness of Christ, then the unity of body and soul could be undermined. This is because this spiritual development might imply that the image is only situated in the soul. For example, the English Reformed theologian Colin Gunton (1941–2003) argued that this manner of understanding the image of God encouraged the belief that it was only in reason or the mind that this image could be found.[41]

In this, Gunton is among many contemporary theologians who believe that it was mistaken to believe in any artificial distinction between the image and likeness of God in humankind since it is not supported in Scripture.[42]

In addition, Calvin believed that it was not just the original spirit of human beings that was lost in the Fall but that their original talents or abilities were also distorted and perverted.[43] Accordingly, though the image of God was not wholly lost, human beings by themselves could not contribute anything at all to this image in the presence of sin.[44] As the American Protestant theologian Anthony Hoekema (1913–88) explains: 'Man's fall into sin did not result merely in the loss of something additional to his existence, but involved the total corruption of his entire being.' Thus, in contrast to many early theologians, a number of contemporary Christian thinkers suggest that a true concept of the image of God cannot be defined in the rationality of humankind.[45]

For example, the Protestant theologian Richard Middleton suggests that up until the Middle Ages most Christian writers seemed to have ignored the human body as such. Because of this, he believes that a dualistic view of human beings became accepted which restricted the image either to some characteristics in the soul or to the relationship of a Christian with God while diminishing the role of the human body.[46]

Similarly, Barth believed that the image of God in humankind cannot be restricted to anything a person is or does, nor to any anthropological description of the being of a human, his or her structure, disposition or capacities such as the intellect or reason. By examining Genesis 1.27, 'So God created mankind in his own image, in the image of God he created them; male and female he created them', Barth argues:

> Could anything be more obvious than to conclude from this clear indication that the image and likeness of the being created by God signifies existence in confrontation, i.e., in this confrontation, in the juxtaposition and conjunction of man and man which is that of male and female ...?[47]

For Barth, the fact that the man and the woman are confronted with each other means that it is in this kind of relationship that the image of God is expressed. The image is seen in terms of 'I and Thou' in confrontation[48] which also expresses the kind of relationship that exists between God and human beings.[49]

In addition Barth believed, with respect to the humanity of the Son of God, that Jesus was the image of God incarnate and that it was important to look at the humanity of Jesus to understand this image. His arguments suggest that it is Jesus who is true humanity and that it is in him that the image of God can truly be seen.[50]

Another Swiss theologian, Emil Brunner (1889–1966), argued in a similar way that because Christ is the only true image of God, the restoration of the image means existence in Christ, the Word made flesh:

> Jesus Christ is the true *Imago Dei*, which man regains when through faith he is 'in Jesus Christ'. Faith in Jesus is therefore the *restauratio imaginis* [restoration of the image], because he restores to us that existence in the Word of God which we had lost through sin. When man enters into the love of God revealed in Christ he becomes truly human. True human existence is existence in the love of God.[51]

For Brunner, Calvin's belief in a 'relic' of the image of God after the Fall is problematic. This is because it expresses too much and too little. It says too much because it implies that there is some core element in humanity's nature that remains untouched by sin; and it says too little because, even after the Fall, human beings must stand before God since they were created for a relationship with God.[52]

In more specific terms, Brunner held the position that the universal image of God in human beings exists because they were created to have an inalienable standing before God and the rest of humanity in their responsibility. Moreover, this image is not only spiritual but bears reference to the human body. It is in his or her whole being that a human person is created for relational love with God and neighbour. This is the true meaning and purpose of his or her existence.[53]

In this way, Brunner sought to retain the Reformed tradition, differentiating between the 'formal' and the 'material' image. The 'formal image' is common to all humanity and originates in human beings standing before God as responsible persons. On the other hand, the 'material' image can be recovered in redemption and reconciliation through the love of Christ.[54]

Interestingly, there is a surprising amount of agreement between Barth and Brunner. They both accepted that the image of God cannot be found in isolation but in an active relationship between a human being and God as well as between a human being and his or her neighbours. They also agreed that the image of God is universal in that it cannot be completely destroyed by sin.[55]

The Anglican theologian David Atkinson usefully summarizes this emphasis on relationships:

> To be in the image of God, then, is not primarily a matter of our capacity to do anything. It is a matter of the relationship to himself which God confers on us. It is not our addressability; it is to be addressed as Thou by the divine I.[56]

In addition, the Dutch Reformed theologian Gerrit Berkouwer (1903–96) believed that it is possible to understand the meaning of the image of God by looking to Jesus Christ, the perfect image of the invisible God (2 Cor. 4.4; Col. 1.15). According to him, in looking at the life of Christ, it is his amazing love that shines through most remarkably and it is this that best reflects the perfect image of God in contrast to just 'reason' or 'intellect'. This also means that for a person to be restored in the image of God entails becoming increasingly more like Christ (Rom. 8.29; 2 Cor. 3.18).[57]

Similarly, Hoekema considered that it was impossible to reduce the image of God in humankind to any specific particularity: 'Since the image of God includes the whole person, it must include both man's structure and man's functioning.'[58] As with a number of other Reformed theologians, he also emphasized that the image of God was not lost through the Fall but had merely been distorted or perverted:

> According to the biblical evidence ... fallen man is still considered to be an image-bearer of God, although other evidence shows that he no longer images God properly, and therefore must again be restored to the image of God. Thus, there is a sense in which fallen man is still an image-bearer of God but also a sense in which he must be renewed in that image. We ought not therefore to say that the image of God has been totally lost through man's fall into sin; we ought rather to say that the image has been perverted or distorted by the Fall.[59]

This same theme is taken up by John Stott in a good summary of historical Protestant thinking:

> The image of God in us has been defaced, so that every part of our humanness has been tainted with self-centeredness. Yet God's image has not been destroyed. On the contrary, both the Old Testament and the New Testament affirm that human beings still bear God's image and that this is the reason why we must respect them.[60]

Convergence Between the Christian Denominations

Over a number of years, important controversies remained between Eastern Orthodox, Protestant and Catholic theologians in their understanding of the image of God in humankind. For example, Protestants were uneasy with what they considered to be a reduction, by Catholic theologians, of the image of God to a static concept of human nature and human beings' need for God. On the other hand, Catholics were uncomfortable with what they believed to be the Reformers' tendency to deny the very existence of the image of God in human beings, as such. They were concerned that Protestant theology was maybe overemphasizing the relationship with God as the most important aspect of the image of God. Moreover, Catholic theologians considered sin as a wounding of the image of God in human beings while the Reformers argued that the image of God was corrupted by sin.[61]

More recently, however, a convergence has taken place between Christian theologians from different denominations who now generally agree that the image of God in human beings cannot be completely hidden by sin because it expresses the whole of human nature. Accordingly, though hidden or obscured by sin, the image of God in a human being remains despite the presence of sin in the life of this person. Under the reign of sin, the relational aspect of the image of God is disrupted in its orientation towards the perfect image of God, Jesus Christ,[62] but is not entirely and irremediably broken.

The Image of God from a Contemporary Christian Perspective

In contrast to all other animal species, the Bible indicates that human beings have been created in the image of their Maker (Gen. 1.26–27). As T. F. Torrance says, human nature has 'a sacred status by its singular openness to God, and to a transcendent ground of rationality',[63] though nothing about humanity being made in the image of God abolishes the essential distinction between the creator and the created.[64]

But what is distinctively Christian is the reality that the humanity of Christ is the 'image of the invisible God' (Col. 1.15). This means that the image of God found in humankind reflects in some way God's very own being and nature. Torrance argues: 'To deface or mutilate the image of God in man in any way is to sin against the created order grounded in the love of God, and is tantamount to an affront upon God.'[65]

Similarly, any being that reflects the image of God cannot simply be considered as biological material. Humanity as well as the whole of the created natural order cannot be understood merely from a naturalistic perspective. They can only be appropriately investigated, defined and appreciated when they are considered from the perspective of a transcendent and creative Word of God without which human nature and the natural order would cease to have any meaning.

Moreover, and as already noted, Epiphanius argued that it is the whole human being, in his or her entirety, who is created in the image of God.[66] It follows that this image cannot be reduced to some feature of human nature, such as human genetics, or to any human qualities – such as intellect or rationality – or function, such as the dominion of humankind over the earth. Every human person, from a biblical perspective, is a whole body and soul forming a unity which cannot be separated into parts: a unity that also reflects the image of the unity in love of the divine persons of the Trinity.[67]

It is also important to recognize in contemporary theology that the image of God can refer to the concepts of both status and standard. With respect to status and what human beings actually are, the inherent dignity of all human beings only really exists because they are created by God with his image. This dignity, moreover, is not something that can ever be lost or taken away throughout the lifetime of the individual and is not dependent on any function or capacity. Gunton explains that, 'as created, the image of God is in a sense something given, even though it can finally be perfected only eschatologically, and through redemption. That something given cannot be taken away, except by God, because it is part of what it is to be a created human being.'[68]

It is this very strong concept of status that affirms that human beings actually are the image of God (1 Cor. 11.7). Understanding the image of God in terms of standard, on the other hand, means looking at what human beings should be as well as how they should live and is generally presented in biblical passages of the New Testament. This standard is what God intends human beings to become through their renewal and transformation in order to conform to his character and will (Eph. 4.24; Rom. 8.29).

According to this reasoning, while all human beings have the same status of the image of God which gives them their inherent dignity and equality, the degree to which they measure up to the standard of the image of God can vary quite significantly. As Mitchell et al. argue:

The significance of the Fall for the image of God does not rest in any damage done to the image ... but rather in the fact that those created with the status of God's image no longer measure up to the standard of what God's image should look like – even though they retain the status of being the images of God.[69]

One of the advantages of considering the image of God as a status and standard is that both concepts are unrelated to the effects of sin. This is important, as Mitchell et al. again emphasize:

A common feature of both the image as status and the image as standard is that they are thoroughly positive and uncompromised. Accordingly, theological claims that the image of God is 'tarnished' or 'diminished' after the Fall are biblically inaccurate and therefore misleading. Nowhere does the Bible indicate that either the image as status or the image as standard can be compromised.[70]

As the American Protestant theologian John Kilner further explains: 'The dignity of all who are in God's image, humanity's dignity, neither depends on particular human attributes nor diminishes with sin.'[71]

Contemporary theologians would also recognize that the image of God in humanity reflects the reality that God created human beings in such a manner as to be able to have a relationship with them through Christ.

Whether it will ever be possible to explain the image of God in this way remains an open question, but what is certain is that the image of God must be understood as reflecting, in some way, concepts that exist in the uncreated God as expressed in Jesus Christ. As T. F. Torrance says:

> Quite basic is the biblical teaching that man has been made in the image of God. In Christian theology, however, this is regarded as recast and strengthened by the fact that in Jesus the Son of God himself has become man among us, which implies that the image of God in which man has been created is related to God's own being and nature in an ontologically closer way.[72]

Furthermore, the very being of human persons includes both their creatureliness and their nature, which enables them to relate to God, and their very orientation towards God. This means that the image of God must be considered in both a static and a dynamic manner. For example, Hoekema suggests that the divine image must be considered both as a noun (image) and as a verb (imaging).[73] In this way, human persons stand before God as beings who are created and confronted by, but also mirroring, God.

Accordingly, any dynamic perspective of the image of God must take into account the purpose of humankind. Since human beings are oriented towards God, they are also directed towards his loving restorative purposes for them. As Gunton explains:

> To be in the image of God is not, therefore, to have some timeless quality like reason, or anything else, but to exist in a directedness, between our coming from nothing and our being brought through Christ before the throne of the Father.[74]

Likewise, it is important to remember that the image of God in human beings is not just reflected by the manner in which they exist on this earth. It must also express what Christians will become after death.[75] This is a destiny which is in the presence of Christ, filled with the love of Christ and clothed with the righteousness of Christ. As the British Catholic ethicist Pia Matthews concludes: 'The teaching of the image of God in humans then is principally a theological message of creation, relationship and salvation.'[76] Human beings are made in the image of God and are destined for a sharing in eternal life in friendship with God. Each human being is created to be an eternal child of God.[77]

A more developed theological perspective is given by Kilner, who explains:

Image involves connection and reflection. Creation in God's image entails a special connection with God and intended reflection of God. Renewal in God's image entails a more intimate connection with God through Christ and an increasingly actual reflection of God in Christ, to God's glory. This connection with God is the basis of human dignity. This reflection of God is the beauty of human destiny. All of humanity participates in human dignity. All of humanity is offered human destiny, though only some embrace and will experience it. Christ and humanity, connection and reflection, dignity and destiny – these lie at the heart of what God's image is all about.[78]

Of course, this special connection with God, which forms the very basis for understanding the image of God, will probably never be completely characterized. But it does certainly include God's love in his creation of, and continued relationship with, his human children.

Kilner also emphasizes that it is a mistake to believe that God's image has been damaged by sin, and thereby rejects Gregory of Nyssa's statement that the full image could not be retained due to sin. He also disagrees with Luther, who believed that the image of God is almost completely lost with only a 'relic' remaining, and with Calvin's statement that the image is nearly lost with only 'traces' or a 'remnant' being left.[79]

Instead, Kilner argues that the Fall hides but does not destroy the image of God. He explains: 'While the Bible consistently avoids indicating that the image of God is either lost or damaged in human beings – now or in any day – all too many people are learning today that such loss or damage has occurred.' And he adds: 'The result has been an understanding, influential in Protestant circles, that sinful human beings have virtually lost God's image.'[80]

For Kilner this is unfortunate since it is the recognition of the full image of God in human beings, though hidden by sin, which is the greatest defence against any destruction of human beings.[81]

This brief overview of the image of God in human beings has sought to emphasize the important features included in the concept although, of course, it has sometimes meant overemphasizing one feature at the expense of another. But the final conclusion can only be that the divine image in humankind cannot be reduced to certain characteristics or abilities but reflects, instead, humanity's very nature. Human beings do not simply bear the image of God; they are the image of God. As such, every human person is endowed with a distinctive moral status which calls for special protection (Gen. 9.6).

At this stage in seeking to develop the concept of the image of God, it may be useful to comment on the significant parallels that exist between this image and being a person. As will be shown, the notions of creature-liness and relatedness are, here again, interrelated. It is also important to emphasize the need to consider the concepts of both being and becoming, together, in seeking to grasp these key notions.

Notes

1 For a helpful discussion see Henri Blocher, 1984, *In the Beginning*, Leicester: InterVarsity Press, pp. 79–94.

2 Blocher, *In the Beginning*, p. 79; David Cairns, 1953, *The Image of God in Man*, first edition, London: SCM Press, p. 16.

3 Claus Westermann, 1984, *Genesis 1–11: A Commentary*, London: SPCK, pp. 206, 207.

4 Westermann, *Genesis 1–11*, p. 155; similarly Colin Gunton writes that 'questions about the … image, such as that concerning human dominion over the remainder of the creation, are secondary and consequent, rather than constitutive of the image'. Colin Gunton, 1998, *The Triune Creator: A Historical and Systematic Study*, Grand Rapids: Eerdmans, p. 200.

5 Anthony A. Hoekema, 1986, *Created in God's Image*, Grand Rapids: Eerdmans, pp. 78–9.

6 The Greek version of the Old Testament, produced in the third century BC.

7 The Latin translation of the Bible, produced by Jerome from 382 to 404 AD.

8 Francis Brown, S. R. Driver and Charles Briggs, 1907, *Hebrew and English Lexicon of the Old Testament*, New York: Houghton Mifflin, p. 853.

9 C. Ben Mitchell, Edward D. Pellegrino, Jean Bethke Elshtain, John F. Kilner and Scott B. Rae, 2007, *Biotechnology and the Human Good*, Washington, DC: Georgetown University Press, p. 71.

10 Gerhard von Rad, 1961, *Genesis*, London: SCM Press, p. 58.

11 Driver and Briggs, *Hebrew and English Lexicon*, pp. 197–8.

12 Ascribed to Luther in Carl Friedrich Keil and Franz Delitzsch, 1861, *Biblical Commentary on the Old Testament, Vol. 1, The Pentateuch*, trans. James Martin, Edinburgh: T&T Clark, p. 63.

13 Hoekema, *Created*, p. 13; Mitchell et al., *Biotechnology*, p. 69.

14 Denis R. Alexander, 'Cloning humans – distorting the image of God?', *Cambridge Papers, Jubilee Centre* 10:2 (June 2001), http://www.jubilee-centre.org/document.php?id=32 (accessed 20 December 2011).

15 David Cairns, 1973, *The Image of God in Man*, second edition, London: Fontana Library of Theology & Philosophy, p. 41.

16 For a detailed discussion of the different interpretations of the *imago dei* throughout Christian history see Stanley Grenz, 2001, *The Social God and the Relational Self: A Trinitarian Theology of the Imago Dei*, Louisville: Westminster John Knox Press.

17 Colin Gunton disagrees with this: 'While there may be some evidence that Irenaeus sometimes speaks like that [drawing a distinction between likeness to God, which has been lost at the Fall, and the image, which has not] … that is not generally his view, which is to treat the two as synonymous.' Gunton adds: 'Additional confirmation that Irenaeus is not guilty of a dualistic interpretation of the image is found in his view that for him both image and likeness are lost in Adam, both restored in Christ.' Gunton, *Triune Creator*, Grand Rapids: Eerdmans, pp. 196–8.

18 Irenaeus, *Against Heresies* V.6.1.

19 Hoekema, *Created*, pp. 33–4; Brendan McCarthy, 1997, *Fertility & Faith*, Leicester: InterVarsity Press, p. 128.

20 Irenaeus, *Against Heresies* V.16.2, in Alexander Roberts and James Donaldson (eds), 1953, *Ante-Nicene Fathers, Vol. 1*, Grand Rapids: Eerdmans, p. 532.

21 Cairns, 1953, *Image of God*, first edition, p. 81.

22 Hoekema, *Created*, p. 35.

23 Tertullian, *Baptism* V.6.7.

24 Letter LI. From Epiphanius, Bishop of Salamis, in Cyprus, to John, Bishop of Jerusalem. http://www.ccel.org/ccel/schaff/npnf206.v.LI.html (accessed 1 July 2016).

25 Epiphanius of Salamis, *Panarion*, 70, Patrologia, Series Graeca, J. P. Migne, 42, 344B.

26 Gregory of Nyssa, *On the Making of Man* II.

27 Augustine, *On the Trinity* 12.7.12.

28 Augustine, *Confessions* I.1.1; *On the Trinity* 14.6

29 Thomas Aquinas, *Summa Theologica* I, q. 93. a. 9; Hoekema, *Created*, p. 36.

30 Hoekema, *Created*, p. 37.

31 Aquinas, *Summa Theologica*, I, q. 93. a. 2 and I, q. 93. a. 6

32 Plato, *The Timaeus*, 90 C; Aristotle, *De Anima*, Bk 1, 408b, also *Nic. Ethics*, Bk 10, 1177b.

33 Hoekema, *Created*, p. 37.

34 John Calvin, *Commentary on Genesis* 3.1.

35 John Calvin, *Institutes of the Christian Religion*, ed. John T. McNeill, trans. Ford Lewis Battles, Philadelphia: Westminster Press, 1960, I.15.3.

36 Calvin, *Institutes* III.7.6.

37 Cairns, 1973, *Image of God*, second edition, p. 146.

38 Cairns, 1973, *Image of God*, second edition, p. 137.

39 Thomas F. Torrance, 1949, *Calvin's Doctrine of Man*, London: Lutterworth Press, p. 36.

40 Calvin, *Institutes* I.15.3.

41 Colin Gunton, 1991, 'Trinity, Ontology and Anthropology: Towards a Renewal of the Doctrine of the Imago Dei', in Christoph Schwöbel and Colin Gunton (eds), *Persons, Divine and Human*, Edinburgh: T&T Clark, pp. 47–61.

42 Hoekema, *Created*, p. 35; McCarthy, *Fertility & Faith*, p. 128.

43 Hoekema, *Created*, p. 45.

44 Cairns, 1973, *Image of God*, second edition, p. 141.

45 Hoekema, *Created*, p. 35.

46 J. Richard Middleton, 2005, *The Liberating Image*, Grand Rapids: Brazos Press, pp. 18–19.

47 Karl Barth, 1960, *Church Dogmatics*, Edinburgh: T&T Clark, Vol. III.1, p. 195.

48 McCarthy, *Fertility & Faith*, p. 134.

49 Hoekema, *Created*, pp. 49–50.

50 McCarthy, *Fertility & Faith*, p. 134.

51 Emil Brunner, 1953, *The Christian Doctrine of Creation and Redemption*, trans. Olive Wyon, Philadelphia: Westminster Press, p. 58.

52 Emil Brunner, 1939, *Man in Revolt*, London: Lutterworth Press, p. 96.

53 Cairns, 1973, *Image of God*, second edition, p. 157.

54 Brunner, *Creation and Redemption*, pp. 59–61, 77–8; John F. Kilner, 2015, *Dignity and Destiny: Humanity in the Image of God*, Grand Rapids: Eerdmans, p. 212.

55 Cairns, 1973, *Image of God*, second edition, p. 184.

56 David Atkinson, 1987, 'Some Theological Perspectives on the Human Embryo',

in Nigel M. De S. Cameron (ed.), *Embryos and Ethics*, Edinburgh: Rutherford House Books, pp. 46–7.

57 Gerrit C. Berkouwer, 1962, *Man: The Image of God*, trans. Dirk W. Jellena, Grand Rapids: Eerdmans, pp. 107–12.

58 Hoekema, *Created*, p. 69.

59 Hoekema, *Created*, p. 72.

60 John Stott, 2006, *Through the Bible Through the Year*, Oxford: Lion Hudson, p. 18.

61 International Theological Commission, Communion and Stewardship, *Human Persons Created in the Image of God*, The Vatican, 2002, paragraph 17, http://www.vatican.va/roman_curia/congregations/cfaith/cti_documents/rc_con_cfaith_doc_20040723_communion-stewardship_en.html#_edn1 (accessed 3 February 2011).

62 International Theological Commission, Communion and Stewardship, *Human Persons*, paragraph 46. For further discussion relating to the concept of the image of God in the different Christian denominations, see: Thomas Albert Howard (ed.), 2013, *Imago Dei: Human Dignity in Ecumenical Perspective*, Washington, D.C.: The Catholic University of America Press.

63 Taped lecture given by T. F. Torrance, 'Ethics and Embryos', at Rutherford House, Edinburgh, recorded by Andrew Rollinson. Cited in Andrew R. Rollinson, 1994, 'The Incarnation and the Status of the Human Embryo', a thesis submitted for the degree of M.Litt. with the Religious Studies Department of Newcastle University, p. 58.

64 Gunton, *Triune Creator*, p. 205.

65 Thomas F. Torrance, 1984, *Test-tube Babies: Science – Morals – and the Law*, Edinburgh: Scottish Academic Press, p. 10.

66 Epiphanius of Salamis, *Panarion*, 70.

67 International Theological Commission, Communion and Stewardship, *Human Persons*, paragraph 9; John Bryant and John Searle, *Life in Our Hands: A Christian Perspective on Genetics and Cloning*, Leicester: InterVarsity Press, 2004, pp. 40–1.

68 Gunton, *Triune Creator*, p. 204.

69 Mitchell et al., *Biotechnology*, pp. 70, 74.

70 Mitchell et al., *Biotechnology*, pp. 70–1.

71 Kilner, *Dignity and Destiny*, p. 314.

72 Torrance, *Test-tube Babies*, pp. 9–10.

73 Hoekema, *Created*, p. 65.

74 Colin E. Gunton, 1992, *Christ and Creation* (The Didsbury Lectures 1990), Exeter: Paternoster Press, p. 102.

75 Hoekema, *Created*, p. 96.

76 Pia Matthews, 2010, 'Discerning Persons: How the early theology can illuminate contemporary bioethical approaches to the concept of person', doctoral thesis, Saint Mary's University College, p. 160.

77 Pia Matthews, 2013, *Pope John Paul II and the Apparently 'Non-acting' Person*, Leominster: Gracewing, p. 73.

78 Kilner, *Dignity and Destiny*, p. xi. Kilner also explains that: 'people are "in" or "according to" God's image; God's image is undamaged by sin; not only are individuals in God's image but humanity as a whole is as well; God's image has to do with people as a whole rather than with particular human attributes.' John Kilner, 2017, 'Grounding Significance in God', in John Kilner (ed.), *Why People Matter*, Grand Rapids, MI: Baker Academic, p. 144.

79 Kilner, *Dignity and Destiny*, pp. 67, 159, 164, 166.

80 Kilner, *Dignity and Destiny*, pp. 174, 164

81 Kilner, *Dignity and Destiny*, p. 21.

3

Being a Person from a Christian Perspective

By its very nature the concept of personhood is associated with a moral dimension. This is because a person is a being who ought to be treated as having the same full moral status as any other person.[1] It is even possible to state that an appropriate understanding of personhood is essential for the very existence of ethics[2] and, as a result, for any discussion relating to the moral status of the early embryo. The crucial question then becomes, 'When does a human person begin to exist?' It is, for example, at this stage that the maxim of the German philosopher, Immanuel Kant (1724–1804) becomes effective, in that a person should always be treated as an end and never only as a means.

Some contemporary ethicists, of course, such as the American philosopher Michael Tooley, would suggest that, although the concept of personhood is important, the crucial element for a moral judgement is whether a being has a 'right to life', which is related to whether the being has an interest in, or claim on, continued life.[3] But for the majority of Christian ethicists it is the crucial concept of personhood that is morally relevant.

Being a Person from a Historic Perspective

There was never any clear understanding of personhood in the ancient world. In Greco-Roman philosophy the concept is not clearly defined, with Greek Platonic thought describing an 'individual' as being secondary to the reality of essential forms. It was a human being's immortal soul that was essential, in contrast to his or her body which was seen as less important.[4] For example, in Aristotle's philosophy the soul is the 'organizing principle' of the body and both together make up an individual.

The first time the term 'person' (*prosopon* in Greek) appears is in the theatre where it was associated with an actor's mask. Although it was eventually related to an actor's role and identity, a human being's essential being (*hypostasis* in Greek[5]) was never identified with this role or with the word 'person'. This was similar to the Roman understanding in which *persona* was associated with the role that an individual played.

These Greco-Roman understandings of what actually constituted a human person were also a reflection of the manner in which the ancient world considered the cosmos. In Greek thought a complete, unified whole existed in which everything, including God, the universe and all individuals, formed one single system defined as the cosmos.

It was only when Judeo-Christian beliefs began to expand the biblical perspective that this monist cosmology was supplanted by the understanding that a creator God was radically different and distinct from his creation – a creation which was created *ex nihilo*, from absolutely nothing, and therefore a contingent, not a necessary, creation. This enabled the very nature of the existence of the individual to be defined within creation.

Such an emphasis came as a result of the reflections of the Church Fathers when seeking to express the Christian faith in a triune God. The Greek Orthodox theologian John Zizioulas states that what happened could be considered as a conceptual revolution.[6] He begins his (1985) book *Being as Communion*: 'Although the person and "personal identity" are widely discussed nowadays as a supreme ideal, nobody seems to recognise that historically as well as existentially the concept of person is indissolubly bound up with theology.'[7]

By identifying the essential being or reality of an individual (the *hypostasis*) with the *person,* a new perspective was given by the early Christian scholars. But it also resulted in the unfortunate and well-documented confusion between the Eastern and Western churches. Tertullian, in the West, used 'persons' to characterize the Trinity as 'three Persons, one Substance' (*una substantia, tres personae*).[8] But precisely because, in Greek thought, the concept of 'person' lacked any ontological content (representing instead just an actor's role), it was deemed heretical. For the Eastern Greek theologians, this characterization of God was unacceptable because it reflected back to the Sabellian notion of God in three 'roles' which denied the distinctiveness of the three persons of the Godhead.

In the East, the Trinity was considered as three hypostases which, for the Western theologians, was uncomfortably close to tri-theism since they were accustomed to identifying *hypostasis* with *substantia*. In other words, the West was concerned that God was being represented by the Eastern theologians as three essential realities with three substances.

Importantly, it seems to have been just such a misunderstanding that led the Greek Fathers to identify 'person' with *hypostasis*. Zizioulas and the English philosopher Clement Webb (1865–1954) both agree that it was the Roman theologian Hippolytus (170–235) who first used *prosopon* for the Trinity and identified it with *hypostasis*, thereby bringing East and West together.[9]

God is personal and each member of the Trinity is personal although the personalness of God can be distinguished from the persons in the Trinity. Since the Council of Constantinople in 381, the concept of 'three hypostases in one ousia' (three persons in one being) became the orthodox doctrine of the Trinity in Christianity.

This meant that the 'person' was no longer 'an adjunct to being' but was itself the hypostasis of being[10] and was what constituted being. In other words, the person was the being and the term could no longer be considered as simply describing the being with a certain role. Thus a person, defined in this way, cannot be determined qualitatively and is not simply 'an appearance' or a mask but is the individual himself or herself, including his or her history and continuity of identity. This was the ground-breaking legacy of Trinitarian theology concerning what it means to be a person, and can also be considered the most important challenge to the contemporary interpretation of personhood.[11]

This Christian understanding of being a person can, moreover, be emphasized in two complementary manners.

First, because of the Trinitarian being of God, the West emphasized God's unity in that God is one substance (*una substantia*). On the other hand, the Greek Church emphasized God's essential being, with the *hypostasis* (person) of the Father 'initiating' both the generation of the person of the Son and the procession of the person of the Spirit. In this way, the one substance does not exist in a 'naked' state and without the three hypostastic persons of the Trinity.[12]

Second, when the Council of Chalcedon in 451 defined Jesus Christ as 'one person with two natures', this meant that the concept of 'person' comes before the concepts of 'natures' or 'attributes'.

When early arguments were then made suggesting that the identity of the Word made flesh resided either in a human soul or mind, or in a divine soul or mind, problems with the Chalcedonian understanding of the person of Christ immediately became evident. Indeed, it is impossible to fully understand the identity of Jesus Christ in any qualitative manner. Here again, an emphasis on the *hypostasis* had to be seen as the solution. In other words, the essential being and substantial reality of Christ must come before his nature or attributes. This is similar to the Roman philosopher Boethius' (*c.* 480–*c.* 524) famous definition of 'person' as 'the individual substance of rational nature' (*Persona est naturae rationabilis individua substantia*).[13]

Again, what comes first is the substance and essential being (*hypostasis*) of a person, with the attribute of rationality coming second. As O'Donovan comments, 'the distinctive qualities of humanity are attributable to persons, not persons to the qualities of humanity'.[14] This means that being a person comes before any attributable characteristics. Moreover, that a person has a rational nature does not entail that he or she must display or express the capacities of a rational life. The infant and the unconscious patient are also persons since they possess and share the nature of rational beings.[15]

This means that a human person is an individual rational substance of body and soul where the soul may be defined as the life-giving and integrating principle.[16] As D. A. Jones et al. say: 'Throughout the history of the Church, Christians have used the language of "body and soul" to understand the human being in such a way as not to deny the unity of God's creation.'[17]

In attempting to clarify this human unity, the fourteenth-century Ecumenical Council of Vienne accepted the doctrine that the soul was 'the form of the body' (forma corporis),[18] meaning that which gives life to the body. As the Catholic theologian Peter Bristow puts it: 'The soul is the principle of life and unity of the soul/body composite which unites the different organs and parts that make it up, and, in turn, works through the organs and senses of the body to produce unitary actions.'[19]

In the specific case of humanity (in contrast to other kinds of non-human persons) the rational nature is also that of the human being as such. Aquinas expanded on Boethius' definition by clarifying: 'It belongs to every man to be a person as much as every subject in a human nature is a person.' He added: 'The words "individual substance" appearing in the definition of person signify a complete substance, subsisting in its own right and separately from others.'[20] According to this view, it is beings who belong to the whole individual substance of a rational nature who can be considered as persons.[21] As D. A. Jones explains, the rational nature on which Boethius focuses 'is shared by all members of the same species, rather than the powers someone possesses at a particular time. According to this understanding, a human person is nothing more or less than a living human being.'[22]

With this Boethian definition, the following three characteristics can be emphasized: a person (1) is an individual and exists in and by him- or herself and not in another while maintaining his or her identity through change, (2) is a unity of body and soul, and (3) is distinguished from animals and objects by potentiality for rationality and free will.[23]

Another concept that arose from the early Church's understanding of incarnational theology is found in the meaning of the Greek word ekstasis,[24] defined as God's love in the community and fellowship of the triune Being. In his essential being, God is a community in whom love is being shared in the persons of the Trinity. As Rollinson writes: 'Ekstasis must be put alongside hypostasis as the two grand formative contributions of Trinitarian theology.'[25] In other words, the very being of the Trinity must always be associated and integrated with the love that binds the persons of the Trinity together in oneness.

According to the Church Fathers, therefore, an appropriate understanding of being a person can only be based on (1) particularity through otherness and (2) communion through relationships.[26] As Zizioulas observes: 'The mystery of being a person lies in the fact that here otherness and communion are not in contradiction, but coincide.'[27]

It was Augustine, in his *De Trinitate*, who very much focused on the importance of a relational understanding of personhood. Instead of emphasizing the causal origins of the persons in the Trinity, as did some of the Greek Fathers, Augustine refused to recognize the persons of the Trinity in terms of generation or procession, but as being inherently in relationship with one another. He sought to explain the Trinity as an analogy of 'the lover', 'the beloved' and 'love itself' flowing between the two.[28] Because of this, Augustine was uncomfortable with the term 'person', only using it when he had no other option,[29] since he considered 'person' as being appropriate only in the context of 'essence' and not relations.[30]

Yet Augustine's focus is both his strength and his weakness. It is his strength because he focuses on relationships, and it is his weakness because it may give rise to the temptation of identifying personhood with the relationships themselves. For example, Gunton argued that Augustine did not appropriately emphasize the essential persons, as such, who are in relationship with one another.[31]

In other words, it is important to affirm that although a relational concept of person reflects a search of identity in a given context, being a person is more than just a role or function. According to this view, the German Reformed theologian Jürgen Moltmann says, in explaining the relationship between Father and Son, 'It does not constitute existence of Father and Son, it presupposes it.' Being a person and relationships must be accepted together in a simultaneous manner. Moltmann goes on to explain: 'There are no persons without relations, but there are no relations without persons either.'[32]

This proper understanding of what it means to be a person was also re-emphasized by T. F. Torrance when he stressed how the very notion was derived from early Christian theology through the doctrine of the Holy Trinity: that is, from 'God as an eternal communion of three hypostatic realities or Persons who are who and what they are in their eternal coinherent relations with one another'[33] – namely, through their interrelations in being and acts with one another. He added:

While that notion of 'person' applied originally and strictly to the Triune nature of God, it came to be applied to creaturely human beings, in such a way that the relations between human beings constitute what they are as persons. Persons are what and who they are in the inter-personal relations of their one being with each other.[34]

As such they also reflect and image the transcendent relatedness or community in oneness inherent in the Trinity.[35]

In other words, since the likeness to God involves the triune God, in the communion of the Father, Son and Holy Spirit, and since, in Genesis, human beings are portrayed not as existing alone but as existing in relation to others, being a person in the image and likeness of God also involves existing in a relationship. This means that each human being is individually like God, as a rational and free being, and each in his or her common humanity is called to mirror the communion of love that is in God.[36]

But ever since about the sixth century, the notion of being a person has been split into two independent historical directions. One remained loyal to the theology of the early Church which stressed the 'individual substance' of Boethius' definition and of personhood as such. The other, however, slowly departed from this Christian understanding, focusing instead on the 'nature', the attributes or the qualitative dimensions of personhood.

In this context, Zizioulas bemoans what he believes is a Western understanding of personhood which even in modern theology has often characterized the person as an individual. This has, either explicitly or implicitly, led modern thought to assimilate the person to a thinking, self-conscious, rational and autonomous individual. For Zizioulas, the Eastern Fathers' insight is a better reflection of the reality whereby a true person can only exist in a loving relationship with others, not in an individualistic isolation from others.[37]

O'Donovan also laments this development, observing: 'The history of the concept of "person" is the history of how "nature" takes over from "substance", the secondary feature of the definition displacing the primary one.'[38] In other words, the person in his or her substantive otherness is slowly reduced to what the person can do.

This change in focus was further exemplified in the writings of the French philosopher René Descartes (1596–1650), for whom the only concept that was certain to exist was a human being's thoughts. It follows that self-consciousness became the very essence of personhood[39] in a dualistic understanding of human persons who were divided up into different characteristics.

This focus on self-consciousness was also emphasized by the English philosopher John Locke (1632–1704), who defined personhood as 'the ability to think combined with self-consciousness'.[40]

Similarly, the Scottish philosopher David Hume (1711–76) suggested that personal identity was a series of human experiences. He argued that a person was 'nothing but a bundle or collection of different perceptions, which succeed each other with an inconceivable rapidity, and are in a perpetual flux each moment'.[41] This kind of thinking was supported, as well, on the European continent by individuals such as the German philosopher Christian Wolff (1679–1754), considered to be the Schoolman of the Enlightenment, who defined a person as a thing that is conscious of itself (*Ein Ding das Sich Bewusst ist*).[42]

Another manner in which personhood was discussed without any reference to Christian theology came from Kant, who emphasized the central role of 'practical reason'. He maintained that the most important part of mental activity was not cognition but the will, with the 'rational willing agency being the essential characteristic'.[43] O'Donovan contrasts Kant's 'practical imperative' – 'Act so that you treat humanity, whether in your own person or in that of another, always as an end and never as a means only' – with the Council of Chalcedon's definition written in the year 451: 'one person in two natures'. Indeed, for Kant what was crucial was not 'being a person' with a rational nature but what is 'in a person' (the rational nature itself), whereas for Chalcedon what was central was Christ's being a person but 'in two natures'. Again, for Kant nature has taken over from substance.[44] As Zizioulas comments: 'It is all too often assumed that people "have" personhood rather than "being" persons.'[45] This means that what becomes important in more modern philosophy is what an individual is able to do, rather than his or her very being and substantive otherness. It is this substitution, which arose from losing contact with the Trinitarian roots of being a person, which has resulted in the regrettable contemporary understanding of personhood. In all the philosophical thinking of Descartes, Locke and Kant, human persons are only a subgroup of human beings who can do something. This also means that some human beings could actually be considered as non-persons or only partially persons.

Interestingly, with respect to the moral status of the embryo, this view – that the very existence of a person is dependent on what he or she can do – stands in a historical tradition. In Aristotelian embryology, the proposal of a gradual development from vegetative, to animal, to rational human life, leading to a view of delayed animation, reflects this gradual ability to do more things. As already mentioned, this theory, which was also accepted by Aquinas, led to the suggestion that ensoulment took place 40 days after fertilization for male and 90 days after fertilization for female embryos.[46] Unfortunately, though this gradualist argument was never used as a reason for undertaking an abortion, it has been very influential in promoting the idea that human life and being a person are different.

But it may be appropriate at this stage to present a more cautionary interpretation of Aristotle and Aquinas. Indeed, the philosophical theory of hylomorphism, developed by Aristotle, describes the concept of being (*ousia*) as a compound of matter and form. Thus matter and form may be interpreted in a more integrated manner, with the soul being considered as the form of the body though both are holistically united to one another. Had Aristotle and Aquinas not been constrained by a limited understanding of embryology, it is very likely that their thinking might not have been restricted to the concept of delayed animation where the human soul came into existence after the body.[47]

Indeed, it is possible that early dualistic understandings of personhood as body and soul were also the result of seeking to integrate more Platonic perspectives of individual souls into the Aristotelian schema, with the later body–soul dualism of Descartes coming to reinforce such a view, although it should be noted that, in the Middle Ages, there was a strong perception that the body and the soul were integrated together.[48]

Unfortunately, however, Cartesian dualism is still very much in evidence in contemporary discourse. For example, the Australian ethicist Peter Singer argues that the concept of 'person' could be defined as 'a being possessing, at least at a minimal level, the capacities distinctive of our species, which include consciousness, the ability to be aware of one's surroundings, the ability to relate to others, perhaps even rationality and self-consciousness'.[49]

Similarly, for the British ethicist John Harris it is only what can be immediately experienced that is important:

> A person will thus be any individual capable of valuing its own life. Such a being will, at the very least, be able to conceive of itself as an independent centre of consciousness, existing over time with a future that it is capable of envisaging and wishing to experience.[50]

He further states that 'it is not because an individual is a person that its life is morally valuable, rather it is because it has those features that make life morally valuable that it is a person'.[51]

But according to this kind of reasoning, not all human beings are persons. For example, Singer and the Australian bioethicist Helga Kuhse take their arguments about personhood to the logical conclusions when they state:

We must recall, however, that when we kill a new-born infant there is no person whose life has begun. When I think of myself as the person I now am, I realize that I did not come into existence until sometime after my birth. At birth I had no sense of the future, and no experiences which I can now remember as 'mine'. It is the beginning of the life of the person, rather than of the physical organism, that is crucial so far as the right to life is concerned.[52]

With respect to human embryos, this argument would mean that they would become persons (and be protected as such) only at some developmental stage after conception, or even after birth, when their lives become morally valuable. This also implies that individuals may cease to be persons at some stage before the human body dies. In addition, it would mean that the personhood of an individual can increase or decrease according to its attributes. As the British philosopher Jonathan Glover commented, 'being a person is a matter of degree'.[53]

Fortunately, this whole manner of thinking has now been challenged, especially from the more classical, non-empirical and non-dualistic traditions of continental Europe, with an emphasis that human beings cannot simply be considered as physical bodies in which personhood can exist at a later stage. Human bodies are not mere objects or containers which enable the existence of a rational consciousness. A human being is a person. Indeed, the Holy See's *Instruction on Respect for Human Life* asks, 'How could a human not be a human person?'[54] It then focuses on the unitary nature of human beings consisting of an in-dissociable body and soul.

A person, as the Irish philosopher Teresa Iglesias argues, is 'an entity of *a kind* to which it is proper to ascribe a number of specified attributes',[55] but where it will never be possible to reduce its existence to a number of specific characteristics.

In the correct understanding of a person, therefore, abilities and special characteristics are secondary and do not have to be displayed at a point in time. Having a rational nature (in the context of Boethius' definition of a person as an individual substance of rational nature) does not mean that rationality must always be present. This is what happens, for example, with neonates or the unconscious adult. What is important is having the constitution of beings of a human kind, rather than being able to express such a nature.[56] It is a reflection of the Thomist principle, *operari sequitur esse*: 'our behaving and characteristics flow out of who we essentially are'. In other words, the embryo's potential to grow and develop arises out of what it essentially is.

This 'natural kinds' theory has also been supported by Iglesias: 'What makes us persons is the kind of beings we are ... if we can attain self-consciousness at some stage, we must already be the kind of beings that can attain it.'[57] From a theological perspective, such a stage where self-conscious rational thought is attained may also include, or indeed may only be (in certain pre-natal, newborn or severely mentally disabled persons), the stage of existence after death.[58] As Zizioulas has pointed out, the concept of being a person is, in the end, an eschatological concept 'in that true personhood will be realised only in the final Kingdom of God'.[59] This means that God sees his children as persons just as much after death as on earth.

A holistic body–soul perspective is also supported by an understanding of both Scripture and tradition. In the creation account, the soul is not portrayed as being an independent element of a living human being. God 'breathed into his [man's] nostrils the breath of life; and the man became a living being' (Gen. 2.7). In the Greek Septuagint this was described as *psyche* or soul. Thus Adam did not *receive* a soul, he *became* a living soul – a complete and whole person. In Barth's term 'man is embodied soul and besouled body'.[60] The soul as form of the body constitutes the human being as a human being. The Christian belief of the person as 'a being composed out of union of soul and body into one form of the beautiful',[61] in addition to belief in the resurrection of the body, confirms that the body shares in the beauty of creation in the image of God.[62]

Being a Person from a Contemporary Christian Perspective

Because of the growing separation between personhood and the human body in modern society there is an increasing tendency to consider the body as raw material in its efforts to produce goods for consumption. But enormous dangers lie behind the application of such criteria to humanity. When the human body comes to be used as raw material in the same way as the bodies of animals, such as in the experimentation on embryos and foetuses, society will inevitably experience a dreadful ethical defeat.[63]

Fortunately, in contemporary Christian theology, being a person has not been considered in this dualistic manner. Instead, the body and the person have been seen as united with an immeasurable and irreducible value and worth. Moreover, there have never been 'half persons' and human beings have always been considered as full persons. As D. A. Jones writes:

> The idea of an embryo or foetus as meriting some proportion of the respect due to a person seems to imply that respect for persons could be present in proportion. This is reminiscent of the discredited

compromise of the Philadelphia Convention of 1787 where a slave counted for 'three fifths' of a free citizen. To be counted as three fifths of a person is surely a denial of respect.[64]

Such an understanding of personhood would quickly lead to a demise of civilized society. At present every human being, no matter what characteristics he or she may have, is equally considered as a person without exceptions. Karol Wojtyla (the future Pope John Paul II) concluded:

> Man is a person 'by nature', by which he is entitled to the subjectivity proper to a person ... The fact that sometimes the human subject does not manifest the characteristics of personal subjectivity does not authorise doubts concerning the foundations of this subjectivity.[65]

This unitary approach may imply that the embryo person grows at the same time as the embryonic and foetal body. In other words, the development of the soul cannot be considered as completely separate from the whole developmental process since it is integrally bound up with such a process.

But it is important to note that the concept of being a person is always associated with the notions of completeness and wholeness. Since there can never be a partial or incomplete soul, there can never be a partial or incomplete person. This means that, although an embryo's body and soul may develop with time, his or her personhood does not change in time to any degree since the embryo is complete and whole. As a result, the early human embryo can never be diminished to just a partial person or even just a 'pile of cells', as is so often the case in modern bioscience.

This implies that personhood must be recognized from the creation of the embryo onwards. The emphasis is on the development *of* a person in contrast to the development *into* a person.[66]

It is also noteworthy that the themes presented by a theological examination of the divine image and those of being a person inevitably come together. In both, purely qualitative characteristics, such as human capabilities, are inappropriate to define the concepts. If they were, no member of the species *Homo sapiens* could be considered as having the same moral status.

Instead, both notions, of being a person and of the divine image, have converged on an understanding of being created from outside the cosmos as well as in humanity's relatedness to God, other persons and creation as a whole. These concepts are at the heart of the very existence and meaning of human nature.

This means that a physical person can be defined as a being who reflects the image of God with all the complexity and meaning that this image represents. To be in the image of God is to be created by God as a person. Both concepts and their discussions are intrinsically related.

But as already indicated, this was to be expected since it was because early Christian thinkers began to reflect on the Christian doctrines of the incarnation of Christ and the persons of the Trinity, who exist in the Godhead, that they started to understand what it means to be a human person.[67] T. F. Torrance summarized one of the main outcomes of such an investigation:

> In the strict sense God alone is Person, complete, self-sufficient Person, who as such is the creative source of all other personal being ... Hence the Incarnation means that all God's relations with us within human being are acutely personalised, and that it is through his person-creating relations with us that we are unceasingly sustained in our personal being day by day. Jesus Christ as the incarnate Son of God, therefore, is personalising Person, whereas we who draw our personal being from him, are personalised persons. From being static, human personal being is continuously dependent on and dynamically upheld by God's person-creating relations with us.[68]

Moreover, since a human being is a living whole created by God in his image and personalized by him, it will never be possible to completely define or fully understand what it means to be a human person and why others are persons, since God cannot be defined. Because of this, O'Donovan argues that it will be impossible ever to demonstrate that a person exists through scientific examinations for attributes, functions or capacity, and that it is futile and even perilous even to seek to do so. Instead, 'we discern persons only by love, by discovering through interaction and commitment that this human being is irreplaceable'.[69]

Human beings are created in such a manner as to transcend their creation and be able to think of what is beyond themselves in their relationship with their creator.[70] As Gunton emphasizes: 'To be a created person is, first, to be in the inescapable relation to God ... who will not, this side of eternity, cease to hold and direct those created in hope.'[71]

It is the incomprehensible love of God for human beings and which he shares through human beings that makes them real, wonderful but incomprehensible persons. As the German Protestant Theologian Helmut Thielicke (1908 – 1986) explains, the dignity reflected in humankind has an origin which is external to humanity. He states: '[I]t is not man's own worth – his value for producing "good works," his functional proficiency ... – that gives him his dignity, but rather what God has "spent upon him," the sacrificial love which God has invested in him (Deut. 7:7f.)'.[72]

It is because of this love that a person can be defined as a being with a full inherent dignity reflecting the image of God.

Notes

1 A. C. Danto, 1967, 'Persons', in Paul Edwards (ed.), *The Encyclopaedia of Philosophy*, New York and London: Macmillan, quoted in Egbert Schroten, 'What Makes a Person?', *Theology* 97 (1994), pp. 98–105 (p. 99).

2 David Jenkins states: 'People who refuse a proper concern for people are immoral as human beings and wrong as judges of matters of fact.' David Jenkins, 1967, *The Glory of Man*, London: SCM Press, p. 3.

3 Michael Tooley, 1988, 'In Defence of Abortion and Infanticide', in Michael Goodman (ed.), *What Is a Person?*, Clifton, NJ: Humana Press.

4 Zizioulas states: 'The Platonic soul of a human being, far from safeguarding the survival of the particular eternally, could be reincarnated in other beings, even in animals.' John D. Zizioulas, 1991, 'On Being a Person – Towards an Ontology of Personhood', in Christoph Schwobel and Colin E. Gunton (eds), *Persons, Divine and Human*, Edinburgh: T&T Clark, p. 36.

5 *Hypostasis* may be interpreted in two different ways. The first expresses the originally objective or substantial reality. The second describes the unique reality or personal subsistence of the three 'persons' in the one being of God. Since the Council of Constantinople in 381, the concept of 'three hypostases in one ousia', i.e. 'three persons in one being', became the orthodox doctrine of the Trinity in Christianity.

6 Zizioulas, 'On Being a Person', p. 36.

7 John D. Zizioulas, 1985, *Being as Communion*, London: Darton, Longman and Todd, p. 27. C. C. J. Webb wrote: 'Not only has the concept of personality been profoundly affected by the discussions which were carried on in the Christian Church concerning the mutual relations of the persons of the Trinity and the union of the divine and human natures in the person of Christ, but that philosophical discussion of the nature of human personality is posterior in time to these theological discussions. Nay, it may even be said that it was the religious and theological rest in the personality of Christ, conceived as being at once God and man, which actually afforded the motive and occasion of undertaking the investigation of the nature of personality in men generally.' C. C. J. Webb, 1919, *God and Personality* (Gifford Lectures 1918 & 1919), London: Gifford Lectures, p. 20.

8 Tertullian, *Against Praxeas*, 11–12, Patrologia, Series Latina, J. P. Migne, 2, 1670D.

9 Zizioulas, 'On Being a Person', p. 38.

10 Zizioulas, 'On Being a Person', p. 39.

11 Andrew R. Rollinson, 'The Incarnation and the Status of the Human Embryo', a thesis submitted for the degree of the M.Litt. with the Religious Studies Department of Newcastle University, November 1994, p. 164.

12 Zizioulas, 'On Being a Person', p. 41.

13 Boethius, *Contra Eytychen et Nestorium C. 3*, quoted in Webb, *God and Personality*, p. 47, fn. 21.

14 Oliver O'Donovan, 1984, *Begotten or Made?*, Oxford: Clarendon Press, p. 54.

15 Peter Byrne, 1988, 'The Animation Tradition in the Light of Contemporary Philosophy', in G. R. Dunstan and Mary J. Seller (eds), *The Status of the Human Embryo: Perspectives from Moral Tradition*, Oxford: Oxford University Press, p. 95.

16 Peter Bristow, 2009, *Christian Ethics and the Human Person*, Oxford: Family Publication, p. 76; Jean Boboc, 2014, *La grande métamorphose: Éléments pour une théo-anthropologie orthodoxe*, Paris: Les Éditions du Cerf, p. 320.

17 David A. Jones et al., 'A Theologian's Brief: On the Place of the Human Embryo Within the Christian Tradition and the Theological Principles for Evaluating Its Moral Status', *Ethics & Medicine* 17:3 (2001), pp. 143–53 (p. 148).

18 Council of Vienne, in Norman P. Tanner (ed.), *On the Catholic Faith*, Decrees of Ecumenical Councils, London: Sheed & Ward, 1990, p. 361.

19 Bristow, *Christian Ethics*, pp. 75–6.

20 Aquinas, *Summa Theologica* III, q. 16 a. 12, ad. 1.

21 Norman M. Ford, 1991, *When Did I Begin?*, Cambridge: Cambridge University Press, p. 84.

22 David A. Jones, 2004, *The Soul of the Embryo*, London: Continuum, p. 242.

23 Bristow, *Christian Ethics*, p. 75.

24 Zizioulas, 'On Being a Person', p. 91.

25 Rollinson, 'Incarnation and Status', p. 166.

26 Colin E. Gunton argues that 'space', as well as relationship, is important for an understanding of person. Colin E. Gunton, 'Augustine, the Trinity and the Theological Crisis of the West', *Scottish Journal of Theology* 43:1 (1990), pp. 33–58.

27 Zizioulas, 'On Being a Person', p. 106.

28 'Behold, then, there are three things: he that loves, and that which is loved, and love.' Augustine, *On the Trinity*, trans. A. W. Haddan, Edinburgh: T&T Clark, 8.10.14.

29 'What therefore remains, except that we confess that these terms sprang from the necessity of speaking, when copious reasoning was required against the devices or errors of the heretics.' Augustine, *On the Trinity* 7.4.

30 In contemporary theology, Barth has taken a similar emphasis, and also eschewed the term 'person', preferring 'mode of being' (*Seinswesen*). For Barth 'person' implies the modern 'self-consciousness' concept, and thus leads towards tritheism. His equating person and personality may, however, be unfounded.

31 Gunton argued that Augustine's weakness is due to two main factors. First, through his neo-Platonic heritage, he has a weakened understanding of incarnation. Second, Augustine never really appreciated the Cappadocian meaning of *hypostasis*. Gunton concludes: 'He had prepared the way for the later, and fateful, *definition* of the person as a relation.' Gunton, 'Augustine, the Trinity' pp. 33–58 (pp. 42–3).

32 Jürgen Moltmann, 1980, *The Trinity and the Kingdom of God*, London: SCM Press, p. 172.

33 Thomas F. Torrance, 1999, *The Soul and Person of the Unborn Child*, Edinburgh: Scottish Order of Christian Unity/Handsel Press, pp. 17–18.

34 Thomas F. Torrance, 2000, *The Being and Nature of the Unborn Child*, Edinburgh: Handsel Press, p. 8.

35 Torrance, *Soul and Person*, pp. 17–18.

36 Pope John Paul II, 1988, *Mulieris Dignitatem*, 7.

37 Patricia Fox, 2001, *God as Communion*, Collegeville MN: Liturgical Press, pp. 41–2.

38 O'Donovan, *Begotten or Made?*, p. 54.

39 Descartes, *Meditations* (1642).

40 Locke further defined a person as 'A thinking intelligent being, that has reasons and reflection, and can consider itself as itself, the same thinking thing, in different times and places.' John Locke, 1690, *An Essay Concerning Human Understanding*, London: Collins (1964), ii 27, pp. 8–9.

41 David Hume, 1739, *A Treatise of Human Nature*, B1.4.6. R. Trigg also comments: 'Many philosophers have felt that the nature of the self can never be fully captured by any empiricist theory, and that no experience can ever wholly reveal the intricacies of oneself.' R. Trigg, 1988, *Ideas of Human Nature: An Historical Introduction*, Oxford: Blackwell, pp. 74–5.

42 Webb, *God and Personality*, p. 58.

43 Immanuel Kant, 1785, *The Metaphysics of Morality*, 276.

44 O'Donovan, *Begotten or Made?*, p. 58.

45 Zizioulas, 'On Being a Person', p. 33.

46 Aristotle, *Historia Animalium* 7.3.

47 Teresa Iglesias, 1990, *I.V.F. and Justice*, London: Linacre Centre for Health Care Ethics, pp. 101–09. Iglesias comments that: 'It can reasonably be argued that if Aristotle and his followers had had the biological knowledge we possess today, they would have had to claim, in virtue of the principles they held about matter and form, that the substantial change that occurs when generative human material becomes a human being must occur at fertilisation and not at any other later stage.' T. Iglesias, 1984, *Test Tube Babies – A Christian View*, Oxford: Unity Press, p. 86.

48 Caroline W. Bynum comments: 'The theological writings of the thirteenth and fourteenth centuries came to treat the relationship between body and soul as much tighter and more integral than it had earlier been understood to be. It seems reasonable to suppose that the extraordinary importance given to body, especially female body, in thirteenth to fifteenth century religion ... owe something to the fact that the theorists in the High Middle Ages did not see body primarily as the enemy of soul, the container of soul, or the servant of soul; rather they saw the person as a psychosomatic unity ... A concept of person as soul and body undergirds scholastic discussions on such topics as bodily resurrection, miracles, embryology, asceticism, Christology and the Immaculate Conception.' Caroline W. Bynum, 1989, 'The Female Body and Religious Practice in the Late Middle Ages', in Michel Feher, Ramona Naddaff and Nadia Tazi (eds), *Fragments for a History of the Human Body*, Part 1, New York: Zone, pp. 190–1.

49 Peter Singer and Deane Wells, 1984, *The Reproductive Revolution: New Ways of Making Babies*, Oxford: Oxford University Press, p. 90.

50 John Harris, '*In Vitro* Fertilisation: The Ethical Issues', *Philosophical Quarterly* 33:132 (1983), p. 225.

51 John Harris, 'Book Review: *A Philosophical Disease: Bioethics, Culture and Identity*, Carl Elliott', *British Medical Journal* 320 (2000), p. 1611.

52 Helga Kuhse and Peter Singer, 1985, *Should the Baby Live? The Problem of Handicapped Infants*, Oxford: Oxford University Press, p. 133.

53 Jonathan Glover, 1990, *Causing Death and Saving Lives*, London: Penguin, p. 127. Scott Rae explains, however, that a capacities understanding of human value and worth results in serious difficulties for Christians. He states that 'if being in God's image is capacities based, then it is also degreed. Such an understanding stands in stark contrast to the biblical teaching that human significance is not degreed – an absolute that holds regardless of a person's functional abilities'. Scott Rae, 2017, 'More than meets the eye', in John Kilner (ed.), *Why People Matter*, Grand Rapids, MI: Baker Academic, p. 98.

54 Congregation for the Doctrine of the Faith, *Instruction on Respect for Human Life in its Origin and on the Dignity of Procreation*, Catholic Truth Society, 1987.

55 Teresa Iglesias, 1987, '*In Vitro* Fertilisation: The Major Issues', in Nigel M. de S. Cameron (ed.), *Embryos and Ethics*, Edinburgh: Rutherford House Books, pp. 21f.

56 Byrne, 'The Animation Tradition', p. 95.

57 Iglesias, 'In Vitro Fertilisation', p. 21.

58 Calum MacKellar and David A. Jones (eds), 2012, Chimera's Children, London: Continuum, p. 174.

59 John Zizioulas, 1989, The Forgotten Trinity, Volume 1, The Report of the British Council of Churches Study Commission on Trinitarian Doctrine Today, London: British Council of Churches, p. 22.

60 Karl Barth, 1961, Christian Dogmatics, ed. G. W. Bromiley and T. F. Torrance, Edinburgh: T&T Clark, Vol. III.2.

61 Pope John Paul II, 1997, Theology of the Body: Human Love in the Divine Plan, Boston: Pauline Books, p. 342.

62 Pia Matthews, 2013, Pope John Paul II and the Apparently 'Non-acting' Person, Leominster: Gracewing, pp. 63–4.

63 Pope John Paul II, 1994, Letters to Families, n. 19.

64 David A. Jones, 'The "Special Status" of the Human Embryo in the United Kingdom', Human Reproduction and Genetic Ethics 17:1 (2011), pp. 66–83 (p. 72).

65 K. Wojtyla, 1991, 'The Person, Subject and Community', quoted in James J. McCartney, Unborn Persons: Pope John Paul II and the Abortion Debate, Bern: Peter Lang, p. 96.

66 Keith Ward, 1990, 'An Irresolvable Dispute', in J. Dyson and J. Harris (eds), Experiments on Embryos, London: Routledge, p. 8.

67 Pia Matthews, 'Discerning Persons: How the early theology can illuminate contemporary bioethical approaches to the concept of person', doctoral thesis, Saint Mary's University College, 2010, p. 341.

68 Thomas F. Torrance, 1984, Test-Tube Babies: Morals – Science – and the Law, Edinburgh: Scottish Academic Press, p. 11; Torrance, Soul and Person, p. 116.

69 O'Donovan, Begotten or Made?, p. 59.

70 Torrance, Soul and Person, p. 105.

71 Colin Gunton, 1998, The Triune Creator: A Historical and Systematic Study, Grand Rapids: Eerdmans, p. 210.

72 Helmut Thielicke, 1964, The Ethics of Sex, Cambridge: James Clarke & Co. Ltd., p. 231. See also: Helmut Thielicke, 1970, 'The Doctor as Judge of Who Shall Live and Who Shall Die', in Kenneth Vaux (ed.), Who Shall Live? Medicine, Technology, Ethics, Philadelphia: Fortress Press, p. 172. Similarly, D. Gareth Jones writes: 'The value of human life in God's sight leads to the concept of the dignity of human beings. This dignity ... stems from our creation by God and is revealed supremely in the redemption made possible in Christ. It rests not on what human beings can accomplish in material or social terms, but on the fact of God's love. Consequently, human dignity is always based on what individuals are in the light of God and never on what they can do for society, for mankind, or even for God.' D. Gareth Jones, 1987, Manufacturing Humans: the challenge of the new reproductive technologies, Leicester: InterVarsity Press, p. 70.

PART II

The Image of God, Personhood
and the Embryo

As previously discussed, ever since the very early Church, many conver-
sations have taken place about what it actually means for humanity to
be made in the image of God, with countless books being written on the
subject over the centuries. In seeking to define better what the concept of
the image of God expressed, Christian scholars have generally focused
on a number of notions which, for them, emphasized the reasons why
human beings were so unique in creation.

But some general themes seem to return regularly in many discussions.
As the South African Reformed theologian Wentzel Van Huyssteen
suggested:

> One of the most important and widely accepted categorizations is the
> focus on a three-phase development that historically leads from sub-
> stantive interpretations, to functional interpretations, to relational
> interpretations of this crucial, canonical concept. In addition, the well-
> known triad has also been modified and amplified to include existential
> and eschatological interpretations of the imago Dei.[1]

But many other aspects have been suggested which can and should be
considered as complementary to each other while, at the same time,
remembering that a purely empirical or descriptive manner of defining
humanity is inappropriate. If humanity cannot be reduced to biology it is
impossible to use the biological sciences, by themselves, to define what is
'human'. Dunstan maintains that if an important part of being human is
'the invasion, moulding and transformation' of nature, then nature itself
cannot dictate what it is to be truly human'.[2]

In the following chapters, therefore, a study will be attempted to
understand the image of God from five of the most relevant perspectives
as they relate to the embryo, although, because of their complementarity,
it will sometimes be impossible to completely separate their positions
from one another.

These five perspectives will be examined because they can either be seen as the most helpful in considering the image of God in the embryo, as with (1) the concept of creation and (2) the doctrine of the incarnation, or because they are the most common and have already been studied by scholars, as with (3) substantive, (4) relational and (5) functional positions. Moreover, since discussions relating to certain functionalities of the embryo have been the basis of extensive debate, a section examining these functionalities is included at the end of the book in order to seek to address some of the arguments.

Of course, it should again be stressed that this study is not exhaustive. There are certainly other ways of understanding this image of God in the embryo.

In each chapter, the topic of the image of God and being a person will be developed using as a basis the previous general study of these topics before going on to explicitly apply these two concepts to the moral status of the human embryo. However, because the first two notions (creation and incarnation) may be seen as more helpful in recognizing the image of God in the embryo, they have been developed more extensively than the other sections.

Notes

1 J. Wentzel Van Huyssteen, 2006, *Alone in the World? Human Uniqueness in Science and Theology*, Grand Rapids: Eerdmans, p. 126.
2 Gordon R. Dunstan, 1974, *The Artifice of Ethics*, London: SCM Press, p. 61.

4

Creation and the Embryo

The Theology of Creation

Creation, defined as 'mak[ing] out of nothing or bestow[ing] existence upon',[1] has been the source of some of the most complex theological, philosophical and scientific discussions down through the ages. It is indeed a most fascinating concept for human beings to contemplate. Creating entails bringing forth something that did not previously exist in time and space; there is a kind of 'magical moment' before which nothing existed and after which existence is present. There is also a mystery at the heart of creation, with the very concept of creation itself being meaningless if the cosmos and humanity were not created.

A secular definition of the concept of creating may be presented as a type of 'making' in which a new subject or object is brought forth into existence. But care must be taken in the use of the term. For example, it is often understood that artists are the creators of their art-work though they do not create beauty. Instead, their art reveals the 'beautiful', pointing beyond itself to the creator of beauty. Good art points through itself to the source of beauty and is greater than itself.[2]

For Christians, only God is creator and he alone can create something out of the absence of existence of anything (*ex nihilo*) and without being subject to an outside agenda. In this context, and because God's creative act will always remain a mystery, the creation accounts in Genesis and their later use in the Bible are not seeking to answer the question about how the world came into existence but are providing, instead, a development of the meaning of the created order. Accordingly, the following assertions can be made or inferred with respect to such a meaning.

Creation Is of God

The creation accounts in the Bible are a clear exposition that the whole of creation is of God. As a result, any meaning in creation cannot be found in itself but must necessarily be found outside of the cosmos, namely in God, the creator. Even though the cosmos does witness to its

Maker (Ps. 19.1–4; Rom. 1.20), creation cannot reveal itself as God's creation all alone. It is God revealing himself as creator, preserver and saviour that enables the cosmos to be recognized as a creation of God and more specifically of a Trinitarian God. As Moltmann stressed, 'creation exists in the Spirit, is moulded by the Son and is created by the Father. It is, therefore, from God, through God, and in God.'[3] In addition, this Trinitarian emphasis of the creator God includes the notion that God both transcends but is also present in the world.

As a result, since the created cosmos originated in God it is inherently rational since God is the source of all order and rationality in creation. The Church Father and Bishop of Alexandria, St Athanasius (296/8–373), in his *Contra Gentiles*[4] represents this order in an artistic fashion as a great symphony. The whole cosmos is therefore an expression of an original rational harmony that reflects the love of God.

Only God Creates

The act of creation by God describes the specific activity or initiation of God which only he can do. In addition, it is an act in which the word and act of creation are one (Gen. 1.1; Ps. 148.5). Interestingly, it is through speech that creation is portrayed as being brought into existence in Genesis and not through any other means. It is also through words that a reply is called for even if this reply is silent. In a way, when God creates he is talking to himself and responding to his own discourse by indicating that what he has spoken into existence, during each day of creation, is good.[5]

The word and act of creation is generally characterized by the special Hebrew verb *bara* which is used when God created the cosmos out of nothing (Gen. 1.1). A comprehensive examination of the use of *bara* leads to the conclusion that, in nearly all cases,[6] it refers to activity uniquely performed by God and includes the concepts not only of command and execution[7] but also of (1) the performance of bringing forth and (2) making a new subject or object.[8]

This is emphasized in that when God created humankind, represented by *Adam* with the specific name *Haadam*, in his own particular image, the word *bara* was also employed (Gen. 1.27; 5.1).

This means that a powerful and intrinsically divine act of creation took place in the *bara* creation of humanity. But what makes human beings so special is that they are created in the image of God. As Christian biologist John Bryant and physician John Searle emphasize:

What makes human life special, and separates us from the rest of the creation, is not what *we* do but what *God* has done, namely that he made, created, formed us to be in his likeness. Therein lies the essential dignity of every man and woman.[9]

God creates (*bara*) and makes (Hebrew *asah*); the latter has a similar though more general meaning with a manual connotation expressing the notion 'to fashion' or 'to make'[10] in Genesis 1—5, though the author appears not to have two different concepts in view. For example, in Genesis 1 the author states God's intention to make (*asah*) humanity (v. 26) and then describes God acting on that intention by saying that God created (*bara*) humanity (v. 27). Moreover, in Genesis 5, when the author looks back to God's bringing humanity into existence (v. 1), both *bara* and *asah* describe that action.[11]

Creation out of Nothing

To correctly understand the notion of creation it is important to accept that God made the world *ex nihilo*, out of nothing. This is a crucial concept since, as the English theologian Maurice Wiles (1923–2005) succinctly states, 'Creation is creation out of nothing or is nothing.'[12] This is implied by the first verse of Genesis: 'In the beginning, God created the heavens and the earth. Now the earth was formless and empty, darkness was over the surface of the deep, and the Spirit of God was hovering over the waters', and more specifically in Romans 4.17: '... the God who gives life to the dead and calls into being things that were not'.[13]

This shows that creation itself is not divine but results from a specific decision expressing God's will. It implies that the cosmos is not the outcome of some pre-existent matter and that the divine bringing into existence was not 'out of something'.[14] Though there is still some discussion about whether this creation *ex nihilo* is originally a Jewish concept,[15] the notion of 'out of nothing' was the result of a theological understanding of creation by the Church Fathers who resisted Gnostic theology.[16]

In ancient Jewish tradition God created from what the Hebrew characterizes as *tohu-bohu*. The word *tohu* represented an unformed nothingness or a sort of 'desert' uninhabited and uninhabitable in which references of space and time are impossible, while the word *bohu* meant a state of 'void', 'emptiness', or more exactly of mist. So defined, *tohu-bohu* is a 'nothing' independent of any organized order characterized by measurements of space and time.[17]

In contemporary theological discussions, creation *ex nihilo* is contrasted with some concepts originating in process theology in which creation came about out of chaos, rather than out of nothing. In such an understanding, creation is reduced to the making of something out of 'not yet actualized primordial matter'. In other words, it becomes the moulding and ordering of 'nothing', instead of the 'bringing into being from nothing'. But as Moltmann emphasizes, this is unacceptable since it would imply that the 'process' must be as uncreated and eternal as God himself.[18] The term *ex nihilo* is, therefore, important in Christian theology in order to distinguish creation from shaping or forming something out of something else.

Creation out of Love

Though God creates *ex nihilo*, this does not mean that he did not create out of his personalness, love and image, although this does not imply any necessity in God. As Barth explains:

> He wills and posits the creature neither out of caprice nor necessity, but because He has loved it from eternity, because He wills to demonstrate His love for it, and because He wills not to limit His glory by its existence and being, but to reveal and manifest in it his own coexistence with it.[19]

This implies that God created his children out of his love to be loved. In other words, God decided to expand his love by creating other new personal existences whom he could love. As Gunton puts it:

> To be love, there must be a distinct being to love. Creation is the bringing to be of that object of love. God creates that which he may love; and a world on which he may love it. That is the point ... of the creation account in Genesis 1.[20]

This means that only through the creation by God of an 'other' can God love this 'other' person. He thus created the wonderful, personal human 'other' to communicate his reality of *being* love which expresses itself onto and with this personal 'other'. God created freely out of his love for the sake of the persons he created so that he could share his love with them.[21] Made in the image of their creator, human beings are made out of love and for love.[22]

In short, for the relationships of love to be multiplied, the existence of personal 'others' must also be multiplied. And both these multiplications are sourced in the original love of God. Moreover, it is because the personal 'others' (his children) know that they are created from God's unconditional love that they may recognize their own call to love and to return to their creator.

It is on this basis that the creation of the cosmos and humankind should be understood – a foundation of self-giving, free and inestimable love. As Moltmann says, 'His love is literally ecstatic love. It leads Him to go out of himself'.[23] God created out of the sheer generosity of his love; an act which went beyond what was required or expected. Barth further states that 'the doctrine of creation answers that God, who does not need us, created heaven and earth and myself, of "sheer fatherly kindness and compassion, apart from any merit or worthiness of mine"'. He adds, 'Creation is grace ... God does not grudge the existence of the reality distinct from himself.'[24]

In this way, the doctrine of creation expresses the amazing grace of God. Creation *ex nihilo* reflects a transcendent, free and intentional, loving God acting, without necessity or imperative for himself, towards the manifestation of the fullness of his engaging love with others.[25] As Bristow emphasizes:

> God is 'Creator' and 'Love' at the same time. And we are the 'image of God' so that these two characteristics are also shared in by us. In God they are not separated, and thus love or superabundance of goodness, is the reason for the creation.'[26]

All this is eloquently summarized by John Paul II in his General Audience of January 1980:

> 'In the beginning God created the heavens and the earth,' to Genesis 1:27, 'So God created man in his own image.' God reveals himself above all as Creator. Christ referred to that fundamental revelation contained in Genesis. In it, the concept of creation has all its depth – not only metaphysical, but also fully theological.
>
> The Creator is he who 'calls to existence from nothingness,' and who establishes the world in existence and man in the world, because he 'is love' (1 John 4:8). Actually, we do not find this word in the narrative of creation. However, this narrative often repeats: 'God saw what he had made, and behold, it was very good.' Through these words we are led to glimpse in love the divine motive of creation, the source from which it springs. Only love gives a beginning to good and delights in good (cf. 1 Corinthians 13). As the action of God, the creation signifies not only calling from nothingness to existence and establishing the existence of the world and of man in the world. It also signifies, according to the first narrative, *beresit bara*, giving. It is a fundamental and 'radical' giving, that is, a giving in which the gift comes into being precisely from nothingness.[27]

This love of God, like all real loves, however, is intrinsically vulnerable through God's self-limitation in the contingent freedom of the created cosmos and order. This ultimate self-limitation by God in the incarnation, crucifixion and atonement of Jesus Christ is therefore a demonstration of the true fulfilment of self-sacrificial love.[28]

Creation Depends on God

A rational consequence of the concept that God created *ex nihilo* is that the created order is a contingent order. This means that it depends entirely on God for its origin and continuation. There was no necessity in God to create the universe but he chose to do so out of his own free rational will expressed in love. Gunton explains: 'This enables it to be said that the creation is contingent, in the sense that it does not have to be. It might not have been, or God might have chosen to create a different world.'[29]

This is also reflected by the English theologian Neil Messer:

God's creative activity is characterized by an expansive, generous love. God does not create as a matter of necessity or in order to meet any divine need ... But this does not mean that it is the product of an arbitrary divine decision.[30]

As a result, the cosmos is endowed with a contingent rationality which is dependent on, but distinct from, God's rationality. As T. F. Torrance points out:

The reason for the creation is theologically traced back to the free, ungrudging will of God's love to create a reality other than himself which he correlates so closely with himself that it is made to reflect and shadow forth on its contingent level his own inner rationality and order.[31]

This means that since the rationality of creation is a contingent rationality dependent on God and is not self-sufficient, scientific questions about meaning must be set in the context of transcendent theological concepts.[32] It liberates any examination from the restricted bonds of fate and determinism. Before the arrival of Christianity, the general understanding of cosmology arising from Greek philosophy was of an all encompassing monist whole. In such a view, there could be no creator–creature distinction and the very existence of the cosmos was considered as necessary.[33]

It was only when a Christian understanding of creation *ex nihilo* started to develop that Greek theologians began to revise their understanding and that the very existence of the world became free from necessity.[34]

Finally, God's decision to create was not only rational and free, it was a wonderful expression of his self-giving love. God created not only 'out of freedom', but 'out of love'. These two concepts are, of course, intrinsically connected since, without freedom, there is no love and there is no necessity in real love. This also means that, because of the divine communion of love between the Father, Son and Holy Spirit, there is no necessity in God to create the cosmos or humanity. Creation is a free expression of God's love.[35]

The Communion of Creation

When God created the cosmos and humanity it was not only the Father who participated in this wonderful action but all three persons of the Trinity – Father, Son and Holy Spirit – unified by the three relationships of love between them. In other words, creation resulted from both (1) the three persons, and (2) the three relationships of love between these persons of the Trinity. As the Scottish theologian David Fergusson writes: 'Creation is thus consistent with the eternal love and being of God. It is not a random act of the will but a free expression of the personal love within the triune being.'[36]

In more specific terms, the creation of existence by God can never be understood outside of his love or in a static or passive way. Creation is a dynamic action of God characterized by his love.[37] Moreover, the dynamic activity of God's love and creation is expressing relationships between the personal othernesses of the Triunity. This means that the essence of God's being is to exist in a creative relationship of love and mutual belonging between the communion of the Triunity of Father, Son and Holy Spirit.[38]

In the same way, humankind was created in the image of God in that it expresses and echoes the most central relatedness of all, which is to be found in the relatedness of the Father, Son and Holy Spirit, expressing a Trinity in unity, and a unity that is trinal.

Moreover, because God created the world and his children from his love, a deep sense of belonging continues to exist between himself and his children bonded by a profound reality of love. There is always a sense of communion, together with the experience of a deep bond, between a personal creator and the personal creatures brought forth through this creation. God's children cannot but feel that they truly belong to their original creator. They also know that but for their creator they would not exist.

This is reflected in the word 'nostalgia', which comes from the Greek words *nostos* meaning return home, and *algos*, meaning pain. It expresses a feeling of homesickness whereby individuals want to return to where they really belong – to find the source of love that brought them into existence and to be unconditionally loved by this source, which gives them a place and meaning in existence. No matter how much God's created children may seek to fill their lives with other things, the deep longing inside all of them for him is never satisfied until they finally recognize and accept his unconditional love from which they were created.[39]

Even when humankind revolted against this relationship and was estranged from God through sin, he did not abandon his creation to go and create another and better cosmos with more obedient children. The mystery and awesome reality of creation, including human beings belonging to God because he created them, can only be realized in its most profound sense by the events that took place on the cross.

God Is Involved in Creation

Another element which is necessary to appropriately understand the meaning of creation is to remember that God is continuously involved in what he has created. The transcendent creator God is the immanent God who continuously upholds, sustains and preserves the created order. As Aquinas asserts:

> As it depends on the will of God that he produces things into being, so it depends on his will that he preserves them in being, for he does not preserve them in any other way than by always giving them being; hence, if he withdrew his action from them, all things would be reduced to nothing.[40]

Moltmann bemoans the fact that many commentators have often reduced creation to *creatio originalis* and made little of *creatio continua* and *creatio nova*. He notes Calvin's concern: 'To make God a momentary Creator, who once for all finished his work, would be cold and barren.'[41]

Thus it would be preferable to recognize a God who is actively and continuously involved in creation, which also better reflects contemporary scientific understanding of an ever-changing cosmos. On the one hand, the apparent created rationality is expressed, for example, in the regular scientific laws of the created order. On the other hand, science recognizes that there is a very real dynamic perspective to the cosmos in which many elements are in continuous and persistent change.[42] The English theologian and biochemist Arthur Peacocke (1924–2006) argued: 'Any notion of God as Creator must now take into account, more than ever before in the history of theology, that God is continuously creating, that God is *semper Creator* [God is always creating].'[43] Hence both *creatio ex nihilo* and *creatio continua* may be accepted together.

Nonetheless, it is important to differentiate God's initial act of creation from his continuing preservation, in that *creatio continua* is the upholding of all that he has made and is different from *creatio ex nihilo*. As Brunner stresses:

> The danger zone has already been entered when Creation and Preservation are identified with one another. For anyone who does not admit the distinction between the creation and the preservation of the created world does not take the fact of creation seriously.[44]

Creatio continua, however, while distinguishable from *creatio originalis*, may involve more than preservation. *Creatio continua*, which includes some elements of creation such as the creation by God of human children, may be seen as an ongoing process in which the mysterious creative action of God in time still has its origin in the mysterious initial act.

This may be what Augustine was trying to express:

> In the seed, then, there was invisibly present all that would develop in time into a tree. And in this same way we must picture the world, when God made all things together, as having had all things together which were made in it and with it when day was made. This includes not only the heaven with sun, moon, and stars ... but it includes also the beings which water and earth produced in potency and in their causes before they came forth in the course of time as they have become known to us in the works which God even now produces.[45]

God remains faithful and sustains his universe which he has created, and does not retreat out of any involvement with his creation.

Nevertheless, care is required concerning the manner in which some commentators use the concept of *creatio continua*. For example, any use of the concept to reflect the optimistic suggestion that this present world will one day be perfected through creative and redemptive acts of transformation by both God and humankind does not have any substance in biblical theology.

Creation Affirms Moral Order

Finally, an appropriate understanding of creation asserts that there is a moral order to the cosmos. God's creation is not disorganized and does not result in chaos. As the Canadian Catholic theologian Janet Soskice emphasizes: 'Creation in the Old Testament is above all, order – and it comes from God ... Creation is the triumph of order over chaos, and because creation is order, it is law-abiding.'[46]

This means that God's creation cannot be reduced to the bringing into existence of matter, out of which the universe is constructed, but must also include the creation of order and rationality which sustains the universe. Thus creation is not just about the substance of entities but about their relatedness.[47] In fact, the very creation order is not arbitrary since there is no order without love and no love without relatedness. This means that the whole of the order manifest in creation is a reflection of God's unconstrained love which is the ultimate source of all order.[48]

Creation and the Son of God

At this stage it is important to examine, as a short excursus, the manner in which the Son of God participates in creation, although a fuller study of the incarnation will be presented in later chapters. This is necessary because an appropriate Christian understanding of creation is possible only when the relationship between Jesus Christ and creation is examined.

The Scottish theologians Iain Torrance and William Storrar develop the doctrine of creation by explaining that it is immeasurably enriched through the doctrine of the Trinity which, of course, is presupposed by the doctrine of incarnation.[49] Both creation and incarnation are even parts of the same divine and unique action of love and grace. It is in Christ that 'all things have been created through him and in him' (Col. 1.16) and that: 'Through him all things were made; without him nothing was made that has been made. In him was life, and that life was the light of all mankind' (John 1.3–4). It is because Christ is the Lord of creation but also part of it,[50] like humankind, that he is able to reconcile the world, separated by Adam's Fall, to God.

The central relationship between creation and incarnation is further revealed by Calvin, who argued that, without the knowledge of God as the creator and redeemer of humanity, human persons are unable to know themselves as they truly are.[51] But this knowledge of God can only be known through the self-disclosure of God in creation and the incarnation. As the Church of Scotland Board of Social Responsibility affirmed in 1999:

> If we turn to the creed, we confess that we believe in one God, the Father Almighty, Maker of heaven and earth ... It is similar when we speak of God as Father. When we dare to do this, we do so not in a neutral or abstract or anthropomorphic sense, but we mean that he is the God and Father of our Lord Jesus Christ. We do not, and cannot, know God as Father in himself, or as our Father, apart from his only Son Jesus Christ, in whom, and through the Holy Spirit, God gives us access to himself.[52]

In other words, it is impossible to fully appreciate Christ's Lordship of creation without a full understanding of the Trinity. In this manner, Christology and creation are intrinsically associated in five important ways.[53]

1. Christ Is Lord of Creation

From the perspective of the New Testament, Christ's position in relation to creation is that he is Lord of Creation. Accordingly, creation is through and to Christ, which means that it is structured by the very one who became incarnate and thus part of the created order.[54]

Through the incarnation, God demonstrates that he is sovereign over all that was created. Even the miracles over nature, such as the calming of the storm (Mark 4.35–41) and the turning of water into wine (John 2.1–11), are confirmation of Christ's authority over the physical and spiritual worlds.

2. Christ Is Agent of Creation

Though creation is from God, the origin, it takes place through Christ, the agent. The Apostle Paul's Christological hymn in Colossians states that 'in him [Christ] all things were created, things in heaven and on earth, visible and invisible' (Col. 1.16). Similarly, John the Apostle asserts, 'He was in the world, and ... the world was made through him' (John 1.10). This means that the agent of creation is the one who continuously upholds and sustains it (Heb. 1.3). As the American Lutheran bioethicist Gilbert Meilaender explains:

> In those opening verses of the Gospel of John, Jesus is identified as the Word – the *logos* – of God. All things, the Gospel says, were created through that Word, through the One in whom the love of God is expressed and revealed ... God's own creative power is never exercised apart from his love – the Word, who is Jesus.[55]

As a result, a Trinitarian understanding of creation usually emphasizes the Father's creation, which takes place through the Son and is mediated and fulfilled by the Holy Spirit.

Such an understanding of Christ as agent of creation is very different from a number of contemporary discussions concerning this concept. For example, Peacocke, seeking to bring together evolutionary theory with biblical theology, disagrees with the pre-existence of Christ: instead, Christ, as 'the agent of creation', is simply reduced to revealing 'the intentions of God in creation'. Peacocke adds: 'It is not in any sense that ... the man Jesus is the agent of creation, but that he mediates to us the meaning of creation.'[56]

Peacocke then develops his thinking by suggesting that Christ, through his very creativity and openness to God, uniquely reveals the One who is 'continuously creating and bringing his purpose to fruition in the order of energy-matter-space-time'.[57] Of course, Jesus Christ is witness to God's involvement and continuous creativity in the cosmos but this must ultimately mean that he is also pre-existent and takes part in creation.

3. Christ Is Part of Creation

The New Testament's presentation of Christ depicts him not only as Lord over, and agent of, creation but also as part of creation. The non-created Son of God became a creature, a human being, whose birth, life and death all emphasize his genuine humanity. He is the Eternal Word made flesh.

Through the reality that Christ shares in creation, the incarnation is a positive affirmation of all creation and a wonderful confirmation that God's creation 'was good'. This means that the Platonic/Aristotelian suggestion that matter is evil cannot be sustained. As T. F. Torrance observed: 'The Incarnation had the effect of sanctifying the physical universe for God.' The very fact that the Son of God took on human flesh highlights the integrity and unity of all that was created by the divine creative act. Through an appropriate understanding of incarnation, creation is shown to have a new solidity and stability. In all creation's fragility and temporality, the universe is anchored to the unchangeable nature and constancy of God's wisdom and love.[58] God is therefore very much present and involved in all aspects of his creation through the 'Word made flesh'.[59]

4. Christ Is the Saviour of Creation

Because of the Fall, the whole of creation was alienated from God. But Christ came to reconcile this creation to God through his death on the cross, with the New Testament emphasizing that it is the whole of creation that is redeemed and not just humanity. In this way creation, which is groaning to be liberated, awaits 'the freedom and glory of the children of God' (Rom. 8.21).

This saving and transforming power of Christ over the whole of creation is crucial to understanding the final aim not just of humanity but, as will be discussed later, of all the other kinds of personal beings who may be only partially human and who are, unfortunately, being brought into existence in this fallen world.

5. Christ Is the Goal and Consummation of Creation

The Apostle Paul's vision of the ultimate finality of the cosmos is that, one day, all things will be reconciled under the sovereignty of Christ (Eph. 1.10). Though the incarnation expresses a real vulnerability of the creator, it is also a confirmation of a wonderful promise for his Church. Christ's death and resurrection has brought into existence a new beginning for humanity (2 Cor. 5.17): a new creation which will find its consummation in the transformation of all the created order with a new heaven and a new earth (Rev. 21.1).

Moltmann makes the point that creation began with nature and reached its culmination with the bringing into existence of humanity while the eschatological re-creation, at the end times, reverses the order. It begins with the redemption of human beings in order to conclude in the deliverance of all of nature.[60] Humankind's liberation through the life and death of Jesus Christ signifies the beginning of the liberation of all creation. Humanity is not, therefore, advancing by itself to an unknown 'omega point' representing its ultimate transformation without God but is, instead, moving forward from the cross towards its ultimate goal of becoming truly and genuinely human, defined in and with Christ, the Word made flesh.

God's Creation of Human Beings

Before continuing to examine the theological interpretation of the reality and wonder of God's creation, and especially in the context of creating personal beings, it is essential to return, once again, to studying the initial acts of creation in Genesis.

As already indicated, when God created the cosmos the Hebrew verb *bara* was used, signifying a unique and specific activity of initiation by God. It also expresses the incomparable creativity of God, in which word and act of creation are one (Gen. 1.1; Ps. 148.5). However, this is not the only time the word *bara* is used in the biblical context. When God created humankind, represented by *Adam*, in his own particular image, the word *bara* was also employed (Gen. 1.27; 5.1), in contrast to the Hebrew *asah* which has a more manual connotation and means 'to fashion' or to 'make'.[61]

Because of this, Westermann concluded that, when the context of the use of the word *bara* in Genesis is carefully studied:

> [T]he meaning is indisputable. Man in his entirety ... is to be designated as a creature in God's image ... [It] serves to underline the uniqueness of man's creation. The creation of man is something far different

from the creation of the rest of the world. One can almost say that this ruptures the framework of the course of creation in which all the other works of creation are included.[62]

Therefore, a specific, powerful and intrinsically divine act of creation is found in *bara* for both the cosmos (space–time dimensions) and human persons who were the crown of God's creative action of the cosmos out of nothing. The cosmos and human beings are thus, in some profound way, unified in their essence and reality, which suggests the presence of a unified rationale of creation in God.

As D. A. Jones et al. write:

The beginning of each human being is therefore a reflection of the coming to be of the world as a whole. It reveals the creative act of God bringing about the reality of this person (of me), in an analogous way to the creation of the entire cosmos. There is a mystery involved in the existence of each person.[63]

The same authors cite a significant passage expressing the mysterious connection between Genesis and embryogenesis in the deutero-canonical book of Maccabees, in which a mother speaks to her children:

I do not know how you came into being in my womb. It is not I who gave you life and breath, nor I who set in order the elements within each of you. Therefore the Creator of the world who shaped the beginning of man and devised the origin of all things, will in his mercy give life and breath back to you again.[64]

It is also worthy of note that, although the existence of the universe and human personalness both originate from the same wonderful and all-powerful God, they both begin as extremely small physical entities in which it is difficult to ignore the sense of vulnerability and even humility. At the same time, though they may begin their existence as points in space, they are still completely whole. They grow in size and complexity while never losing their wholeness.

Moreover, it is interesting that this growing process is present in (1) humanity in general, (2) the cells of the human body, and even (3) the life of the Christian, all of which also find their origins in God. Growth in time is something that God has ordained. Moreover, there is a progression in this process in that God is the origin of the universe, which is the origin of all cells, which are the origin of humanity, which is the origin of individual persons, who are the origin of Christian children who are born again.

In summary, the creative acts of God of the cosmos and of human persons have their source in the same intrinsic divine love. But, as already indicated, it is more than just a source or an origin! In a mysterious way, creation of the cosmos and of autonomous personal human beings is an expression of profound and real love. In other words, creation and love are aspects of the same action in God.

The reality that creation and love are wonderful mysteries of the essence of God is reflected in the way Jewish tradition affirms that no one can completely understand this love and the beginning of all things. It belongs exclusively to the realm of God.[65]

Interestingly, this theological situation is very similar to the present understanding in modern astro-physics of the beginning of the cosmos in which there is a boundary, defined as the Planck-wall, limited by 5×10^{-35} metres in space and 5×10^{-44} seconds in time, beyond which it is physically impossible to gain any prior knowledge.[66]

Such a point in space–time, like the beginning of the cosmos, is an example of what scientists call a singularity in which the laws of physics break down. In short, a singularity is a point in space–time which scientists are certain of never being able to completely understand.

From a theological perspective, singularities can also exist when a specific act of God has its incomprehensible source in God which humankind will never be able to fathom. Theologians suggest, in this respect, that the incarnation of Jesus[67] and *bara*-creation by God can also be considered as singularities.

This may be of assistance when considering the ever-present question in bioethics of when life begins. If it is possible to compare the *bara*-creation of the cosmos with that of a person, other 'Bio-Planck-walls' in time and space may be considered beyond which it is physically impossible to gain any prior knowledge. In other words, it would correspond to the point in space–time before which it would be impossible to understand the beginning of human life. Of course it may be possible to come ever closer to this point but one would never be able to finally reach the creation moment.[68] These biological points in time would exist, for example, when considering the point in space–time of fertilization when the two pronuclei containing the chromosomes of the sperm and egg come into contact with each other. Moreover, these values would be different for reproductive cloning and twinning (when an already existing embryo splits apart to give twin embryos), in which cases the new personal lives would be limited in their origins by other Bio-Planck-walls beyond which one would not be able to gain any prior knowledge.

But even though it will never be possible to fully understand the creation by God of the cosmos and of each human child, a glimpse of God's purpose may be obtained by examining what is required for love to exist.

Indeed, as already indicated, the fullness of love in, and emanating from, God has a mysterious pressure to expand into more personal otherness such as in the creation of his human children.

Moreover, because each and every human being is created from the three persons of the Triniry who are bound by love, each human child of God cannot but express the love existing in the Trinity of God. This is the real wonder of human beings. Every human child is, to a certain extent, a real reflection of the wonderful and infinite love in God made other while also being made flesh.

This means that when God looks upon one of even the smallest of his children on earth, the magnificent image of the wonderful and divine love that binds the Trinity, from which he or she was created, is reflected back to him.[69] In other words, to be made in the image of God is to be made from the personal love of God.

However, care must be expressed here, in that the likeness to the divine communion can only be approximate. This approximation is implied in the biblical text itself since its imprecision on the content of 'image' and 'likeness' expresses the limitations of human language and comparisons.[70]

Human Procreation

Procreation is the process by which new human beings are brought into existence by existing human beings. But *pro* in Latin means 'on behalf of' or 'for', thus children are not only procreated 'for' the parents but also 'for' the child's sake, since he or she is begotten and is endowed with the same moral status, nature and essence as his or her human procreators.

From a human perspective, procreation generally assumes that a number of persons (usually two parents) are involved in the bringing into existence of the child through a loving relationship. As Meilaender writes: '[I]n distinctively human procreation the child is not simply a product of the will or choice of its progenitor. It is, instead, the internal fruition of an act of marital love.'[71]

For Christianity, moreover, human persons participate in the creation act of God in bringing forth children. According to Genesis 4.1, when Eve gave birth for the first time she said: 'With the help of the Lord I have brought forth [*qana*] a man.' In other words, since in the Hebrew Bible only God can create (*bara*) she does not use the verb *bara* but *qana*, which means 'to acquire' or 'to bring forth'.

What is particularly significant about this 'procreation' – this 'creation for' – is that it is a creation that is not only 'for' the sake of parents or the sake of the child but ultimately for the sake of God. In addition, procreation generally entails the presence of a relationship of love between procreators and the creator God which opens out towards the procreated being.

In Christianity, it is also recognized that, in God's creation of a child through procreation, this must involve another person made in the image of God. Only through a person can a new person be procreated, only images of God can procreate other images of God, which means that non-persons cannot procreate persons all by themselves.

These concepts are expanded in paragraph 43 of *Evangelium Vitae* in which John Paul II writes:

A certain sharing by man in God's lordship is also evident in the specific responsibility which he is given for human life as such. It is a responsibility which reaches its highest point in the giving of life through procreation by man and woman in marriage. As the Second Vatican Council teaches: 'God himself who said, "It is not good for man to be alone" (Genesis 2:18) and "who made man from the beginning male and female" (Matthew 19:4), wished to share with man a certain special participation in his own creative work. Thus he blessed male and female saying: "Increase and multiply" (Genesis 1:28).'[72]

By speaking of 'a certain special participation' of man and woman in the 'creative work' of God, the Council wishes to point out that having a child is an event which is deeply human and full of religious meaning, insofar as it involves both the spouses, who form 'one flesh' (Genesis 2:24), and God who makes himself present. As I wrote in my Letter to Families: 'When a new person is born of the conjugal union of the two, he brings with him into the world a particular image and likeness of God himself: the genealogy of the person is inscribed in the very biology of generation. In affirming that the spouses, as parents, cooperate with God the Creator in conceiving and giving birth to a new human being, we are not speaking merely with reference to the laws of biology. Instead, we wish to emphasize that God himself is present in human fatherhood and motherhood quite differently than he is present in all other instances of begetting "on earth". Indeed, God alone is the source of that "image and likeness" which is proper to the human being, as it was received at Creation. Begetting is the continuation of Creation.'[73]

Thus, a man and woman joined in matrimony become cooperating partners under God, the sole creator, in an act of bringing forth new human life through procreation.[74] This was re-emphasized by Pope Benedict XVI:

Human generation can never be reduced to the mere reproduction of a new individual of the human species, as happens with any animal. The arrival of each person in the world is always a new creation. The words of a Psalm recall this with profound wisdom: 'For it was you who created my being; knit me together in my mother's womb ... my body held no secret from you when I was being fashioned in secret' (Psalm 139[138]:13,15).[75]

It is also important to recognize that it is from his existing love that God creates his children whom he loves through the participation of the love of the parents. As Paul Ramsey says when commenting on Ephesians 5:

> It is out of His love that God created the entire world of His creatures ... Of course, we cannot see into the mystery of how God's love created the world. No more can we completely subdue the mystery (which is but a reflection of this) contained in the fact that human acts of love are also procreative ... Nevertheless, we procreate new beings like ourselves in the midst of our love for one another, and in this there is a trace of the original mystery by which God created the world because of His love. God created nothing apart from His love and without the divine love was not anything made that was made.[76]

This means that God's love is always behind the creation of a human child and this love always continues towards the child. There is never a moment in all the existence of the child (even at the very beginning of his or her existence) wherein he or she is not loved by God.

God always intended men and women to express their love and communion, through the acts of procreating with him, a symbol and reality of their union of love made flesh in a child. Though it would have been perfectly possible for God to create, at the very beginning, millions of sterile, sexless human persons to populate the Earth, God chose to share the essence of his creative love by making it possible for a man and a woman to procreate with him new children. These children, being then created out of, and representing, the communion of love between all three actors (God and the two human parents), participate in the creative action while also becoming, for these actors, the collective focus of new relationships of love. The *bara*-creation by God continues through the involvement of the parents. The act and gift of procreating, in this way, becomes one of the most wonderful and mysterious expressions of real unifying love. In fact, procreating a child is one of the most extraordinary and exciting participatory acts that can ever be contemplated by human persons because it is so close to a divine act of creation. Procreating human life is also incomparably wonderful because it is participating in the creation of eternal life.

God always intended parents, in this way, to share and recognize a glimpse of the wonder and celebration of his creation of the cosmos and his human children by procreating their own children.

The creation of another person by God through a human couple expresses in the most profound manner an act of unity of love in the Triunity. The creation of a child becomes, in this way, the symbol and reality of the love and unity of the Father, the Son and the Holy Spirit participating in the act of creation. As already mentioned, it means that love is the source of creation reflecting the existence of love between the persons in the Triunity. Because such love exists between the personal othernesses of the Godhead, the wonderful result is the creation of yet more personal othernesses in human children. This means that the acts of creation and love express the same action.

But what is wonderful is that this creative power of love in the Triunity takes place at the level of humankind in the same form. As God the Triunity of the Father, Son and Holy Spirit created the universe and humankind, he continues to create through the trinity of God and his two created procreators (the husband and the wife) the ever-increasing family of his children.

According to this view, the incredible power of love through pro-creation is recognized through the possibility of human persons becoming procreators with God. Indeed, God always intended men and women to express their love and communion through the acts of pro-creating a symbol and reality of their oneness in a child. In other words, God chooses to share the essence of his creative excitement and love by enabling his created man and woman to procreate with him independent and free children whom all three different independent actors can love and mutually belong to.

Moreover, in the same way as God looks upon his children and sees the amazing love of the Trinity and his image being reflected back to him, God always intended that parents should be able see their image and all their love for each other and for God being reflected back to them when they look upon their children.

This is reflected in Genesis 5.3: 'When Adam had lived 130 years, he had a son in his own likeness, in his own image; and he named him Seth.' Here, the same Hebrew terms, *demuth* and *tselem*, are used concerning the fathering of Seth by Adam as in Genesis 1.26 when God creates humanity in his image. Since in Genesis 5.1 the author has just reaffirmed the creation of humanity in God's image the implication is clear: as humanity is in God's image, so is Seth also in Adam's image.[77]

This is the magnificent meaning of procreation for human parents and its relationship to the creation of God. In this context, a Christian under-standing of God's creation is important for Creationism, the theological doctrine that God creates a person as an embodied soul and ensouled body as soon as a new human being is brought into existence.[78] In the same way as the soul of Adam was directly created by God when he created his body, as the Church Fathers universally agreed, the soul of a human embryo is also created by God when he creates its body.

Creationism is thus opposed both to the idea of a pre-existence of the soul[79] and to the theory of Traducianism whereby all persons are, somehow, created entirely and uniquely by God in one single act 'at the beginning'. In Traducianism children are simply being propagated like the branches of a tree down the generations, which can only be con-sidered as mistaken[80] since any participation by the human procreators in God's creation is sadly impossible.[81]

Creation and the Image of God

Interestingly, those involved in bringing into existence a person always know that it is from themselves (their own existence) that this new creature was brought into existence. This is as true of God, when he created Adam and humanity, as of Adam when he assisted in the bring-ing into existence of Eve.[82]

From this perspective, one of the aspects of the image of God which has probably been most overlooked in theology is the notion that this image can be transmitted through the very act of creation by God. This omission may be the result of early theologians rightly seeking to high-light that God is wholly 'other' than his creation. But this emphasis may have concealed the very fact that it was God who created his children made in his image. Had it been some existing being other than God who had created humanity, then human persons would not have been cre-ated in the image of God. This is highlighted in that, when God created humankind in his image, there is a reflecting back to himself and his image: 'Then God said, "Let us make mankind in our image, in our like-ness ..."' (Gen. 1.26). In more specific terms, there was something of the image of God in his children because he created them.

In addition, because of the (correct) insistence that God created *ex nihilo*, from absolutely nothing and without any necessity, the central reality that God created out of his love may also have been underempha-sized. This is unfortunate since it is one of the most important and indeed wonderful aspects of God's children. As already noted, each and every human person is created from, and represents, both the beautiful unity of all three persons of the Trinity and also the amazing love that binds them in communion. God also gives of himself completely in love in creating his children. In short, it is because God (1) created his children and (2) in a very specific manner that they bear his image.

An important description of this divine image, with a strong creational and relational emphasis, is the one suggested by Westermann, who maintains that the emphasis of the text in Genesis is not only on persons, as such, who bear the image of God, but on the process of creation itself. This means that the expression 'in our image' is there to clarify the verb 'let us make'. There is a special kind of God-reflecting divine creative activity taking place in the creation of human beings: a special activity or a particular way of creating by God of humanity which brings all human beings into a special relationship with their creator. In this way, the image of God does not only define humanity but also describes the creative manner in which God made humankind different.[83]

But Westermann asserts that the text in Genesis 1.26–30 can be considered as having an additional emphasis. For him, the important theological meaning of the image of God becomes 'a question of human existence as such and not as something over and above it'.[84] The image of God in human beings is something far beyond any ability or characteristic, since it originates in the very special creative manner in which humanity was brought into being by God.

This means, according to Westermann, that the image of God is present and equal in all human beings because they are created in the same way. Whatever characteristics human beings may have, they are all made as God's counterparts (in the image of God) because they are made by him in a special manner. He insists: 'The relationship to God is not something which is added to human existence; humans are created in such a way that their very existence is intended to be their relationship to God.'[85]

Thus, to state that humankind is created in the image of God refers to the reality that God brings into existence a particular being among all the other created beings to stand in a particular and unique kind of relation with him.[86] This is emphasized by the Anglican theologian Christopher Wright:

We should not think of the image of God as an independent 'thing' that we somehow possess. God did not give to human beings the image of God. Rather it is a dimension of our very creation. The expression 'in our image' is adverbial (that is, it describes the way God made us), not adjectival (that is as if it simply described a quality we possess). The image of God is not so much something we possess, as what we are. To be human is to be the image of God.[87]

A further affirmation that the image of God is intrinsically related to the creation by God of human beings is emphasized by Barth:

> It does not consist in something that man is or does. It exists because man exists himself and, as such, exists as God's creature. He would not be man, were he not God's image. He is God's image by being man.[88]

By recognizing that each and every person is a reflection and an image of who God really is, it is then possible to understand how important and valuable each person actually is to God. It strongly suggests that one of the crucial aspects of the notion of the image of God in a person is that it is God who created this person in a special manner. As the International Theological Commission of the Holy See states:

> The doctrine of *creatio ex nihilo* is thus a singular affirmation of the truly personal character of creation and its order toward a personal creature who is fashioned as the *imago Dei* and who responds not to a ground, force or energy, but to a personal creator. The doctrines of the *imago Dei* and the *creatio ex nihilo* teach us that the existing universe is the setting for a radically personal drama, in which the triune Creator calls out of nothingness those to whom He then calls out in love. Here lies the profound meaning of the words of *Gaudium et Spes*: 'Man is the only creature on earth that God willed for his own sake'.[89]

How this creation of every child by God takes place will always remain a mystery. But it does take place and will continue to take place even if the child, as discussed later, is no longer human or only partly human. In other words, these new beings will in some way continue to reflect the image of God because he created them.

Creation and Personhood

Since relatively little has been written relating to the manner in which the image of God is present in human beings because he created them, there is also very little discussion about how being a person is related to the manner in which human individuals are created. But as already indicated, a person is a being who bears the image of God, an image that is present because it was God who created this person out of his love.

In this regard, it is interesting to note that created persons can also procreate (in participating in God's creation) other real persons (their children) whom they can love. But only persons can do this.

In more specific terms, it is only because God first loved and created his human children, as persons, that they can procreate other persons and love them (1 John 4.19).

Moreover, it is only God and other created persons who can create or procreate persons, respectively. From a human perspective, persons do not simply come into existence since they are either planned by their parents or are 'accidents'. But it is always persons who have participated in their creation/procreation. Created persons can only be brought forth by other persons. From God's perspective, moreover, every single human child is welcomed and known by name. As John Paul II states: 'At the origin of each human person there is a creative act of God: no man comes into existence by chance; he is always the result of the creative love of God.'[90]

This emphasis on God's knowing each one of his children is also wonderfully reflected in Psalm 139.13–16:

> For you created my inmost being; you knit me together in my
> mother's womb.
> I praise you because I am fearfully and wonderfully made; your works
> are wonderful, I know that full well.
> My frame was not hidden from you when I was made in the secret
> place, when I was woven together in the depths of the earth.
> Your eyes saw my unformed body; all the days ordained for me were
> written in your book before one of them came to be.

The wonderful love of God is always present when a new person comes into existence. Would this also mean that human–nonhuman interspecies embryos could be considered as persons because God created them? Of course, it may be impossible this side of eternity ever to know whether they are, in reality, persons. For example, it may be impossible ever to determine whether an embryonic (or adult) human–chimpanzee chimera is a person. Only God would know. But in these cases, the only acceptable alternative may be to give these beings the benefit of the doubt and consider them as if they were persons. It should also be remembered that it will never be possible to demonstrate scientifically, this side of eternity, that any being (whether human, nonhuman, adult or embryonic) is a person, since the concept of being a person transcends the created laws of physics and logic and is something that reflects the creator.

In short, though the bringing into existence of nonhuman or only partially human beings can never be seen as God's will, because of the absence of appropriate love between the actors, if they are brought into existence and God does consider them as persons (even if humanity remains agnostic as to the moral status of such beings), they will be loved by God and made in his image.

Creation and the Moral Status of the Embryo

The importance of creation by God in relation to the moral status of the human embryo is crucial when considering the manner in which persons are created and by whom.

As already indicated, only God creates with the other actors (his human children) merely participating in this wonderful act. Moreover, God creates from his wonderful and immeasurable love. Seen from this perspective, no matter how large or small the living being is, there is never a moment in time after the instant of creation where this being ceases to be a representative and expression of this amazing divine love. This is because he or she was created from the continuous love of God and is, in many ways, an expression of this relationship of love found in the divine Trinity. As Pope Francis explains:

> Saint John Paul II stated that the special love of the Creator for each human being 'confers upon him or her an infinite dignity'.[91] Those who are committed to defending human dignity can find in the Christian faith the deepest reasons for this commitment. How wonderful is the certainty that each human life is not adrift in the midst of hopeless chaos, in a world ruled by pure chance or endlessly recurring cycles! The Creator can say to each one of us: 'Before I formed you in the womb, I knew you' (Jer. 1:5). We were conceived in the heart of God, and for this reason 'each of us is the result of a thought of God. Each of us is willed, each of us is loved, each of us is necessary'.[92]

The suggestion, therefore, that a human embryo is created by the amazing love of God, but then ceases to be loved by God until some later stage of biological development, is difficult to accept rationally. There can be no discontinuity between the love of God who brought this embryo into existence and the same love of God who continues to love this embryonic person.

This perspective is crucial since it remains true whether or not any potential functionalities or any other characteristics are later present in the created being. It is because God created the being from his incredible love, and that it reflects his image, that this being has full moral status.

This would, then, for example, include human embryos and infants, but also those who are severely mentally disabled. It is because God created them that they are made in his image. They can, therefore, be considered as having full moral status.

This basis is the same for any whole and complete organism or entity in both time and space, even if they are only partially human, as in the case of human–nonhuman combinations, and who can be considered as persons (or given the benefit of the doubt).

At the Beginning of Human Life There Is a Special Creative Act of God

As already indicated, for Christians, the act of creation is not just a cold biological bringing into existence of a being. Instead, it involves a wonderful and divine action in which God pours out his love into the new existence. But in a mysterious way, creation of personal existence is also an expression of God's love. The act of creating personal existence is in some way intrinsically related to the act of loving.

Those who believe that the moral status of the human embryo is the same as that of a child or adult accept, therefore, that there is no discontinuity between the love found in God and the love God has for his children which he created and who are whole and complete in space and time. God creates from his existing love and bestows this love to the personal existence. But at the same time, he confirms and illuminates this act of creation by bestowing his image upon this person which he loves.[93]

As already noted, some scholars have suggested that for most of Christian history in the West (until 1869 when, in the document *Apostolicae Sedis*, Pope Pius IX declared that the penalty for abortion would be excommunication) the human embryo was considered to possess only a relative value,[94] a value that could, for example, be seen as less important than essential biomedical research. But in more recent years, other scholars have suggested that this view may be misleading since it is possible to accept that Christianity has always recognized a sacred value to the human embryo and foetus. What is more, in spite of all the theological controversies regarding the precise moment of ensoulment, it was never seen as legitimate in Christianity to harm the embryo at any stage.[95]

The key argument supporting the full protection of the embryo, as soon as it is created, is that a personal being may be recognized as already present from the very beginning of its existence (or given the benefit of the doubt). From this point onwards there may be a person, made in the image of God, with whom God can have a relationship of love even though this existence may not yet be (or ever be on this earth) in a position to respond to this love. In this way, the created personal existence can be considered as having the same moral dignity as a person who has been born.

The image of God inheres in the very existence of the being because God loves this child whom he created through the parents.

It is possible that no other person apart from God will ever be aware of the existence and life of this embryonic being, but this does not affect the amazing dignity bestowed upon this child through the love of God.

As argued by Pope Paul VI in *Gaudium Et Spes*: 'For man would not exist were he not created by God's love and constantly preserved by it.'[96] This was re-emphasized by John Paul II who declared:

Human life is sacred because from its beginning it involves the creative action of God, and it remains forever in a special relationship with the Creator, who is its sole end. God alone is the Lord of life from its beginning until its end: no one can, in any circumstance, claim for himself the right to destroy directly an innocent human being.[97]

Furthermore, God does not create his human children only for his own sake but also for their own sakes; so that they may experience and receive his love for them. It is because of this understanding that Christian tradition stresses so emphatically that human life is sacred. As the American Orthodox theologian John Breck explains, sacredness

originates with God and is accorded purely as an expression of his love. As such, it is wholly derivative. It is a gift: the gift of God's own life and holiness, bestowed upon us independently of any merit, value or achievement of our own. Apart from this gift, life is meaningless, absurd.'[98]

This also means that the kind of love that God has for his children includes gracious love – undeserved love.

Thus, by taking the creation of human existence as the key event in the formation of new human life, it is possible to acknowledge that this point in time is the single most significant moment of biological development.

From a biological perspective, however, it should be recognized that this creation of human existence can take different forms. For example, it can take place through:

- the fertilization of an egg cell by sperm (which takes about 24 hours), which is the manner in which most embryos come into existence;
- the formation of a new embryo from early embryonic cells that fully detach themselves from an early embryo giving rise to identical twins;
- the formation of a new existence from early embryonic cells that partially detach themselves from an early embryo giving rise to conjoined (Siamese) twins with, for example, two heads and a common body; and

- the creation of cloned human embryos through the introduction of a full set of chromosomes from a human adult or embryonic cell into an egg which has been stripped of its own chromosomes.

The Human Person Is Created as a Unity of Body and Soul

Though living sperm and eggs do not have any moral value of their own, as soon as they participate in conception to procreate a person, they take on a completely different meaning. They are no longer just cells but are bringing into existence a new person – a complete and whole person with a body and a soul. They are the means through which two persons (with their own bodies and souls) procreate from their love a new person with his or her own body and soul. The man, woman and child then form a communion of wholes which exists beyond that of the individual persons.

As already noted, many of those who believe that it is the creation of a living being that is determinative for the moral status of the human person do not assume that only a biological creation has taken place. The creation of a human life, as the Church of Scotland 1996 report states, 'is not simply a biological process and cannot rightly be understood exclusively in biological terms'.[99] To reduce human existence to any simple amalgamation of biological material would be an incorrect insight into the manner in which God would consider this existence.

Instead, a person is a created being who is whole and complete from the perspective of both body and soul, but in a non-dualistic manner. From the biblical perspective the soul, or *nephesh* in Hebrew, constitutes the very being as an individual person (Gen. 1.26–27; 2.7). In the Hebrew understanding of the human being, his or her nature is not divided into mutually exclusive parts. When the words 'soul', 'spirit', 'reins' or 'heart' are mentioned it is because one aspect of a human being's life is being emphasized, but it is still the whole human person who is being described.

As Cairns explains:

Where it is the life, or the individuality, or strong desire, then it is the word 'soul' (*Nephesh*) that is used. Where eternal influences, or a power above the individual, then 'spirit' (*Ruach*) is the word. Where intellect, will and conscience are to the fore, then it is the word 'heart' (*Lebh*), and where motive, or that which is known to God but hidden to men, then the Old Testament writers use the word 'reins' [kidneys] (*Kelaoth*).'[100]

Accordingly, one may properly affirm that a human person 'is a soul' rather than 'has a soul'. But this should not be understood as reducing the human being to a mere spiritual principle that 'uses' a body as a simple instrument. Bodily life is integral to the human person and to his or her dignity. In other words, the dignity of the person is inseparable from the dignity of his or her body.

One of the fullest considerations of the beginning of human existence in the light of the coexistence of the soul and body was offered by Gregory of Nyssa. He argued, in line with other leading Church Fathers,[101] that since an individual's being is one, consisting of soul and body, the beginning of his existence must be one as well.[102] This means that soul and body come into being at the same moment when the person is created by God and then grow together.[103]

This is skilfully described by Gregory of Nyssa:

> The form of the future human being is there by way of potential, but it is hidden until the necessary sequence of events allows it to become visible. So also the soul is already there, even though it is not yet visible, and it will be manifested by means of its own proper and natural operation as it advances in growth.[104]

This was developed by T. F. Torrance who pointed out that it is this kind of

> holistic, non-dualistic, conception of the body and soul which ... we must allow to govern our understanding of the unborn child in the oneness of its body and soul, as an embodied soul and a besouled body. This means that we must regard the human embryo as already a human life ... not just a potential human being, but as a distinct, viable human being in which body and soul develop together within the womb of the mother.[105]

From this perspective, there is no room for a dualistic approach in which the body would be created first while the soul, and its associated dignity, would somehow be implanted at a later stage. Instead, God considers the human person as being (1) in existence just as he is in existence, (2) complete just as he is complete and (3) whole just as he is whole. From this perspective, the biological materials and even the dimensions of space and time, in which God is not limited, should not have the last word on the concepts of existence, completeness and wholeness. This is reflected in the Church of Scotland 1996 report which noted that

> much of the current debate highlights, primarily, but not entirely, biological issues and seeks to draw the logical conclusions from the different attitudes adopted toward the human embryo. However help-

ful and important this is, our ethical attitude to the human embryo is not based solely on biological issues and the logical conclusions so drawn. Our ethical understanding is determined by our theology.[106]

It is also worth noting that this report considered the human embryo a 'potential person', but declared that development of the embryo 'is not to be seen as growth into that which it was not before but rather the fulfillment [sic] of that which it already is'.[107] Accordingly, it is not the length of time during which pre-natal or post-natal persons exist that matters. It is the fact that they exist at all, even if they exist for less than just a few seconds, and are complete as well as whole. The issue of whether or not an embryo is viable and able to develop into a child does not have any moral significance. It is whether it exists and is alive that is important.

Notes

1 G. N. Garmonsway, 1980, *The Penguin English Dictionary*, London: Penguin Books.

2 Brent Waters, 'The Future of the Human Species', *Ethics & Medicine* 25:3 (2009), pp. 165–76.

3 Jürgen Moltmann, 1985, *God in Creation*, 1984–5 Gifford Lectures, London: SCM Press, p. 98.

4 Quoted in T. F. Torrance, 1980, *The Ground and Grammar of Theology*, Belfast: Christian Journals, p. 53.

5 Brent Waters, 2009, *This Mortal Flesh: Incarnation and Bioethics*, Grand Rapids: Brazos Press, p. 170.

6 God is generally the subject of the verb *bara*, though in a very few verses in the Old Testament man is also the subject of the verb, such as in Joshua 17.5, 18 and 1 Samuel 2.29, although in these cases *bara* is not translated as 'create'. See Terry Mortenson, 'Did God create (*bara*) or make (*asah*) in Genesis 1?', 15 August 2007, https://answersingenesis.org/genesis/did-god-create-bara-or-make-asah-in-genesis-1/ (accessed 27 November 2015).

7 David A. S. Fergusson, 1998, *The Cosmos and the Creator: An Introduction to the Theology of Creation*, London: SPCK, p. 7–8.

8 Thomas J. Finley, 'Dimensions of the Hebrew Word for "Create"', *Bibliotheca Sacra* 148:592 (1991), pp. 409–23; 'Creativity in the Bible – Creativity: The Reformed View', http://www.worshipinfo.com/materials/creatpt1.htm (accessed 2 June 2008). By way of a human analogy, to make something in the construction dimension would be to write, for example, a musical composition. The performance dimension would then represent the musical performance of the composition.

9 John Bryant and John Searle, 2004, *Life in Our Hands: A Christian Perspective on Genetics and Cloning*, Leicester: InterVarsity Press, p. 42.

10 Ernst Jenni and Claus Westermann, 1997, *Theological Lexicon of the Old Testament*, trans. M. Biddle, Peabody MA: Hendrickson Publishers, Vol. 1, p. 255.

11 John F. Kilner, 2015, *Dignity and Destiny: Humanity in the Image of God*, Grand Rapids: Eerdmans, p. 125.

12 Maurice Wiles, 1986, *God's Action in the World*, 1986 Bampton Lectures, London: SCM Press, p. 16.

13 Here the resurrection of Christ is seen as a sign of a God who can bring life from death; existence out of nothing.

14 The Hebrew word *bara* (create) means the creation of something absolutely new, distinguishable from the Hebrew *asah* (make).

15 Frances Young argues, contrary to T. F. Torrance and others, that *creatio ex nihilo* was not primarily a Jewish concept. Her main reason is the sparseness of references to the doctrine in Jewish texts prior to the Middle Ages. She argues that early Christian writers used the term, but even then it probably has to be interpreted in its Platonic context of creation out of pre-existent matter. The concept, as now understood, came into its own in the third century AD, with St Theophilus and Tertullian both speaking of *creatio ex nihilo* to confront Gnostic views. F. Young sees a possible origin in the slightly earlier writings of Basilides. However, it is significant that F. Young accepts that the Jewish stress on the unique sovereignty of God favours the doctrine; and it would seem that though the implications may not have been drawn out in the earliest centuries, it is still implied from the earliest Genesis account of creation. In other words, Young's argument for a non-Jewish origin needs to be confirmed. Frances Young, '"Creatio ex nihilo": a context for the emergence of the Christian doctrine of creation', *Scottish Journal of Theology*, 44 (1991), pp. 139–52.

16 It found its clearest expression in Irenaeus, who stressed the absolute freedom of God to create. For this to happen there must be creation out of nothing because any existence co-eternal with God would impose a necessity on God. Irenaeus, *Against the Heresies* II.10.4. Quoted in Colin E. Gunton, 1993, *The One, the Three and the Many*, 1992 Bampton Lectures, Cambridge: Cambridge University Press, p. 120.

17 Alain Houziaux, 1997, *Le Tohu-bohu, le Serpent et le bon Dieu*, Paris: Presses de la Renaissance, pp. 37–8.

18 Moltmann, *God in Creation*, ch. 4.

19 Karl Barth, 1957–75, *Church Dogmatics*, ed. G. W. Bromiley and T. F. Torrance, Edinburgh: T&T Clark, Vol. III.1, p. 95.

20 Colin Gunton, 1998, *The Triune Creator: A Historical and Systematic Study*, Grand Rapids: Eerdmans, p. 164.

21 Gunton, *Triune Creator*, p. 118.

22 Brigid McEwen, 1997, 'Fertility, Contraception and the Family', in David W. Torrance (ed.), *God, Family & Sexuality*, Carbery: Handsel Press, p. 120.

23 Moltmann, *God in Creation*, p. 76.

24 Karl Barth, 1949, *Dogmatics in Outline*, London: SCM Press, p. 54.

25 International Theological Commission, *Communion and Stewardship: Human Persons Created in the Image of God*, The Vatican, 2002, paragraph 65, http://www.vatican.va/roman_curia/congregations/cfaith/cti_documents/rc_con_cfaith_doc_20040723_communion-stewardship_en.html#_edn1 (accessed 3 February 2011). William Storrar and Iain Torrance (eds), 1995, *Human Genetics: A Christian Perspective*, The Church of Scotland Board of Social Responsibility, Edinburgh: Saint Andrew Press, p. 40.

26 Peter Bristow, 2009, *Christian Ethics and the Human Person*, Oxford: Family Publication, p. 349.

27 John Paul II, General Audience of 2 January 1980, 'Creation as a Fundamental and Original Gift', http://www.ewtn.com/library/PAPALDOC/jp2tb13.htm (accessed 14 December 2007).

28 Peter T. Forsyth, 1909, *The Person and Place of Jesus Christ*, London: Independent Press, Lecture XII.

29 Gunton, *Triune Creator*, pp. 66, 67.

30 Neil Messer, 2011, *Respecting Life*, London: SCM Press, p. 144.

31 Thomas F. Torrance, 1981, *Divine and Contingent Order*, Oxford: Oxford University Press, p. 35.

32 Torrance, *Divine and Contingent*, ch. 1.

33 John Zizioulas, 1985, *Being as Communion: Studies in Personhood and the Church*, London: Darton, Longman and Todd.

34 Zizioulas, 1985, *Being as Communion*, p. 40.

35 Andrew R. Rollinson, 1994, 'The Incarnation and the Status of the Human Embryo', thesis submitted for the degree of M.Litt. with the Religious Studies Department of Newcastle University, p. 70.

36 David A. S. Fergusson, 1998, *The Cosmos and the Creator: An Introduction to the Theology of Creation*, London: SPCK, p. 34.

37 Thomas F. Torrance, 1994, *Preaching Christ Today: The Gospel and Scientific Thinking*, Grand Rapids: Eerdmans, p. 65.

38 Colin Gunton, 1992, *Christ and Creation*, Carlisle: Paternoster Press, p. 101.

39 This recognition by God's children that they belong to him in love also means that their whole lives belong to him. They are only stewards of their lives and made accountable for the manner with which they use their lives. Human beings are expected and entrusted to use their time on earth properly, restrained by certain limits. Brent Waters, 2001, *Reproductive Technology*, London: Darton, Longman and Todd, pp. 32–3.

40 Thomas Aquinas, *Summa Theologica* ix.2c.

41 John Calvin, *Institutes* I XVI 1.197; Moltmann, *God in Creation*, pp. 208–09.

42 J. Polkinghorne writes: 'The matter revealed in the enquiry of modern science is neither inert nor formless. Its pattern-creating dance is in accordance with laws capable of astonishing fruitfulness in their consequences.' J. Polkinghorne, 1988, *Science and Creation*, London: SPCK, p. 55.

43 Arthur R. Peacocke, unpublished lecture given at the annual Society for Theology conference, 1990.

44 Emil Brunner, 1952, *Dogmatics II, The Christian Doctrine of Creation and Reconciliation*, Philadelphia and London: Lutterworth Press, p. 33.

45 Augustine, *The Literal Meaning of Genesis*, trans. John Hammond Taylor, vols 41 and 42 in the series Ancient Christian Writers, New York: Newman Press (1982), 5.23.45. Similarly, in his answer to the question, 'Whether human souls were created together at the beginning of the world?', Thomas Aquinas did not see any contradiction in human souls being created both with the unborn child 'now' but also at the beginning of the world, which included the creation of Adam's soul. Thomas Aquinas, *Summa Theologica*, question 118, a.3.

46 Janet Martin Soskice, 'Creation and Relation', *Theology* 94 (1991), p. 36.

47 This is a central thesis of Colin Gunton's 1992 Bampton Lectures, in which he argues that only a fully Trinitarian understanding of creation can hold together both unity and particularity. When the creator God is replaced by mere rationality, as at the Enlightenment (and a symptom of modernity), the relationship of particulars cannot be preserved. Gunton, *The One*, pp. 46, 124.

48 Gunton, *Triune Creator*, p. 9.

49 Storrar and Torrance, *Human Genetics*, p. 38.

50 Gunton, *Christ and Creation*, p. 25.

51 Gunton, *Christ and Creation*, p. 74

52 Storrar and Torrance, *Human Genetics*, p. 39.

53 Much of this section is indebted to Gunton, *Christ and Creation*.

54 Gunton, *Triune Creator*, p. 10.

55 Gilbert Meilaender, 'New Reproductive Technologies: Protestant Modes of Thought', *Creighton Law Review* 25:5 (1992), pp. 1637–46 (p. 1644).

56 Arthur R. Peacocke, 1979, *Creation and the World of Science*, 1978 Bampton Lectures, Oxford: Clarendon Press, p. 235.

57 Peacocke, *Creation*, p. 241.

58 Torrance, *Divine and Contingent*, p. 68.

59 The converse of this is seen in deism (where God is 'removed' from the world he has made), which cannot coexist with a full incarnational theology. A thoroughgoing deist such as Newton, for example, rejected Athanasian Christology.

60 Moltmann, *God in Creation*, p. 68.

61 W. H. Schmidt, 1997, in Jenni and Westermann, *Theological Lexicon*, Vol. 1, p. 255.

62 Claus Westermann, 1964, *The Genesis Accounts of Creation*, trans. N. E. Wagner, Philadelphia, PA: Fortress Press, p. 21. Quoted in R. J. Berry and M. Jeeves, 'The Nature of Human Nature', *Science & Christian Belief* 20:1 (2008), p. 29.

63 David A. Jones et al., 'A Theologian's Brief: On the Place of the Human Embryo Within the Christian Tradition and the Theological Principles for Evaluating Its Moral Status', *Ethics & Medicine* 17:3 (2001), pp. 143–53 (p. 147).

64 2 Maccabees 7.22–23, cited in Jones et al., 'A Theologian's Brief', p. 147.

65 Jewish thinking portrays this impossibility of totally understanding creation or the beginning by using the letter *Beth* as the first letter of the biblical narrative and not the *Aleph* which is the first letter of the alphabet. Before the *Beth* there is therefore the *Aleph* which is impossible to determine or understand. Houziaux, *Le Tohu-bohu*, p. 34.

66 Houziaux, *Le Tohu-bohu*, p. 37.

67 Torrance, *Preaching Christ Today*, p. 24.

68 Berry and Jeeves, 'Nature of Human Nature', p. 30. The biologist John Medina also noted that fertilization is far more complicated than often assumed: John Medina, 1991, *The Outer Limits of Life*, Nashville: Nelson.

69 Pope John Paul II, 'Mentally Ill Are Also Made in God's Image', *L'Observatore Romano*, 11 December 1996, p. 4.

70 Pia Matthews, 2013, *Pope John Paul II and the Apparently 'Non-acting' Person*, Leominster: Gracewing, p. 66.

71 Gilbert Meilaender, 'Human Dignity and Public Bioethics', *The New Atlantis* 17 (2007), pp. 33–52 (p. 46).

72 Pastoral Constitution on the Church in the Modern World, *Gaudium et Spes*, paragraph 50, Pope Paul VI, 7 December 1965, http://www.vatican.va/archive/hist_councils/ii_vatican_council/documents/vat-ii_cons_19651207_gaudium-et-spes_en.html.

73 Letter to Families *Gratissimam sane* (2 February 1994), 9: *Acta Apostolicae Sedis* 86 (1994), 878; cf. Pius XII, Encyclical Letter *Humani Generis* (12 August 1950): *Acta Apostolicae Sedis* 42 (1950), 574; John Paul II, *Evangelium Vitae* (25 March 1995).

74 John Paul II, *Evangelium Vitae*.

75 Address given by Benedict XVI to the Members of the Pontifical Academy for Life on the occasion of the 15th General Assembly, Consistory Hall, Saturday, 21 February 2009.

76 Paul Ramsey, 1970, *Fabricated Man: The Ethics of Genetic Control*, Yale: Yale University Press, p. 38.

77 Kilner, *Dignity and Destiny*, p. 151.

78 Different versions of Creationism are suggested, such as (1) a person, including body and soul, is created by God as soon as a human organism is generated, (2) the soul is created by God once the biophysical body reaches a certain stage of development (there is some discussion about when this takes place), and (3) once certain biophysical conditions are obtained a soul is created and substantially changes these biophysical conditions to form a new individual essence forming one single substance. J. P. Moreland and Scott B. Rae, 2000, *Body & Soul: Human Nature & the Crisis of Ethics*, Leicester: InterVarsity Press, pp. 218–24.

79 The Church Father Origen (*c.* 185–254) believed in the pre-existence of souls.

80 Louis Berkhof, 1941, *Systematic Theology*, London: The Banner of Truth Trust, pp. 198–9.

81 Both St Jerome (*c.* 347–420) and John Calvin (1509–64) were opposed to Traducianism, indicating that Creationism was the set opinion of the Church, though Martin Luther (1483–1546), like St Augustine (354–430), was undecided. Lutherans, however, have generally been Traducianists. On the other hand, among the scholastics of the Middle Ages there were generally no defenders of Traducianism, with St Thomas Aquinas (1225–74) writing: 'It is heretical to say that the intellectual soul is transmitted by process of generation.' *Catholic Encyclopaedia*, 'Traducianism', http://www.newadvent.org/cathen/15014a.htm (accessed 13 December 2007). See also David Albert Jones, 2004, *The Soul of the Embryo*, London: Continuum, pp. 102–8.

82 Even in the stories of Frankenstein and Pinocchio, Dr Frankenstein and Geppetto both know that they have brought into existence a person which reflects something of them in their image and to which they are bound by a very powerful bond of mutual belonging.

83 Claus Westermann comments: 'There can be no question that the text is describing an action, and not the nature of human beings.' Claus Westermann, 1984, *Genesis 1–11. A Commentary*, London: SPCK, p. 155.

84 Westermann, *Genesis 1–11*, p. 158.

85 Westermann, *Genesis 1–11*, p. 158; G. Wenham replies to Westermann by pointing out that if evidence is drawn solely from Genesis 1, such a view is possible; but passages such as Genesis 5.3 imply that the image describes a product of creation and not the process. Wenham also asks what would be the distinctive qualities which come from such a process. G. Wenham, 1987, *Genesis Chapters 1–15*, Word Bible Commentary, Waco, TX: Word. However, given these weaknesses, Westermann's masterly exposition stands as a moving testimony to the relational dimension of the *imago Dei*.

86 Gunton, *Triune Creator*, p. 207.

87 Christopher J. H. Wright, 2004, *Old Testament Ethics for the People of God*, Leicester: InterVarsity Press, p. 119.

88 Barth, *Church Dogmatics*, Vol. III.1, p. 184.

89 International Theological Commission, *Communion and Stewardship*, paragraph 66.

90 Pope John Paul II, 'Discourse to Priests Participating in a Seminar on "Responsible Procreation"', 17 September 1983, *Insegnamenti di Giovanni Paolo II*, VI/2 (1983), p. 562.

91 *Angelus* in Osnabrück (Germany) with the disabled, 16 November 1980, *Insegnamenti*, III/2 (1980), p. 1232.

92 Pope Benedict XVI, 'Homily for the Solemn Inauguration of the Petrine Ministry' (24 April 2005): *Acta Apostolicae Sedis* 97 (2005), 71; Pope Francis; 'Encyclical Letter *Laudato Si* of the Holy Father Francis on Care for our Common Home' (2015), The Vatican.

93 Ted Peters, 1997, *Playing God? Genetic Determinism and Human Freedom*, London: Routledge, p. 15.

94 Gordon R. Dunstan, 1988, 'The Human Embryo in the Western Moral Tradition', in G. R. Dunstan and M. J. Sellers (eds), *The Status of the Human Embryo*, London: King Edward's Hospital Fund, p. 55.

95 Jones et al., 'A Theologian's Brief', p. 147.

96 Pastoral Constitution on the Church in the Modern World, *Gaudium Et Spes*, paragraph 19.

97 John Paul II, *Evangelium Vitae*, paragraph 53.

98 John Breck, 2000, *The Sacred Gift of Life: Orthodox Christianity and Bioethics*, New York: St Vladimir's Seminary Press, pp. 19–20.

99 Church of Scotland Board of Social Responsibility, 1996, *Pre-Conceived Ideas: A Christian Perspective of IVF and Embryology*, Edinburgh: Saint Andrew Press, p. 60.

100 David Cairns, 1973, *The Image of God in Man*, second edition, London: Fontana Library of Theology & Philosophy, p. 34.

101 Gregory of Nazianzus, *Orationes* 37.15; Cyril of Jerusalem, *Catecheses* 4.18f.; Epiphanius, *Anchoratus* 55; Cyril of Alexandria, *In Johannem* 1.9.

102 Gregory of Nyssa, *De anima et resurrectione*, Patrologia, Series Graeca, J. P. Migne, 46, 125–8; *De opificio hominis* 28–9.

103 Thomas F. Torrance, 1999, *The Soul and Person of the Unborn Child*, Edinburgh: Scottish Order of Christian Unity/Handsel Press, p. 9; Thomas F. Torrance, 1989, 'The Soul and Person in Theological Perspective in Religion, Reason and Self', in S. R. Sutherland and T. A. Roberts (eds), *Essays in Honour of Hywel D. Lewis*, Cardiff: University of Wales Press, p. 108.

104 Gregory of Nyssa, *De opificio hominis* 29.4.

105 Torrance, *The Soul and Person*, pp. 11–12.

106 Church of Scotland Board of Social Responsibility, *Pre-Conceived Ideas*, p. 9.

107 Church of Scotland Board of Social Responsibility, *Pre-Conceived Ideas*, pp. 60, 56.

5

Incarnation and the Embryo

The doctrine of the incarnation is central to any examination of the moral status of the human embryo because it has a profound theological meaning for the whole of creation. As previously mentioned, 'the Word made flesh' is not an addition but an affirmation and confirmation of creation by God. It is his certificate of approval for all he has made. The incarnation gives worth and value to the whole of the created cosmos[1] while disclosing the important significance of creation. It forms what T. F. Torrance calls 'the great axis of God's relation with the world of space and time, apart from which our understanding of God and the world can only lose meaning'.[2]

The Importance of Incarnation

The Scottish Anglican theologian John MacQuarrie (1919–2007) perceptively noted:

> Part of the trouble with the doctrine of Incarnation is that we discuss the divinity and even the humanity of Christ in terms of ready-made ideas of God and man that we bring with us, without allowing these ideas to be corrected and even drastically changed by what we learn about God and man in and through the Incarnation.[3]

Seeking to understand the incarnation is, therefore, a challenge but it is also fundamental to any consideration of humanity and what it means to be a person, while being central in many theological applications such as in gaining insights into the moral status of pre-natal human life.

The incarnation is of crucial importance because it is God's affirmation of his creation. God, the creator, came to share in his creation. The divine Word, the origin of creation's contingent rationality and freedom, took on human flesh and thereby established, in the very deepest sense, a confirmation of all rationality and freedom. In addition, Christ's coming to this world fulfilled the purpose of redeeming and restoring what was originally 'very good' and has never ceased to be the object of his love.

The incarnation is also God's affirmation that the human being is above all other beings in creation. Though all life forms are to be respected, it is because the Word of God took on humanity that human beings have been confirmed as uniquely valued by God at every stage of development and in every condition.

As the 2007 General Assembly Report of the Free Church of Scotland explains: 'God showed the great value of human life by sending his own Son, Jesus, to give us eternal life. The incarnation, life, death, resurrection and ascension of Christ certify for us the worth of human life in God's sight.'[4] More specifically, Jesus Christ stands before humanity as God's decisive Word on humanity, reflecting human life as God had intended it to be.[5]

Christ, Creation and Humanity

The 1987 Report to the General Assembly of the Church of Scotland characterizes the wonderful occurrence which is the incarnation:

> Both as it is attested in Scripture and as it has been understood by the church, the incarnation took place at the point of the virgin Mary's miraculous conception. That is to say, the human life of Jesus began at the beginning of his mother's pregnancy, when she was 'come upon' and 'overshadowed' by the Holy Spirit of God.[6]

This means that it is in the person of Jesus Christ that divine and worldly realities intersect so meaningfully. It was only when the Church Fathers accepted the full deity and humanity of Christ that it was eventually possible to put aside the Platonic suspicions concerning the value and reality of the material world.

Even more significantly, it is only in the incarnation that hope for a fallen creation can be offered. As T. F. Torrance stressed, it is

> the pledge of [God's] eternal faithfulness that He will never let go what He has made, allowing it to decay and crumble away into nothingness, but will uphold it and redeem it, and consummate through it the purpose of his rational love.[7]

More particularly, it is the resurrection of Jesus Christ which vindicates the original creation and gives hope for the re-creation of all things.[8]

These themes of incarnation, death and resurrection are, of course, central to the Christian message of hope. As the Church of Scotland Board of Social Responsibility expressed it in 1995:

Through the incarnation, God the Son made himself one of his own creatures. He entered and made his own the alienation of creation. Through his life, death and resurrection, he brought the love and power of God to bear on its disorder, restoring it to God's love. As it is in Jesus that we are confronted by God, we understand that it is in Jesus that we really see the mystery of God's creative activity ... In Jesus, the Saviour and Redeemer, we learn as never before how the creator works, and through him, the power of God's love is shown as grace.[9]

If this is the real meaning of the incarnation for the whole of creation then it is also the case for humanity. T. F. Torrance affirms that humanity's status and meaning is not at the mercy of relativist views at a merely horizontal level of the cosmos, for by 'the penetration of the horizontal by the vertical, it gives man his true place, for it relates his place in space and time to its ultimate ontological ground'.[10] This was eventually expressed when the very being of God took on humanity in Jesus Christ, confirming the wonderful value, worth and dignity of all human persons.

Based on this understanding of the profound involvement of Christ in creation, the following important points can be noted.

The incarnation affirms the dignity and status of every human being.
If the incarnation confirms that God created the universe (including everything in it) and that this universe belongs to him, it more specifically affirms the dignity and status of every human being. As the English Anglo-Catholic theologian Eric Mascall (1905–93) comments: 'The Incarnation has not only redeemed man from his fallen state but has also conferred a supreme dignity upon his human nature.'[11] As Gunton notes: 'To be created in the image of God is not simply to be made and upheld by the triune God; it is, more specifically, to be upheld by the Son, that is, through Jesus Christ, who is the true image of God.'[12]

That God put on the nature of humanity in Christ, 'the image of the invisible God' (Col. 1.15), emphasizes and confirms in a very significant manner the image-bearing nature of each and every human being, through all stages of their development during their entire existence.

The life of Christ is in conformity to the moral order of creation.
The life, example and teaching of Jesus Christ in the world were in conformity and necessarily consonant with the underlying moral order of creation. This means that all ethical directions originating in Christ will not contradict a creation ethic. Though the Fall brought sin and disorder to creation, it is still possible to recognize a perfect image of its original goodness in the person of Christ. Moreover, the early Church Fathers maintained that the moral nature of the created order originated from

beyond the cosmos in the Word of God. The incarnation is the highest presentation, in human form, of this rationality in love which expresses the moral order of creation. As O'Donovan says:

> God has willed that the restored creation should take form in, and in relation to, one man. He exists not merely as an example of it, not even as a prototype of it, but as the one in whom it is summed up.[13]

O'Donovan thus suggests that the grounding of all Christian understanding of ethics should be in the incarnation. That God's precepts can be recognized in the life, teaching, death and resurrection of Christ, especially since the incarnation did not oppose but entered into the created moral order to restore and renew the order which the Word had initiated in creation.

O'Donovan makes a useful distinction between moral authority and the authority of divine transcendence. Moral authority is the authority of order, invested in the moral order of creation, and therefore *universal* throughout creation. Divine transcendent authority, on the other hand, is beyond and above the creation order, which is only encountered at the specific point of intersection between the divine and the created order. It is therefore unique and particular, though in the incarnation they are both found together. As God's man, Jesus Christ is particular; as the new paradigmatic, archetypical man he is universal. O'Donovan explains that 'Christ's particularity belongs to his divine nature, his universality to his human nature.' Interestingly, he indicates that this is actually the reverse of what is commonly accepted, whereby the universal is understood as the divine, and the particular as the human. This, he argues, is a product of modern idealism rather than biblical theology.[14]

In summary, an examination of the concepts of creation and incarnation provides a rationale to inquire further into the more specific implication of these notions for the moral status of the early human embryo. This is because creation and incarnation not only confirm human dignity but enable a true understanding of what it means to be fully human.

Christ represents the final goal of humanity.
That the person of Christ expresses the final goal of humanity is reflected in a number of biblical concepts. For instance, the Lordship of Christ over all of creation can be considered as imaging the re-establishment and a bringing into perfection of the lordship first given to Adam and Eve at creation. This is a theological understanding of the Adam–Christ description of Paul.[15] A full theology of creation must also take into account the presence of the Holy Spirit as well as that of the Son of God. It is because the Spirit is present in this world that confident hope can

exist for a glorious and final redemption. Moreover, it is because the Spirit is present in the human Jesus Christ that he can redeem the world.

In this way, the love of God for humanity already has a wonderful conclusion through the work of Christ. In the resurrection God discloses creation's destiny where everything is renewed and reconciled to him.[16] This also means that God's creation and re-creation through Christ is crucial since it enables the concept of 'becoming' as well as that of 'being' for humanity. Perhaps this is what Mascall wanted to express when he wrote:

> Christianity does not believe that God became man simply in order to bring human history to a full stop and to reduce man to the status of a divinely certified fossil. The Incarnation did not only set upon man the seal by which God guarantees man's imperishable importance and inalienable dignity, it brought into the world a new thing and in-augurated a new era of human dignity.[17]

Christ represents the final renewal of all persons.
Until recently, the history of the debate relating to the human embryo always assumed that the human element was well defined, or, at least, that it could be taken for granted. But, as already indicated, because of new developments this is no longer the case (see Appendix). Embryos are already being created which are only partially human with the rest being animal, while scientists and bioethicists are beginning to consider the possibility of bringing into existence post-human individuals where nothing human even remains.

In this context, it is challenging to still speak about the concept of humanity in any real manner, although the new beings may still be con-sidered as 'persons' (or given the benefit of the doubt) and, similarly to Adam, they would still be made from the earth and dust of the ground (*adamah* in Hebrew).

In addition, if any of these new persons were created from already existing human persons, or their successors, it would remain possible for them to trace their 'ancestry' back to the origins of humanity in some way. This is significant since they could then still be considered as part of the 'family of human persons'.

Augustine discussed the hypothetical existence of other humanoid races. Though he was not convinced that such races actually existed, he was concerned to understand the implications should such a species be discovered. He stated:

> I must therefore finish the discussion of this question with my tenta-tive and cautious answer. The accounts of some of these races may be

completely worthless; but if such people exist, then either they are not human; or, if human, they are descended from Adam.[18]

In this regard, there is an urgent need for theologians to begin examining the concept of nonhuman physical persons and what the incarnation of Jesus Christ, as a human being, represents for such beings.

What, for example, does Christ's humanity actually mean for such persons who are only partially human? Would the resurrected body of a person, such as human–nonhuman interspecies being, be restored by the humanity of Christ into a fully human body? These remain open questions. But even if these questions wait to be answered, it is crucial to consider why Jesus Christ came as a human person in the incarnation and not in any other way.

Incarnation and the Image of God

The image of God presented in the Old Testament was to be fully revealed and completed in the image of Christ of the New Testament through the Christological and Trinitarian character of this image of God.[19] As the Church of Scotland Board of Social Responsibility put it in 1995:

> The central importance of the incarnation is the real self-communication of God, in Word and act. In Jesus Christ, God committed himself unreservedly to us in his own Triune being. The doctrines of the Trinity and the incarnation are interlinked, and as we trace out the trajectory of the incarnation, so our understanding of the Trinity is enriched.[20]

The early Church writers often accepted the community of the human race as being self-evident since they did not have difficulties in associating the first man, Adam, with Christ the redeemer of humanity. Adam was the representative person who was created in the image of God while also being the first human person to have a relationship with God. All humanity belongs to this first creation of man through Adam, and the image of God is shared by all human beings.[21] Christ, on the other hand, is the last Adam since it is through him that Christians are able to have a relationship with God and will receive a new human nature. In this way, the image and likeness in Adam and the hope and reconciliation in Christ express the real theology and dignity of all human persons. Jesus Christ brings together and restores all humanity.[22] As the 2002 *Communion and Stewardship* report of the Holy See states:

> In reality it is only in the mystery of the Word made flesh that the mystery of man truly becomes clear. For Adam, the first man, was a type

of him who was to come, Christ the Lord. Christ the new Adam, in the very revelation of the mystery of the Father and of his love, fully reveals man to himself and brings to light his most high calling.[23]

In fact, the central emphasis of the three main New Testament passages, Colossians 1.15, Hebrews 1.3 and 2 Corinthians 4.4, which refer to Christ as the divine image, affirm that Christ is the perfect revelation of the unseen God. As T. F. Torrance writes:

> In Jesus Christ we do not have just an image of God, but God himself revealing and communicating himself to us. In Jesus Christ God has imaged himself for us in such a way that Jesus Christ is both the Image and the Reality of God, and therefore the only Image, the eternal and unchangeable Image, of God ... Jesus Christ is not a mere image empty of reality, just a window through which we look at God, but is himself the very Being of God come to us and at work among us. Hence when we encounter Jesus Christ we have to do with the eternal and unchangeable Will of God embodied in him.[24]

This also means that God can only really be known by self-revelation, and such a self-disclosure is uniquely found in Jesus Christ. This is reflected in John's words, 'No one has ever seen God, but the one and only Son, who is himself God and is in the closest relationship with the Father, has made him known' (John 1.18). The double emphasis of this passage, where Jesus both actively reveals the Father and is one being with the Father, is what is implied when Christ is characterized as the image of God.

It is possible that the 'revelatory' understanding of Christ may have an origin in Hellenistic Judaism and the 'personified Wisdom' theme (found in Proverbs 8.22). In extra-biblical Wisdom literature, the theme of personified divine Wisdom is specifically portrayed as 'the image', the *eikon*, of God's goodness – the one who reveals the goodness of God.[25] On the other hand, the very nature and being of Christ imaging God is expressed in the relationship of the phrase 'the image of the invisible God', with the next title, 'the firstborn [*prototokos*] over all creation', in Colossians 1.15, which refers to Christ's pre-existence.

In ancient understanding, the *eikon* was not considered only to be a reproduction of the object being portrayed but involved, in some way, a participation in the very substance of the object being copied. In other words, it is not just a reflection of the reality, but is that reality. As the British theologian Ralph P. Martin (1925–2013) explains:

Christ as God's image means that he is not a copy of God ... he is the objectivisation of God in human life, the 'projection' of God on the canvas of our humanity and the embodiment of the divine in the world of men.[26]

The Greek word *charakter* (an exact representation or imprint) in Hebrews 1.3 is an even stronger word than *eikon* in articulating the correspondence and identity of the image to the nature of what is being represented.[27] As Kilner explains: 'By using character rather than eikon, the author clarifies that Christ is the strongest form of image – an exact image – of God. Christ is uniquely connected, in fact one, with God.'[28] This means that what God essentially is, has been made manifest in Christ. This is probably the most important element in understanding Christ, the divine image.

At this stage, it is useful to examine in what manner the Christological title 'the image of the invisible God' relates to the anthropological title 'man in the image of God' from a biblical and theological perspective. Four important statements can be made.

The Logos is the foundation on which humankind was created in the divine image.

From a certain perspective, the pre-existent Logos is the foundation on which humanity was created in the divine image. This is hinted at in the book of Colossians where Paul, having affirmed that Christ is the image of the invisible God, characterizes salvation as putting on 'the new self, which is being renewed in knowledge in the image of its Creator' (Col. 3.10). Paul may be suggesting here that the 'Creator' is actually none other than Christ (since he has already stated in Colossians 1.16 that by him all things were made). Moreover, even though Colossians 3.10 is more specifically addressing redemption, Paul may be implying that humankind's original image was fashioned by Christ.[29] It is known that that Hellenistic Jewish philosopher Philo of Alexandria (*c.* 25 BC – *c.* 50 AD), regularly identified *eikon* with his concept of Logos. He also described the first man 'in the image of the Image'. This idea is also explicit in the Prologue of John's Gospel where, through the Word, 'all things were made' (John 1.3). In fact, this was a frequent theme of the Church Fathers which was taken up by Luther and Calvin at the Reformation, as well as by more modern theologians such as Brunner and Barth. For Brunner, humankind was created in the image, and by the agency, of the Second Person of the Trinity, the pre-incarnate Logos. In the theology of Barth, there is an important new perspective in that all human beings were made by, and are continually confronted by, the incarnate Logos. Of course, this must be tempered by remembering that it is also the Trinitarian interrelatedness that is important when discussing the image of God. It is humankind's relatedness to God and to others that is at the very centre of any understanding of the divine image.

Christ is the revelation of true humanity.
Christ is the perfect fulfilment of the intentions of God when he created human beings in his own image. In Christ, it is possible to see not only true God but true humanity. In looking to Christ, one is also able to see the true meaning of what the divine image represents. What is so exceptional about Christ is not only his wisdom but his unique relationship with his Father and fellow human beings, a relationship characterized by his sacrificial love. It is this perfect love, revealed in Christ, which participated in the creation of humanity.

This means that, just as Christ is the perfect image of the amazing love of God in the Trinity, humanity is made in the image of God and is a reflection of this same love of God.

The correspondence between God and humankind enables the incarnation.
The correlation that exists between God and humanity, which is implied in humankind being created in the divine image, makes the incarnation possible. This is frequently emphasized by Cairns, who stresses that the physical cosmos, and humanity in particular, is 'sacramentally' fitted to reveal God's spiritual nature.[30]

The divine image reflects a certain kinship[31] between God and humanity which enables the Word to become a human being.[32] Such a statement is uncontroversial if it is remembered that the pre-existent Logos is himself the mould or template for the creation of humanity.

This understanding is very important in the contemporary debate on the nature of Christ, where the very notion of the incarnation is sometimes considered to be incoherent and irrational. For example, the English philosopher of religion Don Cupitt comments:

> The Eternal God and an historical man are two beings of quite different ontological status. It is simply unintelligible to declare them identical. It reflects Spinoza's comment that to talk of one who is both man and God is like talking of a square circle.[33]

But in response, the English philosophical theologian Brian Hebblethwaite argues that, because both humanity and God simply cannot be completely characterized by definitions (in contrast to circles or squares), it is not feasible to make any pronouncements on the issue of a rational impossibility.[34] Hebblethwaite instead uses the theme of the divine image as a pointer to an actual correspondence[35] in the sense that God is not 'wholly other'. Of course, what is implied in this statement is that God is profoundly concerned with humanity's very existence. As a result, since the divine image is perfectly represented and expressed in the man Jesus Christ, any understanding of the image of God in humanity must also seriously take into consideration the totality of the nature of humankind's existence.

Christ defines and enables the renewal of the image of God in humanity.
Since any mention, in the New Testament, of the image of God takes place almost exclusively in relation to Jesus Christ, this means that the doctrine is not concerned only with the status of this image at creation but also with the redemption of the image after the Fall.[36]

It is Jesus Christ who renews the image of God in redeemed humankind and he does this to restore the concealed image of the creator. In other words, when God re-creates and redeems humanity it is in the pattern of Christ.[37] Jesus Christ becomes the prototype of renewal, both in the foundation and in the continuance of the new humanity.[38]

This means that Christ, the perfect definition of true humanity, is both the agent and the agenda in the renewal of redeemed human beings.[39] This is a focus of the early patristic theology with, for example, Irenaeus writing: 'When the Word of God became flesh ... he showed forth the image truly, since He became Himself what was His image, and He re-established the similitude.'[40]

This theme is emphasized even more strongly by Athanasius in his *De Incarnatione*, in which he understood the incarnation as the Word coming to earth to remind humankind of the original image and to restore this humanity to what it was supposed to become. He illustrated this idea with the example of a portrait (humanity) being defaced (by sin) and the requirement for the original subject (Christ) to sit again for the portrait painter so that he can correct the original.[41] This renewal, moreover, where a relation to God and to others is restored, can only come through the Spirit of Christ in the community of Christ's people.[42]

This all seems to indicate that there is a profound dynamic and cohesion in the relationship between Christ and humanity. As Rollinson comments: 'The Word of God, who first impressed his unique stamp upon humankind in creation, and who then became a human being to reveal and restore the true image ... thereby creates an ontological correspondence between himself, the Word, and humankind.'[43]

It is this correspondence that is particularly important for an appropriate understanding of the value of the human person, and the following points can be made.

First, the incarnation may clarify the concept of the divine image and the manner in which this image is present in human beginnings. This can be seen in three ways:[44]

1 the revelation of the Word of God, incarnate in space and time, which led to
2 an appreciation of the pre-existence of this Word, which led to
3 a clearer understanding that the image of God is based on a particular creating and sustaining relationship which the Word of God has with all humankind.

This relationship is of course prior to any response an individual is able to make. It is part of the very basis of the person's being and is the foundation of the nature of humanity.[45] The concept of a dynamic relationship between creator and creature is also wonderfully presented in Psalm 139.13–16 – a relationship which stretches back to the earliest moments of embryonic existence.

Second, because the Word of God revealed himself as the divine image in human flesh, which was created by God, it is a clear affirmation that the image of God in humankind must also be related to being created. This means that the creative process in the development of a human being must be relevant to any appropriate understanding of the divine image in this human individual.

Third, since a correspondence exists between the incarnation and the image of God in humanity, this entails that any appreciation of the dignity of humanity must be of the very highest order. Because the Word of God took on humanity, this must mean that humanity has immense worth and value to God. In the same way, God is not just paying humanity a compliment by taking on human flesh. There is something in the very nature of humanity which is godlike and Christ-like.

Finally, for a person to seek to destroy a human being, made in the image of God, means that he or she is seeking to destroy the image of God himself. Similarly, to seek to protect and promote humanity, made in the image of God, is to seek to protect and promote the Image himself. In a way, this 'correspondence' may be what Christ was exemplifying in his parable of the sheep and the goats, when he said that 'whatever you did for one of the least of these brothers and sisters of mine, you did for me' (Matt. 25.40). In particular, 'the least of these' may also reflect the profound vulnerability and fragility of the early embryo.[46]

The Incarnation and the Humanity of Human Beings

At this stage, it is necessary to examine the connection between Christ's humanity and that of all human beings. This is important when considering whether Christ's humanity is in any way determinative for a moral evaluation of all human life including its beginnings. What it means to be human is at the centre of many questions in bioethics and its search for what represents normative humanity. For example, the American theological ethicist James Gustafson maintains that 'the major question about moral value in the sphere of biomedical developments is, "What do we value about human life?"'.[47]

In seeking to define normative humanity, a number of different perspectives may be considered.

The first tries to determine, from an empirical study or some other research, a set of agreed conditions for what constitutes 'true humanity'. This may examine the social dimension of human life, the cultural aspects of human living or the unique manner in which human persons can become the subject as well as the object of reflection.

The second perspective seeks to determine true humanity as a perfect paradigm or typical example to which persons should aspire.

A final approach tries to define the very nature of the existence of humanity, what Gustafson calls 'the true nature of man, man as he was created to be, man as his fundamental intentionality and tendency direct him to be'.[48]

These different perspectives are, of course, not necessarily mutually exclusive. But in this chapter it will be the last two options which will be examined since both are reflected in the incarnation.

In this regard, it is only Jesus Christ who can be considered as the 'Proper Man' (to use Luther's famous title) or the paradigm (the ideal model) man and who, as such, is 'the self-definition of human life'.[49] This means that an appropriate understanding of humanity cannot be achieved simply by examining the factual existence of human beings. Empirical studies of humanity based on observation and experience will never be sufficient or adequate. Instead, it is necessary to consider the new humanity in Christ, in whom humanity is re-created and restored.

Humanity Can Only Be Understood through Jesus Christ

To begin this section, it may be useful to examine the theological anthropology of Barth which is entirely based on the person of Christ, and as such is 'revolutionary in content'.[50] The practice of considering anthropology as being derived from Christology, however, can be traced back to the Greek Fathers. From this perspective, human beings were considered as the mediators between heaven and earth with Jesus Christ being the *Theandropos*, the mediator in whom all things are summed up (Eph. 1.10) and held together (Col. 1.17). In this way, Christ's human birth is, in a very meaningful expression attributed to Basil, 'the birthday of the human race'.[51]

From such a perspective, Barth maintained that, though an empirical examination of humankind was not without its usefulness, it is very limited and inadequate since humanity is alienated from its own reality by being estranged from God.[52] This means that any anthropological study cannot understand humanity as it was really meant to be as a creation of God. Instead, any appropriate examination of humanity must turn to the only human without sin, the only human in a full relationship with God, namely the True Man, Jesus Christ. As such, Christ's humanity is similar to that of all human beings in body and soul (he is 'real man') but is also different in that he presents humanity as God intended it to be ('true man').

This theme can be considered in the context of Barth's focus on God's election and covenant. From all eternity, God had decided to bring all humanity into a covenant relationship through Jesus Christ. This relationship between God and Jesus Christ, the true representative of humanity, is 'primal history' and, as such, is the foundation of, and must interpret, all history. This also means that Jesus Christ must take theological priority over Adam. Barth writes: 'Man's essential and original nature is to be found ... not in Adam but in Christ ... Adam can therefore be interpreted only in the light of Christ, and not the other way round.' This implies that God's intent for humanity is prior to humanity's rebellion 'in Adam', who was put aside as a historical figure not so much for scientific or anthropological reasons but as a theological necessity. Thus, according to Barth, 'human existence, as constituted by our relationship with Adam ... has no independent reality, status or importance of its own'.[53] Instead, it is the relationship that exists originally and essentially between Christ and humanity that is central. This theme, among many others, emphasizes Barth's insistence that the true nature of humanity can only be recognized in Christ.

But what does it then mean to be human in looking towards Jesus Christ? To answer this question, it is important first of all to remember that a human being is God's creature. Because of this, a human person can ignore or forget his or her relationship with God but this relationship cannot be destroyed. Every human person, since they are part of creation, is in a covenant relationship with God and is essentially 'a God-connected entity'.[54] Second, the very nature of a human being is to be in fellowship both with God and with his or her fellow humans – a human being is a being-in-relationship or a being-with-the-other. For Barth, true humanity is relational and directed towards God and co-humanity[55] which forms the very essence of the image of God. Barth considers such a relational focus as being external to the scope and breadth of modern human sciences in which, unfortunately, the individual and the independent existence of a human being is emphasized.

Barth writes that 'the humanity of each and every man consists in the determination of man's being as a being with others, or rather with the other man', adding, 'It is not as he is for himself but with others, not in loneliness but in fellowship, that he is genuinely human.'[56]

At this stage, it should be noted that human relationships, which form an essential part of humanity, are also defined by Jesus Christ who binds himself to other human beings in a very real and profound manner. Christ receives all the different possible reactions from his fellow humans. He also lives with them and, most significantly, turns towards them in constant, selfless love.

Moreover, Barth's emphasis on the wholeness of every human being is determined from Christology. A whole human being is made up of a body (creaturely being) and soul (creaturely life) which are to be distinguished but not separated. Even though the human soul is dependent on the creating and preserving work of God's Spirit, it cannot be reduced to spirit and should not be understood as such. Barth notes:

The human subject is man as soul, and it is this which is created and maintained by the Spirit. But the Spirit lives his own superior ... life over against the soul and the human subject. He is not bound to the life of the human subject.[57]

In summary, for Barth, the importance of Christ in seeking to understand humanity is central. He states:

We must form and maintain the conviction that the presupposition given in and with the human nature of Jesus is exhaustive and superior to all other presuppositions, and that all other presuppositions can become possible and useful only in connection with it.[58]

This emphasis of Barth is supported by Scripture in that the Christological motif of the 'second Adam' or the 'last Adam' used by Paul can be considered, to some extent, as reflecting the paradigm man. Another emphasis in this direction is the writer to the Hebrews' use of Psalm 8 in which humanity is considered as having the wonderful dignity of being God's viceroy, though this has been hidden through the Fall. Because of sin, this original image can no longer be recognized, though Hebrews 2.9 asserts, 'But we do see Jesus', which seems deliberately to use his human name in order to stress that, in Christ, original humanity can be seen. Here is paradigm human being, the one who fulfils the anthropological vision of Psalm 8.4–5. 'In the Incarnation', to use Mascall's phrase, 'God ... has sealed human nature with a certificate of value whose validity cannot be disputed.'[59]

The reason why the anthropology of Barth has been highlighted in this section is that it presents a particular expression of a general argument that normative humanity can be defined, and only defined, by Jesus Christ.

Thus, to understand what it means to be 'human' – what 'true humanity' entails – it is necessary to look towards Christ. As such, it is possible to see Christ as a 'pattern' for true humanity. Similarly, it is possible to consider Christ as the 'model', 'prototype', 'paradigmatic case' or 'norm' for what is meant to be human. Yet again, another perspective is to use the term 'ideal' to emphasize that Christ does not represent what people actually are (in their sinfulness) but what God intends them to be. But whatever terminology is used, looking to Christ, the perfect image of God, reveals God's intentions, purposes and goals for humanity.[60]

However, this general theological argument must be critically examined when it comes to being applied. The association between Christ's and a human being's humanity is not one of direct equivalence. This now needs to be expanded.

The Humanity of Jesus Christ and That of His Fellow Humans

The academic Stephen Sykes (1939–2014), who was also Anglican Bishop of Ely (in England), made a distinction between two aspects of 'humanity'. The first he defined as 'aspective humanity', which reflects particular features of a given individual or 'a humanity we can look at, feel, and converse with'. The second he characterized as 'empirical humanity', which refers to a generalization of human beings from a universal perspective or a humanity which can be inferred or constructed from all the different examples of aspective humanity.[61] In this regard, it may well be that Jesus Christ's 'aspective' humanity is not the same as his 'empirical' humanity. There are elements in Christ's humanity as a man that are new while remaining consubstantial with the humanity of his fellow humans (in the language of Chalcedon). But this must be developed.

Three approaches to Christ's humanity can be examined, though they all raise issues relating to the exact nature of the association of Christ's humanity with that of his fellow humans.

Jesus Christ is both a real human being and the true and ideal human being.

The first approach is to consider Christ as both a real human being and also the true and ideal human being. The American theologian Robin Scroggs, in his study *The Last Adam*, maintains that this motif of Paul must be seen in its eschatological context: 'The Adamic Christology speaks of the Exalted Lord, not the historic activity of Jesus.'[62] On the other hand, the Anglican David Jenkins, who was Bishop of Durham, in his book *The Glory of Man* presents a balance when he says:

> Such a real man has never yet existed, save in the defining case of Jesus Christ, but this is the reality of which all men to some extent partake … and in which all men will find the complete fulfilment of their existence.[63]

The first question, therefore, must consider to what extent Christ, as the ideal human being, can act as normative for fallen humanity.

Jesus Christ completely shares in the humanity of human beings.

The second approach is to come back to the inevitable paradox of Christology, raised by Sykes in his discussion of 'aspective' and 'empirical' humanity. The American theologian, John Knox (1901–90), in *The Humanity and Divinity of Christ*,[64] explores the theme further. His arguments are worth developing, not because they are beyond criticism, but because they radically emphasize the dilemma of Christology. Knox seems to experience, in the development of his understanding of Christ, a constant temptation towards Docetism (which suggested that Jesus only seemed to be human and that his human form was an illusion) as he discusses Christ's sinlessness and pre-existence.

The 'poignant dilemma', as Knox defines it, is that Christ must share in the humanity of his fellow humans in order to redeem it, but must also be different from this humanity in order to be a perfect Saviour. Christ's complete sharing in the humanity of his fellow humans entails, for Knox, different ideas.

To be a real man Christ had to be born 'out of and into humanity in the same sense every man is'. He must also have had self-consciousness like any other human being. 'Unless he was human to the lowest depths of his conscious and subconscious life, he was not truly human at all.'[65] What is important to note, at this stage, is that Knox's 'poignant dilemma' is influenced, on his own admission, by his understanding of the doctrine of salvation. In a way, this demands that the aspective and empirical humanities converge in a unique and transcendent Christ.

Similarly, over the centuries, Chalcedonian Christology has always maintained the full humanity and the full deity of Christ in the face of such pressing questions as those presented by Knox. The English Anglican theologian Charles Moule (1908–2007) resorted to the use of paradox.[66] He asserted that Christ's humanity is fully continuous with his fellow humans, yet there is also a discontinuity when his sinlessness is considered.

But if it is possible to concede that Christ's humanity can only be considered as a paradox containing unique elements, it is necessary to then return to the question of how Christ's humanity is normative and determinative.

Jesus Christ is a particular and representative human being.
A third line of questions relates to the dilemma of Jesus Christ being a particular, specific human and yet representatively human. It is obvious that he could not have been human in any meaningful manner unless he was a particular human.[67] In fact, he was a first-century Jewish man who lived in a specific cultural, social, historical and political context. But it is when Jesus' particularity is emphasized that more difficulties arise as to his representative status. For example, the American feminist Catholic theologian Rosemary Ruether expresses concern that certain traditional Christologies, such as the necessary maleness of Christ as taught by Aquinas, can exclude women.[68] Sykes comments: 'The more particularity one admits, the more one is in need of a transcendent category.'[69]

For Moule, such a category could be articulated in the theme of Christ reflecting 'Adam' as expressed by Paul. This would mean Christ being 'Man' in some collective sense. Interestingly, Paul's famous phrase *en Christos* (in Christ) implies inclusive personality.[70]

From a Christian theistic perspective based on the New Testament, human nature cannot be characterized by a reductionist understanding of 'nature' or by abstract concepts of transcendence. Instead, it is grounded in the Christian understanding of the intersection between God and humanity in the cosmos through the incarnation of Jesus Christ. Thus a genuine understanding of human nature cannot be considered from a naturalistic or even transcendentalist viewpoint but can only be examined from an eschatological perspective which puts God's new creation through Jesus Christ at the centre.

As the Scottish theologian Alan J. Torrance writes, one of the important elements of the Christian tradition is

> the perception that in Jesus Christ we are presented not only with God but with what it is to be human in truth – that is, with the one who uniquely defines human nature as it is created and elected to be. It is

in him – rather than in the originally created humanity, represented by the first Adam – that the *telos* of humanity is determined. He is the final or *eschatos* Adam, the true *imago Dei*, or *imago Patris*, and, as such, defines and, indeed, constitutes humanity in its properly functional form as this involves our existing in 'communion' with God.

It follows that, in order to understand what is really meant by 'human', it is necessary to look to the *eschatos Adam*, Jesus Christ, who redeems new humanity. 'Clearly, from a Christian perspective there is indeed a true human nature that must be conceived as invariant and is conceived in terms of participation within the "new humanity".'[71]

This also means that questions relating to the 'human' nature of new persons, such as certain animal–human combinations, can only be seen through Jesus Christ and the new human nature which he has redeemed. Though they may have been denied humanity through sin when brought into existence in this fallen world, these new kinds of human–nonhuman persons will eventually be brought, through death, into the presence of the embodied Christ. They will then put on the true humanity of Christ and be redeemed with the entirely human nature for which they were destined.

Cairns makes an interesting remark in this direction concerning 1 John 3.2: 'Beloved, we are God's children now; it does not yet appear what we shall be, but we know that when he appears we shall be like him, for we shall see him as he is.' In this, he suggests that the glorified believer will have both a spiritual and moral likeness to Christ, including 'a quasi-physical likeness of our spiritual bodies to his'.[72]

The Representative or Definitive Humanity of Jesus Christ

Whether Jesus Christ is the representative or definitive model of humanity is very important to those who understand the incarnation as being determinative for the moral status of the human being. The Scottish-American ethicist Nigel M. de S. Cameron exemplifies this position:

> The human life of our Lord was not simply a particular human life, it was a typical representative human life. The biblical teaching is that it was like ours in every respect except in one respect – that it was sinless. His life had to be like ours in every other respect, or he could not have redeemed us. The manner in which the incarnate Son experienced human existence not only may, but must be seen as a paradigm of all human existence.[73]

This quotation reveals a perspective which, if clarified, could be useful. The issue is the apparent association in Christ of 'representative humanity' and what has been defined as 'paradigm humanity' characterizing exemplary or definitive humanity. Indeed, a difference exists between the two expressions, with the 'representative humanity' of Christ being important in the context of his redeeming work while 'paradigm humanity' reflects a context of the wider creation. As the representative human, it was important for Christ to be a particular human being, to have a particular human life facing particular temptations and to bring about a particular victory through the cross and resurrection.[74] It is this moral and existential particularity which is at the centre of the premise of representation. As the Scottish Reformed theologian John McIntyre (1916–2005) notes, the idea that existence precedes essence may be useful in this context.[75] When the Logos took on human nature Christ entered the human situation, which implies that he made authentic decisions. For example, Christ 'learned obedience from what he suffered' (Heb. 5.8). This clearly means that, as the representative of humanity and as an individual, Christ could have been male or female, black or white, young or old. What mattered was that he was a particular human being who lived a uniquely obedient and loving life. From this representative and redemptive perspective, Christ's pre-natal life, which took place before his moral existential battles began, is less significant.

But a question remains as to the manner in which Christ's particular victory on the cross, in his particular manhood, relates to all of humanity. There must be a relationship between the individual *homo* and the universal *humanitas*. This was the emphasis made by the Archbishop of Constantinople, Gregory of Nazianzus (*c.* 329–389 or 390), when he said, 'What Christ has not assumed he has not healed' (and the corresponding expression, 'What has been united with God is saved').[76]

For Paul, such a relationship in Christ makes him the second Adam (Rom. 5.12–19).[77] In other words, Christ must take on in himself the whole of humanity in order to be able to release it from its bondage to sin. This was a theme that was particularly emphasized by the Reformers and one to which T. F. Torrance continually returned. Christ is the Head of the whole human race, not just the Elect.[78]

The virginal conception of Christ is a very strong testimony to this reality in which he expressed his solidarity with fallen humanity even at the very level of biology.

But is such an understanding of Christ being a 'representative' human being similar to understanding Christ as being a 'paradigm' or ideal model human being seen from the perspective of wider humanity? In a way, the relationship between Christ's particularity and his universal significance parallels the 'aspective humanity' and 'empirical humanity' distinction made earlier by Sykes.

As such, the particularity of (1) Christ beginning his human existence at conception and (2) his redeeming work affecting every stage of humanity, are not being questioned. But does it follow that by being humanity's representative Christ is also, and must be, humanity's paradigm for all stages of human existence? In other words, can Christ's existence on earth, including the very beginning of his human life, have anything to say about all other human lives from the very beginning of their existences?

To answer this question, it is now necessary to examine the relevant arguments suggesting Christ's paradigmatic significance to humanity.

The Word Made Flesh

In examining Christ's paradigmatic significance, it is possible first of all to investigate whether considerations relating to the very nature of existence or being can provide further insights into the mystery of the Word becoming flesh. Barth emphasizes that the incarnation is 'the mystery of revelation'[79] which means that it is impossible to understand the 'how' of God becoming human while simply accepting that it did happen.

Because of this, any theological discussion on this theme must seek to respect its mystery as did the Council of Chalcedon. In this context, the first 'sign' of the incarnation was the virginal conception of Mary which sets the time for this wonderful event. It indicates that at conception, and no other later time, did the Word of God become human.

This also means that the joining of the divine and human natures in the person of Christ must have occurred at the very conception of Jesus Christ. As the Dutch Reformed theologian Herman Bavinck (1854–1921) stated, 'the human nature formed in and out of Mary did not for a moment exist by and for itself – but from the earliest moment of conception was united with, and taken up into, the person of the Son'.[80] This implies that the embryonic beginnings of Jesus Christ must be considered in the context of an already existing divine person starting to exist as a human person.

As Mascall comments, this is similar to the conclusions of Aquinas who believed that, in the special case of Christ, his conception and animation were simultaneous. This happened, Mascall notes, 'on the double ground that the hypostatic union must have taken place at the moment of conception and that the divine hypostasis could not become the subject of a nature that was not yet fully human'.[81]

This is a crucial statement because, for Aquinas and his contemporaries, the moment of animation of all other human embryos was not seen as identical to the moment of conception.

For Aquinas, therefore, Christ's incarnation began at conception but human embryos, on the other hand, only became persons at a later stage.

Aquinas' understanding of Christ's conception does not mean, of course, that the human nature of the embryonic Christ was fully developed bio-logically or mentally[82] but it does seem to imply that he already existed as a human person. Aquinas adds:

> There are two ways of considering the beginning of the breath of life. First, as regards the disposition of the body; and thus the quickening by soul began no differently in the bodies of Christ and of other human beings: the soul is infused as soon as the body is formed, and so it was with Christ. Second, this beginning may be considered just with regard to time: and thus because Christ's body was perfectly formed sooner it was sooner animated.[83]

Hence, for Aquinas, his very clear understanding that Christ was a full human person from the moment of conception did not seem to influ-ence his belief that all other embryos became persons some time after conception. But this discrepancy was probably the result of limitations in understanding the relevant biology and his emphasis on the unique-ness of the virginal conception of Christ rather than on its paradigmatic nature relating to the wider humanity.

Incarnation and Personhood

It has already been possible to highlight, at various stages of this study, how incarnational theology may assist in advancing the debate on the moral status of the human embryo. This will now be developed by first explaining the setting of patristic Trinitarian and incarnational theology in which the very concept of being a person was proposed. Second, vari-ous theological concepts arising from the incarnation will be shown to clarify what it means to be a human person. Finally, the importance of such themes, arising from the incarnation, will be examined in the con-text of contemporary philosophical notions of personhood.

The Theological Context of Incarnation and Being a Person

A useful introduction to the importance of theology in understanding the concept of being a person and the important debates which arise can be presented by Jenkins' (1967) book *The Glory of Man*. In this, he completely reverses the German philosopher Ludwig von Feuerbach's (1804–72) famous dictum 'all theology is anthropology' into his own affirmation that all true anthropology can only arise from an under-standing of theology.[84] Jenkins argues that true personhood can never be defined since a listing of the constituent parts of a person cannot reveal the full truth about the unity of the whole. In addition, a person always seems to be, to some extent, open and incomplete since the intrinsic potential for personal fulfilment of an individual can never be quantified or delineated. As suggested by MacQuarrie, the human person is 'a-being-on-the-way'. Consequently, there is a transcendent element in the human person in the sense that it crosses established limits and goes forward, meaning that a wider perspective must be considered if personhood is not to be limited by reductionist constraints. Jenkins writes: 'Science and technology have, as such, no means of reckoning with humanness and personalness.'[85] He also warns that if science begins to take over all knowledge it may eventually kill, without realizing it, the very concept of being a person.

Interestingly, from a historical perspective there is evidence that once anthropology is dissociated from theology, as happened in the Enlightenment and post-Enlightenment periods, there is a risk that the very notion of being a person becomes an empty and meaningless concept. As Jenkins says, 'the reduction of theology to anthropology was a prelude to reducing anthropology to absurdity'.[86] Without a direction towards God, human beings lose their personhood and their meaning. The 'death of God' became the 'death of the person'. Similarly, Gunton stated that one of the main reasons for the re-questioning of morality in modernity is the removal of God from any understanding of human dignity, and that this displacement 'has not given freedom and dignity to the "many" (i.e. individual persons), but has subjected us to new and often unrecognised forms of slavery'.[87]

Hence, the very foundation of a theology of what it means to be a person must be based on the reality that each person is made for a relationship with a personal God.[88] As Rollinson writes: 'A person is essentially a created being, dependent on the Creator, existing only in relationship to Him.'[89] This means that the important Christian doctrines of the incarnation and redemption are not only the core principles for understanding God in personal terms[90] but are also at the very heart of the relationship between the personalness of God and that of human beings.

In this manner, the incarnation becomes the very basis for every human being's own personhood. Jenkins asserts that the historical reality of the personhood of Jesus Christ is 'definitive for our understanding of persons'. He writes: 'I believe ... that our present comprehension of the concern for persons received its initial shaping from the Christian understanding of the universal significance of Jesus.'[91]

Thus, in the same manner as the Logos associates or relates the rationality of the whole cosmos to humankind's rationality, so this same

Logos associates or relates God's personal being to the personhood of all human beings which is therefore derived personhood. This means that, for Jenkins: 'The defining characteristic of every human being lies in his or her potential personal relationship to God in Jesus Christ, rather than in any general or impersonal classification by status or any other category'; and he adds: 'Jesus Christ is the definition, demonstration and declaration of the reality of man'.[92]

It may be necessary at this stage to pause and ponder the amazing reality of the Word coming as the historical person of Jesus Christ. His humanity is overwhelming in its depth and wholeness while representing the definitive fulfilment of human life through his self-sacrificial love in his total submission to his Father. It is in the person of Jesus Christ that true personhood is defined in his unique creaturely relationship to God and his sinless relationship with all whom he knew. As Rollinson comments: 'All philosophising and theological analysis is dwarfed by the reality and sheer beauty of this truly human being.'[93]

At this point, it may also be important to comment on the possible implications of a 'self-emptying' Christ who is totally submitted to his Father. A number of commentators consider the Christological hymn in Philippians 2.5–12 as a moving poetic perspective of God's self-giving and self-denying love but would not seek to interpret the language as an incarnational exposition.[94] Indeed, it may be possible to turn around this hesitation to use 'self-emptying' language by affirming, instead, that in the divine self-emptying the fullness of God is actually being demonstrated. The God whose very nature it is to impart love reveals himself most fully in the coming of Christ. Christ did not cease to be God when he made himself nothing. The incarnation, therefore, expresses the paradox that the self-emptying also reflects a fullness of self-revelation.[95] It is in Christ's sacrificial and self-emptying love for his Father, as well as his sacrificial love for the world, that his full personhood shines most perfectly.

This understanding of the nature of Jesus Christ means that, for humanity, it is possible to assert that the dignity of human beings arises from the incarnation and the reality that God took on humanity in the person of Jesus Christ. But the manner in which Christ's personhood may be definitive for human personhood and the extent to which this may particularly apply to pre-natal human life remains to be considered.[96]

Incarnation and the Moral Status of the Embryo

The question being considered in this chapter is whether the incarnation, in addition to being a unique and divine affirmation of the humanity of human beings, may also have direct relevance to the important ethical debate concerning the moral status of human embryos. In other words, since it is at the decisive moment of the virginal conception of Christ[97] that the incarnation occurred, can this have implications for the earliest beginnings of all embryonic human life?

As already noted, an appropriate understanding of the argument that uses the incarnation to understand the moral status of human embryos involves an appreciation of the fundamental concept of being a person,[98] which has its historic roots in Christian theology and the doctrine of the Trinity.[99]

In this regard, the argument from the incarnation in addressing the moral status of the human embryo is especially informative since it reflects an important convergence between (1) historical theology and (2) philosophical and ethical inquiry. It establishes a crucial discussion which may be both challenging but also critical for a truly Christian assessment of the status of the human embryo.

According to this perspective, the starting point for theologians, such as T. F. Torrance, is the assertion that in a unique way God alone is the definition and source of all personal being. For him, God is the personalizing Person and his children are the personalized persons.[100] This means that the concept of being a person must inevitably have a direction towards God.

The Virginal Conception of Jesus Christ

Before continuing with this examination, it should be noted that the argument from the virginal conception of Jesus Christ is not universally accepted. Two main arguments are usually presented for mistrusting and even rejecting this virginal conception of Christ as the means for the incarnation.

In the first, the historical fact of the virginal conception is considered with scepticism. For example, modern theology often prefers to interpret this occurrence as a theological legend of the early Church which was promoted for reasons relating to the defence of the core principles of the faith.[101]

In the second argument, even if the virginal conception of Christ is accepted as valid, it is portrayed as biologically unique, in which case it cannot be considered as normative and, consequently, as ethically relevant for other human conceptions and the moral status of embryos. For example, the Christian biologist and bioethicist D. Gareth Jones argues: 'If the conception of Jesus did not involve the fertilisation of an ovum by a sperm, why should his conception as a *biological* phenomenon become the base of a *theological* statement about the status of all normally-conceived foetuses?'[102]

This also reflects the view of the Scottish Protestant theologian Elizabeth Templeton, who writes:

> If the embryo emerging from Mary's fallopian tubes was fertilised without male human sperm, its biological and genetic constitution is so unlike ours that its ethical relevance to ordinary humanness is questionable. If, on the other hand God provided the male, human sperm, that is paganism.[103]

In order to respond to these arguments, however, an analysis of the theological significance of the virginal conception is required.

The Theology of the Incarnation and the Virginal Conception

An appropriate understanding of the theological doctrine of the incarnation reflects the reality that God, the Son, became man in that 'the Word became flesh' (John 1.14). As the Apostles' Creed affirms, Christ was 'conceived by the power of the Holy Spirit and born of the Virgin Mary'.[104]

This means that the theological doctrine of the virginal conception asserts that Christ did not have a human biological father and that his conception was a miracle. But this does not imply that God, the Father, replaced Joseph as the male progenitor who supplied the sperm cell containing the 23 male chromosomes. If this was the case, Christ would not be truly human and truly God but instead a half-human, half-divine hybrid. As Barth explains, 'God takes the stage as the Creator, not as a partner to this virgin.'[105]

The relationship between the two doctrines of the incarnation and the virgin birth can be emphasized by stating that Christ's conception relates to the origins of his humanity in that he did not have a human father, whereas the incarnation relates to the deity of Christ in that he, as 'the son of man', was none other than the Son of God, the second Person of the Trinity.[106]

It follows that the virginal conception of Jesus cannot imply that he was not also fully human in the incarnation. This is because the humanity of Christ is as much a doctrinal issue as is the study of his nature and personhood.[107] Both Christ's full humanity and divinity require faith and theological exposition.

As already discussed, Sykes differentiated between what he characterizes as 'aspective humanity', which means 'a humanity we can look at, feel, and converse with',[108] and 'empirical humanity', which is a humanity that can be inferred or constructed from all the different examples of aspective humanity. This makes it possible to enquire whether, in the case of Jesus Christ, one may directly move from considerations of his aspective humanity to those of his empirical humanity. Sykes suggests that because the patristic writers did not imply such a conclusion[109] then neither should anyone else. This means that there is something special about the humanity of Christ which is not found in empirical humanity as a whole. As a result there is an inevitable ambiguity about using the concept of the 'full humanity' of Christ which needs special attention. Any description of Christ that does not distinguish him from the rest of humanity does not fit with any understanding of Christ in the New Testament.[110] But Christ still remains 'fully human' in any orthodox understanding of his nature.

In other words, great care is required in understanding the humanity of human beings based on that of Christ.

In this context, it should be noted yet again that, though related, the virginal conception and the incarnation should not be confused from a theological perspective. But the very nature of this relationship now needs to be examined.

At this stage, it may be useful to consider Barth's understanding of the incarnation.[111] He maintained that, although the 'mystery' of the incarnation is clearly primary, the mode of that incarnation through a 'miracle' is significant since it is important as a sign. By using, as an example, the healing of a paralytic in Mark 2.1–2, Barth suggested that Christ's healing miracle points to (or signals) and emphasizes his far greater work of redemption.[112] In the same manner, the virginal conception is a witness to, but not the heart of, the incarnation as the empty tomb is a witness to, but not the heart of, the resurrection.

The Dutch theologians Klaas Runia (1926–2006) and Gerrit Berkouwer (1903–96) are unsure, however, whether Barth has actually gone far enough and are uneasy with his poetic/optic distinction. Instead, they see the virginal conception and incarnation as interconnected and knotted together in a far more fundamental manner.[113]

Berkouwer suggests that Barth's illustration of the paralytic healing in Mark 2.1–12 may not be sufficient to express what is happening with the incarnation. Similarly, the empty tomb is far more than just a sign since it is inseparable from the bodily resurrection of Christ. In other words, the virginal conception was not just a necessary sign in the sense that God had to realize the incarnation in this manner, but the fact that God did do it in this way necessitates bringing sign and substance together in the closest possible manner. This implies that the virginal conception is a necessary sign for the incarnation because it both illuminates and guards the doctrine.

In addition, Barth was very careful to emphasize that the virginal conception highlights God's sovereign initiative in the incarnation. God did not become a human being out of divine necessity but because of his loving and free decision. It is similar to the act of creation by God where 'God enters the field and creates with creation a new beginning.'[114] The corresponding emphasis for the virginal conception is that God's initiative and grace deliberately excludes any male, and more specifically any human, initiative. Humanity is limited to standing before God in submission and cooperating as the 'handmaiden' (Luke 1.48). Though this does not mean that humanity is unimportant, it is an expression of its total dependence on God.[115]

This implies that the virginal conception illuminates the mystery of the incarnation. Moreover, to reject this miracle means denying the mystery. The very fact that Christ's conception is unexplainable emphasizes the incomprehensibility of the incarnation. As Rollinson comments: 'It is an appropriate witness to the mystery of the personal union of God and man in Christ Jesus.'[116]

But, far more importantly, the virginal conception is the guardian of a full doctrine of the incarnation. It is, as Barth maintained, 'the watch before the door ... it preserves the very knowledge of the Incarnation'.[117]

It does this in two different ways. First, the virginal conception guards the uniqueness of Christ[118] because of its relationship to the sinlessness of Christ.[119] The virginal conception enables Christ to be both a descendant of Adam (Luke's genealogy)[120] while not sharing in the sin of those 'in Adam'.

Second, the virginal conception defines the boundaries of the incarnation and, more particularly, it defines the timing of the incarnation. This is of crucial importance for the embryonic Christ. While seeking to examine what is meant by the full humanity of Christ, Sykes writes:

> We are now capable of pursuing our descriptive analysis of man much fuller than were the Fathers or even the theologians of the last century. We can particularise about genetic inheritance where they could only guess. Thus, contemporary theology is faced with an apparently new dilemma; can it precisely say at what point the divine 'entered' the human?[121]

This is exactly the question for which the virginal conception of Christ is most meaningful and significant. Though the precise manner in which the incarnation took place will always remain a profound mystery, the miracle of the virginal conception does define the moment in time when the incarnation happened. The British Protestant theologian and physician John Wilkinson (1918–2015) makes the point:

> A denial of the virgin birth makes the Incarnation a blurred indefinite event ... If we deny the miraculous conception ... then we do not know when God became man, except that he did so sometime during the life of Jesus of Nazareth.[122]

More specifically, the American Presbyterian theologian John Gresham Machen (1881–1937) concluded:

> The virgin birth tells us that at no later point in time should the Incarnation be put than at the moment of conception. There, and there alone, did the stupendous event occur ... Our knowledge of the virgin birth, therefore, is important because it fixes for us the time of the Incarnation.[123]

Though this emphasis is seldom made, it is of central importance for an appropriate understanding of the life of Christ. Moreover, it corresponds to Barth's 'theory of bracketing' which asserts that unless the life of Christ on earth is bracketed, at the beginning and at the end, it would not be possible to be confident in the incarnation.

Another writer who supported this reasoning that a historical virginal conception could be determinative in the timing of the incarnation was the Anglican bishop and theologian Hugh Montefiore (1920–2005). But he continued to have questions as to the beginning of human life: 'In the light of modern knowledge, the matter cannot be quite so simple. Presumably God's special presence began at the same time as the human life began. But when does human life begin?' This led him to ask even more probing questions:

> On the supposition that the virginal conception was an historic event, we can hardly suppose a two-stage miracle, first when Mary miraculously conceived, and second when God assumed humanity. If there is a continuing process of human development and no moment when human life begins, surely we cannot say that there was also a process of Incarnation?[124]

Montefiore highlights the key point. Precisely because it is very difficult to rationally consider the incarnation as a progressive process taking place over time, the virginal conception must define the moment when the Second Person of the Trinity assumed humanity.[125]

In short, it is possible to maintain that the virginal conception of Christ serves as a guardian to the radical nature of the incarnation. It also means that God, in Christ, shares the humanity of human beings right down to their biological origins. By becoming human flesh, Christ shares in the created nature of human beings, including its destiny, and this took place in the virginal conception of Christ when the divine intersected the human while being brought forth by the perfecting Holy Spirit.

At this stage, it is important to examine how different Christian writers sought to apply this theology of the incarnation and virginal conception of Christ to the moral status of pre-natal human life.

Theological Perspectives

Interestingly, compared to the huge amount of literature concerning the moral status of the human embryo, only a relatively small number of Christian writers have used the doctrine of the incarnation in their discussions.[126] Among those who have, moreover, the arguments are not always presented in any detail.

The Moral View of T. F. Torrance

Probably the most important exponent of the significance of the incarnation for the status of the human embryo is T. F. Torrance. But before his views on the topic are presented it is necessary to examine his theology, which is heavily influenced by the Church Fathers and the Reformation tradition of Calvin and Barth.[127] It is a theology which is very much engaged and concerned with modern developments and understandings especially in the realm of science. In this regard, three key features of his theology are important.

The first of these is Torrance's understanding of the philosophy of knowledge. What is of crucial importance to Torrance is that theology is embedded in the 'constitutive factors of reality itself'.[128] Things are to be known according to their true natures. This means, first of all, that when God is considered, all knowledge of him must be revealed by him since he is a transcendent God. God's self-revelation 'is not a mute fact'[129] which can be taken for granted. Instead, humanity is called to humbly, obediently and prayerfully listen to the gracious Word of God.[130]

In addition, the manner in which human persons listen to God must be determined by the One who speaks. Human beings cannot begin by asking 'How can God be known?' and then ask 'How far is this factual?' Instead, they must recognize that questions relating to the knowledge of God must be determined, from first to last, by the way in which he is actually known.[131] In other words, it is the very nature of God's being that must determine the nature and scope of knowledge, and not the other way round.

The knowledge of God is presented to human beings through the 'given' of Jesus Christ, which is clarified by the Holy Spirit.[132] Christian belief, therefore, is not to be contrasted with knowledge but is integral to it. This means that there is a genuine correspondence between belief, human thought and reality when what is perceived through the mind is in line with the form of rationality presented by reality.

For Torrance this reflects an important parallel with natural science where the main basis is also the 'given'. This means that both science and theology are to be considered in the same way since they are both 'positive, a posteriori, and empirical'.[133] In both fields, there is a requirement to liberate the inquirer from *a priori* conceptions and distortions in order to let the subject of study open up the mind of the examiner to true and clear perceptions. Both scientific method and theological method can be used to guide and inform each other. However, it may be impossible for human persons ever to be free from these *a priori* conceptions since modern interpretations of reality always take place within a given context. This means that there is an inevitable subjectivity to all objective inquiries.

Another important aspect of Torrance's theology is a strong conviction that both theological science and natural science make known the same 'realism' since they both originate in the same God who reveals himself in creation. Theological knowledge is not interested in knowing God in the abstract but in knowing him as he has revealed himself in the reality of creation. In the same way, there is an intelligibility and rationality to natural science, which is a contingent reality dependent on God because the world and all of physics was created by God. Theology and natural science are thus handmaids to each other.[134]

The third feature to consider is Torrance's requirement of a clear theological anthropology. Because of his emphasis on realism he maintains that human beings should be considered, studied and known according to their true natures and not be examined, instead, as if they were machines or biological specimens. If Barth was right in asserting that human beings exist on the border of two worlds, the visible and invisible as well as the earthly and heavenly, then transcendent considerations which go beyond creation must be taken into account for an appropriate understanding of human nature. Accordingly, for Torrance, a human being's relationship with a personal triune God is especially important for a true understanding of himself or herself as a human person.

The Revelation of God at the Stage of Conception

As already mentioned, T. F. Torrance is one of the most important exponents of the significance of the incarnation for the moral status of the human embryo. Even though his published work on this specific topic is limited to three relatively unknown booklets[135] and some unpublished lectures,[136] it touches a nerve at the very centre of his theology which is extensive and influential.

Though some commentators use the argument from the incarnation in the context of the moral status of the embryo, this is often presented only in a secondary or supportive role. For Torrance, however, the argument from the incarnation is primal for it is the very foundation of all his theology relating to the central nature of Christ. This is because the One who created his universe with the rationality of his Word is the very same One who has entered into his creation as the Living Word. It follows that, for Torrance, the 'investigation of the intelligible reality of the triune God in his creation of the contingent and orderly universe, and in the depth of his relation to the universe of his Son, provides for the natural sciences the vertical and horizontal co-ordinates for the integration of the universe'.[137]

This means that at the very centre of the relationship between humanity's knowledge of God and the natural world is the person of Jesus Christ. All true theology must, therefore, have a Christocentric emphasis.[138] For Torrance, any true understanding of God cannot be achieved in isolation but must be considered from the perspective of the whole of theology and especially from angles of revelation and reconciliation. It is only when humankind's separation from God is bridged through redemption that true enlightenment is possible.[139]

Torrance resists any debate about the historicity of the virgin birth but simply affirms the relevant provisions of the Apostles' Creed: that Jesus Christ, God's only Son, 'was conceived by the Holy Spirit, born of the Virgin Mary'.[140] The important implication of the virginal conception for Torrance and other commentators is that it defines the exact moment of the incarnation.[141] The Word of God chose to start his identification with, and take on, humanity not at birth but at conception, as can be inferred from Luke 1.41–44. As Atkinson explains, 'The Word has become flesh right down to the level of our genes';[142] while Cameron emphasizes, 'Not in a cradle merely has God designed to be "contracted to a span", but in the microscopic dimensions of a fertilised ovum.'[143]

For God to relate his very Being to humanity at the point of human conception, as expressed in the doctrine of the virginal conception of Christ, has momentous and profound implications. As Cameron states:

The life-story of Jesus Christ, God and man, begins in the earliest days of his embryonic biological existence; and the significance of this fact is that the manhood which he took on is our manhood. That is, it cannot be claimed that his case was in this respect unusual, since the entire principle of the incarnation is the taking up of normal, yet sinless, humanity by God. If that is the point at which his human life-line began, it is also the point at which ours begins.

Thus, in the same way that God was able to become a human being because humanity reflects the image of God, he was able to become a human embryo because embryos reflect the image of God.[144] In other words, the early stages of human embryonic life must reflect the divine image.

This is important because the Son's 'assumption' of fallen humanity in order to heal it is a central theme of T. F. Torrance's writing[145] and this 'assumption' begins at the virginal conception. Thus, the atonement began with the virgin birth of Christ, was confirmed though his baptism and reached its culmination in the crucifixion. In this way, the whole of Jesus Christ's life, ministry and death was involved in the work of reconciliation.[146]

Jesus Christ and Humanity's Origins

What has been affirmed up to this stage is that Christ's own embryonic beginnings must be viewed in personal terms if the incarnation is to be taken seriously. This is significant for the moral status of the pre-natal child, since Christ's personhood was demonstrated and expounded through the merging of the divine and human natures from conception onwards. The terminology is, of course, completely limited and static but it has the advantage of emphasizing God's unique relationship with the being of the conceptus: a being that must bear the image of God, otherwise the incarnation would not have taken place. As Cameron comments: 'The Incarnation of the Son of God in the form of a human embryo is possible, because already at this most primitive stage in human existence, man bears the divine image.'[147]

By examining the Gospel passages, Cameron also argues that Elizabeth's words to Mary, 'Why am I so favoured that the mother of my Lord should come to me?' (Luke 1.43), implies an acknowledgement that the unborn Jesus was already the Son of God in flesh and blood.[148] This provides the scriptural basis for further arguments. For example, O'Donovan, for whom the argument from the incarnation is only used in the context of wider discussions on the subject,[149] suggests that the text in Luke, together with the position of the early Church, witnesses 'against the Christological heresy of Adoptionism by insisting that if the Son of God was not present in the life of the foetus, the true assumption of humanity by the Godhead could not have happened'.[150]

This now raises the question whether this unique event of the incarnation is determinative for the rest of humanity in being seen as a parallel in which to consider all human beginnings. The important focus here is the kind of relationship God has with all human beings.

One of the first writers on this topic was the theologian Maximus the Confessor, also known as Maximus of Constantinople (c. 580–662), who insisted that if Jesus is ensouled at the moment of conception, and if he shares the same humanity as all other human beings, then all human beings are also ensouled at the moment of conception. Indeed, since Maximus did not accept that souls and bodies could exist separately, he believed that the incarnation could only happen when the embodied soul came into being as an embryo from conception onwards.[151]

Maximus was aware of the argument that the incarnation and Jesus' conception were exceptional and could, therefore, not be seen as normative since they occurred through a miracle in that no male seed was used. However, he argued that it was possible to differentiate between the manner in which Christ was brought into human existence and his very nature as a person. Jesus came to the world through a unique miracle but his human nature is the same as that of humanity. He was both the Son of man as well as the Son of God. That Jesus shared in the fullest sense the nature of all humanity is actually the basis of the incarnation. This is what was declared in Chalcedon: he is 'of one substance with the Father as regards his divinity, of one substance with us as regards his humanity'. Thus, even though Jesus was conceived in a very special way, because of his humanity his embryonic human nature was no different from that of all human beings. This means that if the embodied soul of Jesus was present from the very instant of his conception, then this must also be the case for all human individuals.[152]

At this stage, it may be useful to return to T. F. Torrance's argument that God, the 'Personalising Person', who uniquely in Jesus Christ expressed his own personalness, is the God who, through the creator–creature relationship, personalizes every human person including his or her very beginnings.

Therefore, the reality of the incarnation in which God took on humanity, at the point of human conception, is of immense and crucial significance for Torrance:

It is surely to him who became a holy embryo in the Virgin's womb, and was born of her to be the Saviour of the world, that we must go, in order as Christians to understand what the unborn child is as an embodied human soul, and as one loved by the Lord Jesus who came to be the Saviour of the human race.[153]

This means that Christ's human beginnings, while not being by direct equivalence normative for other human beings, are nevertheless determinative and serve to define a model for considering humanity's derived personhood. Christ's incarnation as a human conceptus at a particular point in space and time thus bestows a sacred status on all human embryonic life for all time.

That Jesus Christ took on the whole of humanity at whatever developmental stage it is in, including the embryonic stage, is also meaningful in that the healing of all humanity can only take place through him.[154] As Torrance writes:

> [The virginal conception] ... acknowledges as one of the central truths of the Christian Faith that in his Incarnation in which the Lord Jesus assumed our human nature, gathering up all its stages and healing them in his own human life, including conception, ... [God] thereby gave the human embryo a sacred inviolable status from the very beginning of his or her creaturely existence. For Christians this excludes the drawing of an arbitrary line at some stage in the development and growth of human being before birth, marking off a period when tampering with the human embryo in any way is deemed permissible.[155]

This means that the whole of Christ's earthly existence is to be seen as 'a vicarious humanity' in which he puts on humanity on behalf of human beings.[156] As a result, because Christ shares in humanity's embryological beginnings he also confirms the special moral nature of all human embryos.

It is here that a real difference exists between Torrance's theological ethics and the modern philosophical ethics of many contemporary commentators. Real personhood and moral worth are not conferred on human beings by the value judgements of other human beings but by the creator God who is the only real source of value and worth. God's final confirmation of the worth and value of humankind is found in Jesus Christ and the cross: a worth that does not originate only through the life, death, resurrection and ascension of Jesus Christ but from his prenatal earthly beginnings. As Torrance explains:

> In becoming a human being for us, he also became an embryo for the sake of all embryos, and for our Christian understanding of the being, nature and status in God's eyes of the unborn child in his/her body and soul. To take no thought or proper thought for the unborn child

is to have no proper thought of Jesus himself as our Lord and Saviour or to appreciate his relation as the incarnate Creator to every human being.[157]

In a similar fashion, the Church of Scotland 1996 General Assembly report maintained that:

> Christ's conception affirms, confirms and sanctifies every other conception, in the same way that his Incarnation, his taking to himself human nature, affirms, confirms and sanctifies our humanity. As Christ from the moment of conception was divine, creating, redeeming, person, so every other human being from the moment of conception, is a person in Christ, called into personal relationship with Christ, and must be so regarded and treated with sanctity.[158]

In the same way as Jesus became a human being for us and confirmed the immeasurable worth of humanity, he also became a human embryo for us and confirmed the immeasurable worth of the embryo.

Incarnation and Paradigm Humanity

As previously indicated, one constructive and fruitful way forward in discussing the moral status of human embryos is to consider the very nature of the incarnation as it relates to an understanding of being a person and the meaning of the image of God. Because the Word of God related his very being in space and time to a human conceptus, this (1) strengthens the assertion that Jesus Christ took on human personhood from the moment of conception and (2) provides a possible model of the manner in which God relates his very being to humanity more generally. In this way God, the unique Personalizing Being, is the origin of all personhood in human beings from their earliest pre-natal days. In a similar fashion, by studying the meaning of the divine image in human beings, it is possible to consider this image in terms of humanity's creaturely relatedness with God, including in human beings' pre-natal as well as post-natal existence, instead of restricting these terms to particular 'godlike' capacities. The reality that Jesus Christ is the 'image of the Invisible God' (Col. 1.15) means that Jesus Christ was the perfect image of God from conception onwards and implies that all human beings are created in the image of God from this moment onwards. It demonstrates a correspondence between God's own being in Christ at every stage of his human development and every human being at every stage of his or her human development.

In his short (1984) publication entitled *Test-tube Babies*, T. F. Torrance presents his personal response to the publication of the UK 1984

Warnock Report on embryological research, which he confessed 'out-raged my conscience at a deeper level than almost anything else I had read in recent years'. In this document he identified the nature of the human embryo as the central issue, stating that, as a matter of scientific fact, the human embryo from conception is biologically complete and must therefore be treated as a distinctive human being and not simply as a potential human being.[159]

Torrance's ethical position is that the human embryo, at whatever stage of development, has a distinctively moral claim to be considered as a human being. It must never, therefore, be used for destructive experi-mentation or discarded as a means to an end.

> It must be said quite unequivocally that all experimentation on human embryos, however early in their existence, is experimentation on human beings, and all the more reprehensible since it is manipulation and exploitation of human beings at their weakest, when their claim on our protection is morally strongest.[160]

More recently, Cameron is probably one of the writers who has used the incarnation argument most frequently in his treatment of the moral status of the human embryo. He did this by independently coming to the same conclusions as T. F. Torrance, though he was influenced by his theology.[161] Accordingly, Cameron writes that:

> [T]he manner in which the incarnate Son experienced human existence not only may but must be seen as a paradigm of all human existence. And there can be no doubt that his human life, in the sense of his per-sonal and moral identity, began at the point of the virginal conception in the womb.[162]

This is one of the fundamental conclusions, arising from the incarnation, that is used in support of the full protection of embryos. For Cameron, 'It provides a theological argument of an altogether different kind to those which have traditionally been drawn from the Biblical text.'[163]

As already noted, however, great care is required in considering Christ as the paradigm, a typical example, of a normative human being. Indeed, such overarching terms may conceal a need for more theological preci-sion since they are not based on the theological theme that Christ is the representative of humanity. This is because Christ's representative nature refers both to the particular pilgrimage which Christ undertook to save humanity and to Christ's solidarity with humanity so that the benefits of his redemptive achievement could be shared by all.

Thus, when Christ is mentioned as the paradigm human being, this only focuses on the reality that Christ became fully human in all the defining dimensions of humanity, including its pre-natal aspects. As such, Torrance's key argument, that 'Christ relating himself to a human conceptus at a particular point in space and time bestows a sacred status on all embryonic life', is valid. It is this that is central and so important to a Christian understanding of the moral status of the human embryo.

At this stage another argument, coming from a different angle but using the same theme of the incarnation in the context of understanding the status of human embryos, may be presented. This examines the importance of being and becoming.

Incarnation, Being and Becoming and the Personhood of the Embryo

In the context of modern ethical perspectives on personhood and their relationship to the moral status of the embryo, a gradualist viewpoint is often presented in which the protection of early human life is graded according to the stages of its development.[164] This suggests a certain progression of something towards becoming a recognizable reality. Comment is made that individuation and indeed fertilization are not instantaneous biological events but processes.

But in what way does the fundamental theological emphasis on 'being' then relate to this theme of becoming? How is it possible to interpret the developmental nature of pre-natal life from a moral and philosophical perspective?

The English mathematician and philosopher Alfred Whitehead (1861–1947), in his (1929) *Process and Reality: An Essay in Cosmology*,[165] asserts that time, change and process must be taken with utmost seriousness for an appropriate perception of reality. This means that human experience must not be considered as an addition to human nature but seen, instead, as an essential part of it.

The metaphysics commentator Jean Mill emphasizes this approach in responding to a focus on the priority of 'being'. She highlights the distinction between considering God as the 'efficient cause' of a person's being ('that which makes a thing what it is') and as the 'teleological cause' (that for which the thing was made). Mill suggests that God's creative and sustaining role is to be considered from a more teleological rather than an efficient perspective. This means that the creature works towards his or her true being, or essential God-given nature.[166] She argues that, if this is not so, 'God is "done with" the creation of an individual in the first instance of his or her existence. What happens thereafter is irrevocably given' (John 1.14). Merely considering the very existence of a being from an efficient perspective cannot, she suggests, do justice to the developmental nature of human embryos. In other words, 'becoming' must precede 'being'.

Mill's argument may seem convincing. Because of the complexities of embryonic development, including the possibilities of embryonic foetal death in spontaneous abortion as well as twinning or recombination, it is possible to hesitate as to the need for full protection of the early embryo before it has reached a certain development. This means that a concept of 'becoming' which has priority over 'being' is attractive from an ethical perspective. But it entails a number of significant problems and difficulties.

'Being' and 'Becoming'

One of the most important features of all living beings is their ability to grow and develop. This is especially relevant for human beings who have a latent capacity for moral, social, spiritual and biological development. In this context, a careful study of embryonic human life may be considered to emphasize, once again, the changes and developments that occur in every living thing.

But one of the continuing themes of this study is the reality that any understanding of the concepts of being a person and divine image, though based on God's relationship with humanity, cannot be dissociated from human beings' bodily existence. Accordingly, the incarnation is of crucial importance since it repudiates all notions of dualism. The Son of God took on human flesh, and in his life, death, resurrection and ascension declared an eternal unity between his soul and body. This also means that both the creator's continuing relationship with humanity and human beings' relationships with each other are the building blocks of human personal identity.

An appropriate understanding, therefore, of the theology of incarnation cannot be limited to notions of models and theories. Instead, the incarnation asserts that the very real empirical world must be taken seriously. It is into this factual world that God entered, confirming its reality by his very coming. This also means that the real physical character of the developing human embryo must be considered in a serious manner.

From this perspective, it is recognized that (1) the human constitution of a new embryonic being marks the beginning of a new individual being and (2) the continuing human identity of this developing individual being is a sign of continuing personal identity. But does this then mean that the human biological basis for 'being' has priority over 'becoming'?[167]

To begin with, it is true that 'becoming' is important from a social perspective through relationships, including not just the vertical divine

I–Thou dimension but also the horizontal human-to-human dimension. As a result, the manner in which human beings are treated, respected and loved from their earliest days affects the positive development of their full personhood.

An interesting comment on this comes from MacQuarrie who notes that, in the writings of Augustine on the creation of man, Adam is considered as being created as a mature adult. In contrast, Irenaeus considered Adam to have been created as a child who then developed into an adult. MacQuarrie comments that Irenaeus' understanding of Adam reflects the reality that 'there could be no personhood without experience, without history'.[168]

In addition, it is important to note the role in creation of the Spirit, the one who enables renewal and communion thereby stressing the purpose and the intended aim for humanity. Human persons have a spiritual destiny. The clear message of the Bible is that redemption in Christ, through the sanctifying Spirit, has as its objective a full communion in Christ (Col. 1.28) and a complete reflection of the divine image.

But while acknowledging all the previous reasoning, the prevailing affirmation of the incarnation and Christian anthropology is that the very being of persons is far more important and fundamental than developmental perspectives or aims. Moreover, the conception of Jesus Christ, though unique, does provide a model or an illustration of the priority of 'being' over 'becoming'. As Rollinson notes: 'If it is true that at no point from conception onwards, personhood does not apply for Jesus Christ, then for him, and by inference, for us, "being" is to have precedence over "becoming".'[169]

But what does the doctrine of the incarnation then mean for the view presented by Mill (that becoming has priority over being) and the moral status of the embryo?

In reply, it is important to re-emphasize the phrase 'the Word became flesh' (John 1.14) where, in the eternal Being of God, the Son takes all precedence over his becoming human. In other words, the hypostasis (the essential being) of Jesus Christ, the Son of God, takes priority over his human constitution. This also means that if the incarnation affirms anything, it is that 'being' must precede 'becoming' though 'becoming' remains important. As Hebrews 5.8–9 says, 'Son though he was, he learned obedience from what he suffered and, once made perfect, he became the source of eternal salvation.'

Here, in a very real and behavioural manner, is the unfolding of what Christ was in his very being. For the Anglican theologian Alistair McFadyen, it is uniquely in Christ who is, in his very being, 'the exact representation of [God's] being' that the image in all its fullness is expressed and manifested.[170]

Thus, from a Christological perspective, the union of both the divine and the human in the one person of Christ affirms that personhood must be more than mere 'nature'. In other words, personhood must be seen in more than just qualitative terms. If it is true that the eternal, pre-existing person of the Word of God became human, the Word relating himself to the very nature of foetal humanity, then foetal life (for Christ) cannot be dissociated from his being a person. Moreover, what is true for Christ is, in a paradigmatic or exemplary way, also true for God's children. Their very 'being', as persons, is far more than what they can become. This also means that any human being, whether a pre-natal or post-natal being, cannot be defined as a person by simply going through a check-list of characteristics.

Nigel Cameron and the British Christian physician David Short (1918–2005) explain:

> [The image of God's] root lies in man's *being* – human *being* itself in its modelling in creation of the very 'likeness' of the being of God. This point is of great importance over against shopping-list 'definitions' of the image of God, since they are inevitably arbitrary and fit in easily with modern notions of 'personhood' which take their point of departure not in any notion of man's 'being' but rather in modern concepts of 'personality'. They tend inevitably to reduce human nature to what men and women have the capacity to *do*, rather than recognising that its essence and the ground of its dignity lie in what they have been made to *be*.[171]

As God's creatures and made in his indefinable image, human beings are loved, known and sustained by him from their earliest beginnings and throughout their existences. Pre-natal children are 'persons-on-the-way' rather than 'on-the-way-to-being-a-person'. Thus, in a similar way to Christ, 'being' must precede 'becoming' for all human beings; though it is not an issue of 'being' versus 'becoming' but of 'being' and 'becoming'. The moral status of a human embryonic 'being', therefore, must be similar to that of a 'being' who has been born.

The Incarnation Remains Relevant to the Moral Status of the Embryo

Even though early Christian writers were very concerned about human abortion it may be noted that they did not generally use the doctrine of the virginal conception of Christ in their arguments against the practice. As a result, the arguments for the moral status of the human embryo based on the incarnation do not have significant historical precedent.

But this does not mean that this line of reasoning is not relevant or important. The way in which the early Christian Church sought to understand and articulate the central doctrine of the incarnation enabled the subsequent Christian community to work from a wonderfully rich legacy of themes, concepts and perspectives. As T. F. Torrance writes:

> It was because in Jesus the Creator Word of God was conceived by the Holy Spirit in the womb of the Virgin Mary, that Christians came to regard the unborn fetus in a new light, sanctified by the Lord Jesus as an embryonic person.[172]

The very fact that the incarnation enables a parallelism or correlation to be presented between the embryonic personhood of Christ and the embryonic personhood of all human beings, while emphasizing that 'being' must precede 'becoming', is of fundamental importance. These great and wonderful themes are essential in the development of an appropriate theological understanding of the personhood of early embryonic human life.

A final, but very important, Christian idea arising from the incarnation relates to Jesus Christ being Love Incarnate. It is Jesus who presents himself as the one who taught his fellow human beings to love their neighbours as themselves. He did this through being a perfect example of love. As the Parable of the Good Samaritan (Luke 10.30–37) indicates, a neighbour is anyone in need of help, including the weak and defenceless. Clearly this also means that the pre-natal child should be considered as a neighbour. Some ethicists, such as the American theologian and ethicist Stanley Hauerwas, have emphasized this fundamental point by stressing that the unborn being has often become an important example of the 'outcast' who is unfortunately rejected and abandoned by modern society.[173]

Since the very beginning of life represents a life at its most vulnerable, the incarnation of Jesus Christ emphasizes God's exceptional valuing of the weak and defenceless who have no one else to speak for them – a theme which resonates throughout the Bible.

Notes

1 Thomas F. Torrance writes: 'The incarnation made it clear that the physical world, far from being alien or foreign to God was affirmed by God as real even for himself.' T. F. Torrance, 1981, *Divine and Contingent Order*, Oxford: Oxford University Press, p. 33.

2 Thomas F. Torrance, 1969, *Space, Time and Incarnation*, Oxford: Oxford University Press, p. 68.

3 John MacQuarrie, 'The Humility of God', in D. R. McDonald (ed.), *The Myth/ Truth of God Incarnate*, quoted in Thomas Morris, 'Incarnational Anthropology', *Theology* 87 (1984), pp. 344–50 (p. 344).

4 Official Report of the 2007 General Assembly of the Free Church of Scotland.

5 Andrew R. Rollinson, 'The Incarnation and the Status of the Human Embryo', a thesis submitted for the degree of the M.Litt. with the Religious Studies Department of Newcastle University, November 1994, pp. 216–17.

6 Report to the General Assembly of the Church of Scotland, 1987, p. 309.

7 Torrance, *Divine and Contingent*, p. 24.

8 This is the thesis of Oliver O'Donovan, 1986, *Resurrection and the Moral Order*, Leicester: InterVarsity Press, p. 31.

9 William Storrar and Iain Torrance (eds), 1995, *Human Genetics: A Christian Perspective*, Edinburgh: Church of Scotland Board of Social Responsibility/Saint Andrew Press, pp. 40–1.

10 Torrance, *Space, Time and Incarnation*, p. 75.

11 Eric L. Mascall, 1956, *Christian Theology and Natural Science*, 1956 Bampton Lectures, London: Longmans, p. 306.

12 Colin Gunton, 1998, *The Triune Creator: A Historical and Systematic Study*, Grand Rapids: Eerdmans, p. 207.

13 O'Donovan, *Resurrection and Moral Order*, p. 150.

14 O'Donovan, *Resurrection and Moral Order*, p. 142.

15 Colin Gunton, 1992, *Christ and Creation*, 1990 Didsbury Lectures, Carlisle: Paternoster Press, p. 19.

16 Brent Waters, 2009, *This Mortal Flesh: Incarnation and Bioethics*, Grand Rapids: Brazos Press, p. 125.

17 Mascall, *Christian Theology*, p. 314.

18 Augustine, *City of God* 16.8.

19 International Theological Commission, Communion and Stewardship: *Human Persons Created in the Image of God*, The Vatican, 2002, paragraph 11.

20 Storrar and Torrance, *Human Genetics*, pp. 40–1.

21 Gregory of Nyssa, *On the Making of Man*, 16.16–17.

22 Irenaeus, *Demonstration of the Apostolic Preaching* 32.

23 International Theological Commission, *Communion and Stewardship*, paragraph 52.

24 Thomas F. Torrance, 1984, *The Christian Doctrine of Marriage*, Edinburgh: Handsel Press, p. 6.

25 Wisdom 7.25, quoted in Peter T. O'Brien, 1982, *Colossians, Philemon*, Vol. 44, Word Biblical Commentary, Waco: Thomas Nelson.

26 Ralph Martin, 1974, *Colossians and Philemon*, London: New Century Bible, p. 57.

27 Frederick F. Bruce, 1964, *The Epistle to the Hebrews*, New London Commentary on the New Testament, London: Marshall, Morgan & Scott, p. 6.

28 John F. Kilner, 2015, *Dignity and Destiny: Humanity in the Image of God*, Grand Rapids: Eerdmans, p. 67.

29 Frederick F. Bruce and G. K. Simpson refer to Christ as the 'archetypal image' in F. F. Bruce, 1957, *Commentary on Ephesians and Colossians*, New London Commentary on the New Testament, London: Marshall, Morgan & Scott, p. 194.

30 David Cairns, 1953, *The Image of God in Man*, first edition, London: SCM Press, p. 26.

31 Cairns, 1953, *Image of God*, first edition, p. 37.

32 Anthony A. Hoekema comments: 'Presumably, it was only because man had been created in the image of God that the Second Person of the Trinity could assume human nature.' Anthony A. Hoekema, 1986, *Created in God's Image*, Grand Rapids: Eerdmans, p. 22.

33 Quoted in Brian Hebblethwaite, 1988, *The Incarnation*, Cambridge: Cambridge University Press, p. 3.

34 Hebblethwaite, *The Incarnation*, pp. 3–4.

35 Brian Hebblethwaite, 'The propriety of the doctrine of the Incarnation as a way of interpreting Christ', *Scottish Journal of Theology* 33:3 (1980), pp. 201–22.

36 Gunton, *Triune Creator*, p. 196.

37 Charles D. F. Moule, 1958, *Cambridge Greek Testament Commentary, Colossians and Philemon*, Cambridge: Cambridge University Press, p. 120.

38 Martin, *Colossians and Philemon*, p. 108.

39 It is very important not to lose sight of the role of the Spirit in this renewal. This is a distinctive emphasis of Colin E. Gunton; cf. 'In the Image and Likeness of God', in *Christ and Creation*: 'Imaging is therefore a triune act: the Son images the Father as through the Spirit he realises a particular pattern of life on earth', p. 101.

40 Irenaeus, *Adv. Haer.* (Against Heresy) V.16.2. Quoted in Cairns, 1953, *Image of God*, first edition, p. 77.

41 Athanasius, *De Incarnatione*, ch. 14. Quoted in Cairns, 1953, *Image of God*, first edition, p. 92.

42 Gunton, *Christ and Creation*, p. 112.

43 Rollinson, 'Incarnation and Status', p. 207.

44 Rollinson, 'Incarnation and Status', p. 209.

45 This prior 'onto-relation' must be distinguished from our human-to-human relationships. Otherwise we would have to agree with E. Templeton who comments: 'Once you insist that personhood is relational, the foetus, the mother, the family, the community, all become open and fluid identities, not unreal, but mutually interdependent, and defined not by biology or sociology, but by love, by uncoerced relationship.' Elizabeth Templeton, 1987, 'Abortion: Our Painful Freedom', in Church of Scotland Board of Social Responsibility, *Abortion in Debate*, Edinburgh: Quorum Press, p. 22.

46 Rollinson, 'Incarnation and Status', p. 210.

47 James M. Gustafson, 1974, *Theology and Christian Ethics*, Cleveland: Pilgrim Press, p. 232. Gustafson is known for his *theological* ethics, but his theocentrism has been seriously questioned. His conception of God is drawn more from science and human experience than from Scripture and tradition. His main concern is to place human life and ethics in a larger whole, but, because of his weak concept of God, his ethics 'can more appropriately be described as cosmocentric rather than theocentric': Martin Reilly, 'James M. Gustafson's, Ethics and Theocentrism – Has He Made It?', *Irish Theological Quarterly* 57 (1991), pp. 298–309.

48 Gustafson, *Theology and Christian Ethics*, p. 241.

49 Philip Hefner, quoted in A. R. Peacocke, 1979, *Creation and the World of Science*, 1978 Bampton Lectures, Oxford: Oxford University Press, p. 250.

50 Herbert Hartwell, 1964, *The Theology of Karl Barth: An Introduction*, London: Gerald Duckworth & Co., p. 123.

51 St Basil of Caesarea, 'On the Holy Nativity of Christ', Patrologia, Series Graeca, J. P. Migne 31, 1473A. Quoted in Kallistos Ware, 'The Unity of the Human Person according to the Greek Fathers', in A. R. Peacocke and G. Gillett (eds), 1987, *Persons and Personalities: A Contemporary Enquiry*, Oxford: Blackwell.

52 'No definition of human nature can meet our present need if it is merely an asser-

tion and description of immediately accessible and knowable characteristics of the nature which man thinks he can regard as that of his fellows and therefore of man in general ... How does man reach the platform from which he can see himself? ... Who is the man who to know himself first wishes to disregard the fact that he belongs to God?' Karl Barth, 1957–75, *Church Dogmatics*, Edinburgh: T&T Clark, Vol. III.2, p. 75.

53 Karl Barth, 1956, *Christ and Adam: Man and Humanity in Romans 5*, Edinburgh: Oliver and Boyd, pp. 29, 30.

54 Cf. Stuart D. McLean, 1981, *Humanity in the Thought of Karl Barth*, Edinburgh: T&T Clark.

55 Stuart D. McLean explains: 'Man is structurally and essentially, not secondarily or accidentally, related to others.' McLean, *Humanity*, p. 23.

56 Barth, *Church Dogmatics*, Vol. III.2, p. 243.

57 Barth, *Church Dogmatics*, Vol. III.2, p. 364.

58 Barth, *Church Dogmatics*, Vol. III.2, p. 43.

59 Eric L. Mascall, 1959, *The Importance of Being Human*, London: Oxford University Press, p. 22.

60 Kilner, *Dignity and Destiny*, p. 73.

61 Stephen W. Sykes, 1972, 'The Theology of the Humanity of Christ', in Stephen W. Sykes and J. P. Clayton (eds), *Christ, Faith and History*, Cambridge Studies in Christology, Cambridge: Cambridge University Press, p. 55.

62 Robin Scroggs, 1966, *The Last Adam: A Study in Pauline Anthropology*, Oxford: Blackwell, p. 99.

63 'Jesus Christ is not only the demonstration of the ultimate possibility of the emergence and fulfilment of personalness, he is also the definition of the nature of personalness.' David E. Jenkins, 1969, *The Glory of Man*, 1966 Bampton Lectures, London: SCM Press, p. 91.

64 John Knox, 1967, *The Humanity and Divinity of Christ*, Cambridge: Cambridge University Press.

65 Knox, *Humanity and Divinity*, p. 67.

66 Charles F. D. Moule, 1972, 'The Manhood of Jesus in the New Testament', in Sykes and Clayton, *Christ, Faith and History*, p. 102.

67 Donald M. Baillie writes: 'While to speak of Jesus as "a God" is a nonsense from a Christian point of view, it is equally nonsense to say that he is "Man" unless we mean that He is a man.' D. M. Baillie, 1948, *God Was in Christ*, London: Faber & Faber, p. 87.

68 Rosemary Ruether, 1981, *To Change the World: Christology and Cultural Criticism*, London: SCM Press.

69 Sykes, 'Theology of Humanity', p. 68; Eric L. Mascall explains: 'The assertion which one sometimes hears, that if the Incarnation means anything it must mean that there is literally nothing that distinguishes Jesus from any other male human being, would make his uniqueness unrecognisable, if not indeed non-existent.' Eric L. Mascall, 1977, *Theology and the Gospel of Christ*, London: SPCK, pp. 133–134.

70 Moule, 'Manhood of Jesus', p. 109.

71 Alan J. Torrance, 'Is there a distinctive human nature? Approaching the question from a Christian epistemic base', *Zygon* 47:4 (2012), pp. 907, 912, 913.

72 Cairns, 1973, *The Image of God in Man*, second edition, London: Fontana Library of Theology and Philosophy, p. 47.

73 Nigel M. de S. Cameron, 1987, 'Kindness that Kills', in Church of Scotland Board of Social Responsibility, *Abortion in Debate*, p. 13.

74 John Macquarrie states: '[Christ] has attained this representative status not in any magical or instantaneous way, but through striving and the overcoming of temptation.' John Macquarrie, 1990, *Jesus Christ in Modern Thought*, London: SCM Press, p. 374.

75 John McIntyre, 1966, *The Shape of Christology*, London: SCM Press, p. 106.

76 Gregory of Nazianzus, Epistola 101.7, Patrologia, Series Graeca, J. P. Migne, 37, 181.

77 James D. G. Dunn explains: 'The key idea which runs through [Paul's] Christology and binds it to his soteriology is that of solidarity or representation.' J. D. G. Dunn, 1974, 'Paul's Understanding of the Death of Jesus', in R. T. Banks (ed.), *Reconciliation and Hope: New Testament Essays on Atonement and Eschatology, presented to L. L. Morris*, Exeter: Paternoster Press, p. 128.

78 Thomas. F. Torrance, 1984, *Test-tube Babies: Morals – Science – and the Law*, Edinburgh: Scottish Academic Press, p. 10.

79 Barth, *Church Dogmatics*, Vol. I.2, p. 122.

80 Herman Bavinck, 'Geref. Dogmatiek' III, 291, quoted in G. C. Berkouwer, 1973, *The Person of Christ*, Grand Rapids: Eerdmans, ch. 12.

81 Mascall, *Theology and the Gospel*, Appendix I, p. 195.

82 I.e. the Preformationist view that the fully developed physical organism was contained in a microscopic state inside the embryo.

83 Thomas Aquinas, *Summa Theologica* III a, qu. 33, par. 2.

84 David Jenkins, 1967, *The Glory of Man*, London: SCM Press, p. 50.

85 Jenkins, *The Glory of Man*, p. 75.

86 Jenkins, *The Glory of Man*, p. 79.

87 Colin E. Gunton, 1993, *The One, the Three and the Many*, 1992 Bampton Lectures, Cambridge: Cambridge University Press, p. 29.

88 'Personal God' is by no means an uncontested description. As C. C. J. Webb makes clear in his *God and Personality*, it was only in the eighteenth century that God in his unitary nature became described as a person. Webb knows of no instance prior to Schleiermacher. The emphasis in the early Church was on personhood *in* God, rather than the personhood *of* God. Clearly, given God's incorporeality, and the inability of an application of many assumptions about personhood to God, the issue as a theoretical one remains open for debate. Webb writes: 'Whilst the affirmation of Personality in God has been a characteristic of Christian theological terminology since the third century of our era, the great majority of Christian theologians down to quite modern times have not in so many words affirmed the Personality of God.' C. C. J. Webb, 1919, *God and Personality*, 1918 & 1919 Gifford Lectures, London: George Allen & Unwin, p. 65; R. Swinburne can hold that 'God is a person, yet one without a body, seems the most elementary claim of theism'. Richard Swinburne, 1984, *The Coherence of Theism*, Oxford: Clarendon Press, p. 31. Others consider it far from elementary: Keith Ward, 1974, *The Concept of God*, Oxford: Blackwell.

89 Rollinson, 'Incarnation and Status', p. 170.

90 Adrian Thatcher writes, 'Christian theism is the only kind of theism which can substantiate belief in a personal God.' Adrian Thatcher, 1987, 'Christian Theism and the Concept of a Person', in A. R. Peacocke and G. Gillett, *Persons and Personality: A Contemporary Inquiry*, Oxford: Blackwell, p. 188.

91 Jenkins, 1967, *The Glory of Man*, pp. 38, 21.

92 Jenkins, 1967, *The Glory of Man*, pp. 55, 59, 84.

93 Rollinson, 'Incarnation and Status', p. 171.

94 Jenkins, *The Glory of Man*, p. 105.

95 Moule, 'Manhood of Jesus', p. 102.

96 Certainly, David Jenkins would not wish to apply his arguments to a human being's earliest moments, expressing as he does scepticism about a historical virginal conception.

97 The term 'virginal conception' is to be used in preference to the common term 'virgin birth'. This is to avoid any confusion with the distinctively Catholic belief in *virginitas in partu* (i.e. that at birth the hymen was not ruptured).

98 See, for example, Michael F. Goodman (ed.), 1988, *What Is a Person?*, Clifton, NJ and London: Humana Press; James W. Walters, 'Proximate Personhood as a standard for making difficult treatment decisions: Imperilled newborns as a case study', *Bioethics* 6:1 (1992), p. 12.

99 Thomas F. Torrance explains: 'It was only with the formulation of the doctrines of Christ and the Holy Trinity, in which the Church sought to give adequate expression to God's self-revelation to mankind in the Incarnation, that the technical theological concept of person was formed.' Thomas F. Torrance, 1989, 'The Soul and Person in Theological Perspective in Religion, Reason and Self', in S. R. Sutherland and T. A. Roberts (eds), *Essays in Honour of Hywel D. Lewis*, Cardiff: University of Wales Press. As already mentioned, Oliver O'Donovan argues that Boethius' famous definition of a person, 'the individual substance of rational nature', was forged in the historical context of the Chalcedonian definition of Christ, where 'substance' had the particular connotation of 'hypostasis', an individual existence with continuity in history. When this Christological basis was eroded and forgotten the Boethian definition took on a new slant, with a person being merely a particular instance of a rational nature. He concludes: 'The history of the concept "person" is the history of how "nature" takes over from "substance", the secondary feature of the definition displacing the primary one.' O. O'Donovan, 1984, *Begotten or Made?*, Oxford: Oxford University Press, p. 54.

100 Torrance, 'Soul and Person'.

101 This view is classically stated in Hans von Campenhausen, 1964, *The Virgin Birth in the Theology of the Ancient Church*, London: SCM Press.

102 D. Gareth Jones, 1987, *Manufacturing Humans: The Challenge of the New Reproductive Technologies*, Leicester: InterVarsity Press, pp. 131–3, note 38, p. 291.

103 Elizabeth Templeton, 1987, 'Response to Nigel M. de S. Cameron', in Church of Scotland Board of Social Responsibility, *Abortion in Debate*, Edinburgh: Quorum Press, p. 31.

104 This was confirmed in a number of important councils such as the Fourth Ecumenical Council of Chalcedon in 451. It also reflects Mary's own surprise in Luke 1.34 that she was to bear a child: 'How will this be, ... since I am a virgin?'

105 Karl Barth, 1947, *Dogmatics in Outline*, trans. G. T. Thompson, London: SCM. Press, p. 97.

106 Cf. Anthony N. S. Lane, 'The rationale and significance of the virgin birth', *Vox Evangelica* 10 (1977), pp. 48ff.

107 Sykes, 'Theology of Humanity', ch. 4.

108 Sykes, 'Theology of Humanity', p. 55.

109 E.g., Clement of Alexandria denied that Christ had any real physical needs of hunger. Quoted in Sykes, 'Theology of Humanity', p. 56.

110 Sykes, 'Theology of Humanity', p. 66.

111 Barth, *Church Dogmatics*, Vol. I.3:2, pp. 173–202.

112 Mark 2.10: 'that you may know that the Son of Man has authority on earth to forgive sins'.

113 Klaas Runia, 1982, 'Karl Barth's Christology', in H. H. Rowden (ed.), *Christ the Lord*, Leicester: InterVarsity Press, p. 302; Gerrit C. Berkouwer, 1965, The Work of Christ, Grand Rapids: Eerdmans, p. 106.

114 Barth, *Dogmatics in Outline*, p. 97.

115 Barth, *Church Dogmatics*, Vol. I.2, p. 206.

116 Rollinson, 'Incarnation and Status', p. 107.

117 Karl Barth, 1962, *Credo*, 2005 edition, Eugene, OR: Wipf and Stock, p. 69.

118 Alan Richardson comments: 'The doctrine of the virgin birth of Christ is an integral part of the theology of the New Testament ... It is a unique event because Christ is unique.' Alan Richardson, 1958, *An Introduction to the Theology of the New Testament*, London: SCM Press, p. 175.

119 J. Gresham Machen writes: 'Deny or give up the story of the virgin birth, and inevitably you are led to evade either the high biblical doctrine of sin, or else the full biblical presentation of the supernatural person of our Lord.' J. Gresham Machen, 1930, *The Virgin Birth of Christ*, London: James Clarke & Co., p. 395.

120 Luke 3. 22–38. The congruity of the virginal conception with the sinlessness of Jesus has been pointed out in the Church of England bishops' report, 1986, *The Nature of Christian Belief*, Church House Publishing, p. 32: 'Without endorsing any of the older theories which linked human sinfulness with sexual generation, would not the child of human parents inevitably share our imperfect human nature? And are there not difficulties in the belief that God was able to live out his essential character in such a nature? It can fairly be agreed that this view of Jesus' human origins calls for special divine intervention quite as radical as in the traditional account of the virginal conception.'

121 Sykes, 'Theology of Humanity', p. 59.

122 John Wilkinson, 'Apologetic aspects of the virgin birth of Jesus Christ', *Scottish Journal of Theology* 17 (1964), p. 159.

123 Gresham Machen, *Virgin Birth*, p. 394.

124 Hugh Montefiore, 1992, *The Womb and the Tomb*, London: Font, p. 92.

125 Jean Boboc, 2014, *La grande métamorphose: Éléments pour une théo-anthropologie orthodoxe*, Paris: Les Éditions du Cerf, p. 268.

126 Some authors who employ the argument are: David Atkinson, 1987, 'Some Theological Perspectives on the Human Embryo', in Nigel M. de S. Cameron (ed.), *Embryos and Ethics*, Edinburgh: Rutherford House Books, p. 54; John W. Montgomery, 1964, 'The Christian View of the Foetus', in W. O. Spitzer and C. L. Saylor (eds), *Birth Control and the Christian*, Wheaton: Tynedale, p. 87; Teresa Iglesias, 1990, *IVF and Justice*, London: Linacre Centre for Health Care Ethics, p. 104.

127 Thomas F. Torrance, 1988, *The Trinitarian Faith: The Evangelical Theology of the Ancient Catholic Church*, Edinburgh: T&T Clark.

128 Daniel W. Hardy, 1989, 'Thomas F. Torrance', in David F. Ford (ed.), *The Modern Theologians*, Vol. 1, Oxford: Blackwell, p. 75.

129 Thomas F. Torrance, 1969, *Theological Science*, Oxford: Oxford University Press, p. 29.

130 'There is no factual knowledge of God except where He has condescended to reveal Himself in his objectivity.' Torrance, *Theological Science*, p. 55.

131 Torrance, *Theological Science*, p. 9.

132 Thomas F. Torrance, 1965, *Theology in Re-construction: Essays towards Evangelical and Catholic Unity in East and West*, London: Geoffrey Chapman, pp. 90–4.

133 Torrance, *Theological Science*, p. 33.

134 Torrance sees great significance in the historical fact that the flowering of mod-

ern empirical science followed on directly from the rise of modern theology at the Reformation. At the Reformation, theology was set free from the medieval notion of the impassibility of God and an implied eternal coexistence of creator and creation, leading to a blurred distinction between the two. Second, the Reformation clarified the distinction between Grace and Nature. The creator–creature relationship has been established out of pure Grace. God created a world utterly distinct from him; and though entirely dependent on God it has to be interpreted in its distinctness. This freed up natural science to examine the natural world in and of itself, and yet to view it in its relationship to God.

He also comments: 'This distinction between the realm of Grace as the ways of God and the realm of nature as the course of creation in its creaturely distinctness from God bore immense fruit, for it at once disenchanted the world of its alleged divinity, and yet claimed the world of God as His creation, thus denying that it was the product of capricious forces.' Torrance, *Theological Science*, pp. 59, 68.

135 Torrance, *Test-tube Babies*; Thomas F. Torrance, 1999, *The Soul and Person of the Unborn Child*, Edinburgh: Scottish Order of Christian Unity/Handsel Press; Thomas F. Torrance, 2000, *The Being and Nature of the Unborn Child*, Edinburgh: Handsel Press.

136 Rollinson, 'Incarnation and Status'.

137 Hardy, 'Thomas F. Torrance', p. 73.

138 Torrance writes: 'It is the whole life of the incarnate Son, the historical, crucified and risen Jesus Christ that forms the core and axis of the body of Christian theology. It is from that centre that we take our bearings ...' Torrance, *Theological Science*, p. 216.

Baxter Kruger explains: 'This question of the significance of Jesus Christ as God incarnate is the central question of Torrance's theology. The Incarnation of the eternal Son of God is not merely one orthodox doctrine among many for Torrance. It is the heart and logic of his theology.' Baxter Kruger, 'The Doctrine of the Knowledge of God in the Theology of T. F. Torrance', *Scottish Journal of Theology* 43:3 (1990), p. 370.

139 Kruger, 'Knowledge of God', p. 367.

140 Torrance, *Test-tube Babies*, p. 10.

141 J. Foster explains that conception is marked out as the moment of Incarnation. In other words, it is the moment when God took human nature and when Christ began his human life. J. Foster, 1985, 'Personhood and the Ethics of Abortion', in C. H. Channer (ed.), *Abortion and the Sanctity of Human Life*, Exeter: Paternoster Press.

142 Atkinson, 'Some Theological Perspectives', p. 54.

143 Cameron writes of Christ's identification: 'the perilous human existence of the incarnate Son began not in his birth under threat from Herod, but in the hazardous journey of a day-old embryo from out of his mother's fallopian tubes'. Cameron, 'Kindness that Kills', p. 14.

144 Nigel M. de S. Cameron, 1985, 'Image in Embryo', in David C. Watts (ed.), *Creation and the Christian Response to Warnock*, Rugby: The Biblical Creation Society, p. 12.

145 See, for example Thomas F. Torrance, 1998, *Space, Time and Resurrection*, Edinburgh: T&T Clark, p. 53.

146 Thomas F. Torrance, 1959, *Conflict and Agreement in the Church*, Vol. 1, London: Lutterworth, p. 245.

147 Nigel M. de S. Cameron, 'Kindness that Kills', p. 16. As Foster points out: 'For the Son of God could hardly have taken human nature at a point when, in the ordinary case, the human organism would not yet qualify as, or embody, a person.' Foster, 'Personhood', pp. 41–2.

148 Nigel M. de S. Cameron and Pamela F. Sims, 1986, *Abortion: The Crisis in Morals and Medicine*, Leicester: InterVarsity Press, p. 18.

149 O'Donovan, *Begotten or Made?*

150 Oliver O'Donovan, 1973, *The Christian and the Unborn Child*, Bramcote, Nottinghamshire: Grove Booklets on Ethics, p. 15.

151 Maximus the Confessor, *Ambigua* 2.42.

152 David A. Jones, 2004, *The Soul of the Embryo*, London: Continuum, p. 132.

153 Torrance, *Being and Nature*, p. 4.

154 This means that Jesus Christ is to be considered not only as the Head of the Christian Church (which, according to T. F. Torrance, is 'an aberration of classical and biblical theology'), but as the Head of all humanity at whatever stage of development.
   Taped lecture given by T. F. Torrance, 'Ethics and Embryos', at Rutherford House, Edinburgh. Cited by Rollinson, 'Incarnation and Status', p. 56.

155 Torrance, *Test-tube Babies*, p. 10.

156 Thomas F. Torrance, 1971, *God and Rationality*, Oxford: Oxford University Press, p. 158.

157 Torrance, *Being and Nature*, p. 6.

158 Church of Scotland Board of Social Responsibility, 1996, *Pre-Conceived Ideas: A Christian Perspective of IVF and Embryology*, Edinburgh: Saint Andrew Press, p. 62; reflecting the Report to the General Assembly of the Church of Scotland, 1996, paragraph 21/47.

159 'After all, if the human embryo were neither human nor alive it would have no place in research on human beings.' Torrance, *Test-tube Babies*, p. 2.

160 Torrance, *Test-tube Babies*, pp. 3, 5.

161 Nigel Cameron, in personal conversation with Andrew Rollinson. Cited by Rollinson, 'Incarnation and Status', p. 52.

162 Nigel M. de S. Cameron, 'Kindness that Kills', p. 14.

163 Nigel M. de S. Cameron, 1987, 'The Christian Stake in the Warnock Debate', in Cameron, *Embryos and Ethics*, p. 12.

164 Anglican submission to Warnock Committee. Board for Social Responsibility of the General Synod of the Church of England, 1984.

165 Alfred N. Whitehead, 1929, *Process and Reality: An Essay in Cosmology*, Cambridge: Cambridge University Press.

166 Jean M. Mill, 'Some comments on Dr. Iglesias's paper, "*In vitro* fertilisation: the major issues"', *Journal of Medical Ethics* 12 (1986), pp. 32–5.

167 It is also true that individuation is a process and can be complicated (twinning and recombination), and significant changes do occur. The recent, realizable possibility of genetic modification raises important questions. By changing the genetic structure of a conceptus, are the changes to the genetic make-up such that a particular personal identity ceases to exist?

168 John MacQuarrie, 1987, 'A Theology of Personal Being', in A. R. Peacocke and G. Gillett (eds), *Persons and Personality*, Oxford: Blackwell, p. 173.

169 Rollinson, 'Incarnation and Status', p. 223.

170 Alistair McFadyen, 1990, *The Call to Personhood*, Cambridge: Cambridge University Press, p. 46.

171 Nigel Cameron and David Short, 1991, *On Being Human: 'Speciesism' and the Image of God*, London: Christian Medical Fellowship, pp. 4–5.

172 Torrance, *Being and Nature*, p. 4.

173 Stanley Hauerwas, 1981, *A Community of Character*, Notre Dame: University of Notre Dame Press, p. 225.

6

Substantive Aspects and the Embryo

Substantive aspects of humanity in general, and the embryo in particular, are not easy to identify. The Oxford Dictionary definition of 'substantive' reflects the meaning of a 'separate and independent existence' which is also related to the definition of 'substance' as 'the essential material forming a thing'.[1]

From this perspective, and as already noted, the substance or essential material forming humanity is nothing else, in the end, than the dust of the earth. As D. A. Jones et al. comment:

> Often in the Scriptures the forming of the child in the womb is described in ways that echo the formation of Adam from the dust of the earth. This is why Psalm 139 describes the child in the womb as being formed 'in the depths of the earth' (Ps. 139.15).[2]

Substantive aspects of humanity may also reflect what is important in *Homo sapiens* from the perspective of physical human nature or substance, in whatever way this may be characterized. In some cases, it is suggested that this reflects the human body, as such, or the human genetic heritage, but would not usually relate to any human capacities. In other cases, it may reflect human nature in its very constitution, structure and form. For Aristotle, for example, a 'substance' (*ousia*) is an individual entity, such as an individual human being with the substantial form of this entity consisting in its essential properties.[3]

Thus, a clear characterization of these substantive aspects of what makes human nature so important is difficult to define.

Substantive Aspects and the Image of God

From a theological perspective the substantive aspects of the image of God are again not precisely defined. Generally, a substantive understanding of this image in a personal being supports the idea that there is some substantial characteristic in this being that expresses this image, with different interpretations of this substance being proposed throughout history. For instance, this could mean that a kind of 'mirror image' of God's essential nature may exist in human beings or that there may, in fact, be a spiritual commonality with God.

One significant characteristic, however, which has played a fundamental role in understanding the image of God in human beings is in their humanity as such. The American philosopher Robert Wennberg makes a distinction between what he defines, on the one hand, as 'the nature' and, on the other, as 'the status' of the divine image. By 'nature' he means the natural endowment of human capabilities, defining a strict sense of the image of God as 'engaging in acts of intellect, emotion or will', and 'a more elastic sense' as the ability to possess these features only latently.[4] By 'status' he means that the image of God has a unique status conferred by the creator God. However, Wennberg was dissatisfied with this second meaning of the divine image, stating that, by itself, and if unrelated to nature, God could just as equally confer such a status on other animals such as primates. Hence, although he continues to emphasize that the concepts of 'nature' and 'status' should be held together, he unfortunately ends up affirming the importance of nature to the detriment of status, concluding: 'It does not follow that God confers this status on those without the potential for personal life, who cannot ever participate in those purposes.' Wennberg then goes on to admit that the divine image is 'strictly speaking not actualised in infants, but awaits its realisation at a later time with growth and development'.[5] This quote is just an example of the manner in which a misunderstanding of the image of God can be applied to ethical considerations.

The substantive perspective of the image of God also maintains that some characteristic, quality or faculty is uniquely inherent in human beings. It is something in their nature and that they possess which reflects this image.

In the past, this substance was defined as well in a number of other ways, such as humanity's capacity to reason, have free will or have a relationship with God.[6] But this then impinges, somewhat, on the manner in which the image of God can be characterized from relational and functional aspects (especially if this also relates to a capacity for certain activities): this will be examined later.

In order to try to keep the different aspects of the image of God in some sort of category, therefore, the following section on the substantive aspects of this image will concentrate on examining the concept of substance as it relates to the essential nature of humanity. This does not mean, however, that concepts such as a capacity to have a relationship with God, free will and rationality cannot be considered under the substantive aspects. However, in this study, these will be considered under a broader understanding of relational and functional aspects while remembering that no distinct or fixed classification or boundaries exist between all these aspects of the image of God.

The Image of God and Humanity

A lot has already been written relating to the relationship between the image of God and humanity. In the context of the substantive aspects of humanity, Westermann suggests that Genesis does not mention individuals or persons as exemplars of all created personal beings but refers, instead, to human persons who are members of humanity. In other words, the very act of creation by God of human beings means that the image of God in them constitutes them as human.[7] In the words of Genesis 1.27: 'So God created mankind in his own image, in the image of God he created them.' This means that God did not create a being in any random or arbitrary manner but the being was specifically human to reflect his image. There is, therefore, a very deep relationship between the image of God and humanity, as such, which is emphasized in Genesis. As Cameron explains:

> However we construe the scope of its [Genesis 1] biological categories, it is evident that the category 'man' is co-terminous with what we mean by man. It refers to *Homo sapiens* as such, and is not concerned to distinguish between some members of the species and others, whether on the basis of the presence and absence of particular qualities (rationality, the ability to communicate ...) ... What is made in the image of God is man, nothing more, nothing less.

Moreover, when God decided to create in his image he created humankind and not some other animal kind. Cameron observes in this context that: 'The image, with all that it implies, must be species-specific; and any argument which seems to divide biological man from man the image-bearer is revealed as mere sophistry.'[8]

Similarly, Jesus Christ came as a human being and, again, this was not arbitrary. It asserts that it is specifically human beings who are fearfully and wonderfully made (Ps. 139.14) and who are unique among all created beings in God's eyes since they are made in his image.

Even the bread and the wine which Christians take at Communion represent the human body of Jesus. They eat the bread and drink the wine which is eventually incorporated into their human bodies.[9]

Christian anthropology understands human nature, in its very constitution, structure and form, as being defined by God and established by him in the creation of the image of God in humankind.[10] For St Maximus the Confessor, the essential definition of human nature, or its *logos* (which relates to its spiritual, mental and physical reality), was established from all eternity by the Verb in whom it exists as an idea or choice. Human nature as defined and elected by God saw its reality confirmed by the incarnation of the Verb who assumed it and made it completely his own. From a Christian perspective, this divine foundation of human nature, and the transcendent dimension which it receives, enables this definition to be essentially immutable, unalterable and intangible.[11]

There is something in humanity, therefore, which comes from God, which bears God's image and is the grounds for his special relationship with his human children. As Atkinson explains:

> We have been addressed by God, and as it were commanded forth from the whole range of creatures to be distinct in the sense that our whole identity, what it means to be human, is bound up with our calling before God, and with the joy and responsibility of reflecting his glory.[12]

This means that humanity is set apart from all other animals by being created in the image of God. As such, the charge of speciesism made by commentators such as Peter Singer[13] does have a ring of truth to it since it corresponds to the biblical claim. However, this does not mean that the image of God in humanity should be used to denigrate the animal world in what could be termed biological pride or as a mandate (through the directive to 'rule' and 'subdue' in Genesis 1.28) for inappropriate exploitation. Instead, humanity should remember, in a spirit of humility, that the image of God is freely bestowed by God and is a mark of his grace.[14]

Moreover, this image is not based on any individual specificity. It is not the reserve or privilege of only a subsection of humanity. Instead, most Christian commentators accept that the image of God is reflected in the whole of humanity which represents God on earth.[15] The German Lutheran theologian Gerhard von Rad (1901–71) suggests that: 'As earthly rulers ... erect images of themselves in the provinces as signs of their presence, so too has God put human beings on earth in his image and likeness as a sign of his majesty.'[16]

Interestingly, this understanding enables a correspondence to exist between the image of God being reflected by all human beings and the theme of humanity being invited to rule and subdue creation. It is very much in agreement with Psalm 8 and its twin royal themes of all of humankind being 'crowned with glory' and made to rule 'over the works of your hands'.

Such an understanding is important in that it was not the common perspective at the time. For example, ancient Egyptian manuscripts presented kings as being in God's image but never referred to the people, in general, in this way. The Old Testament has, in a way, democratized this idea.[17] Each human being is God's representative in the world, implying that all human life is special (Gen. 9.6) and that every human being, whoever they are and whatever their level of corruption, has an inherent dignity and worth. This is the biblical basis. It is far richer than the Enlightenment reasoning supporting the Kantian imperative which simply maintains that every human individual should be treated as an end and never solely as a means to an end.

The Image of God in Humanity: The Is and the Ought

The statement that humanity is created in the divine image operates both as an assertion of the way things are and as an ideal regulating personal and social conduct. It is both an 'is' and an 'ought'.[18] Cairns states that this image is, first, a quality of man's existence and, second, a purpose of God for man.[19]

Such a dual aspect of the divine image actually corresponds to the biblical perspective. Genesis 5.1 states 'This is the written account of Adam's family line. When God created mankind, he made them in the likeness of God'; and Genesis 9.6, 'Whoever sheds human blood, by humans shall their blood be shed; for in the image of God has God made mankind.'

Neither of these passages suggests that the divine image was lost as a result of the Fall. The ethical imperative of the second passage would be meaningless if the divine image had departed.[20] In the New Testament, the passage from James 3.9, 'With the tongue we praise our Lord and Father, and with it we curse human beings, who have been made in God's likeness', also implies the presence of human sin while acknowledging the continued existence of the image of God in humankind. Other New Testament passages, such as Romans 8.29 and 2 Corinthians 3.18, express an image which is to be revealed, meaning that humanity no longer properly and completely reflects the image of God (though it remains fully present). The biblical evidence thus seems to keep in tension the image as a permanent aspect of human beings[21] and something made unrecognizable through the Fall.

At this stage, two important comments need to be made about the divine image.

The first is that, throughout history, there has been a tendency to interpret the image of God in such a way as to underestimate its creaturely and universal aspects as well as its very existence.

For example, Luther seems to have understood the image in a manner that may have overemphasized the ethical aspects by emphasizing its original righteousness. He argued that humanity now bore only a 'relic' of the image because Adam surrendered humanity's original righteousness which can only be restored though Christ.[22] Such an interpretation, however, may have been motivated by Luther's strong concerns for justification by faith rather than by an objective analysis. In so doing he may have overlooked the reality that the divine image exists, as such, as well as an ethical dimension.

In a similar manner, Calvin sometimes seemed to lose sight of the clear existence of the image of God through his dynamic emphasis. For Calvin, the divine image in humankind is its unique stance in mirroring God's glory.[23] The continued presence of the notion of the 'relic' of the original divine image in fallen humanity in both Luther's and Calvin's theology is a witness to the struggle they experienced in understanding what was actually so unique about humanity.[24]

The second observation is that the very existence of the divine image in each human being is grounded, in part, in his or her bodily existence. This, as already discussed, was emphasized by Irenaeus in his anti-Gnostic writings. Unfortunately, it was the influence of Greek dualistic philosophy on a number of other early writers that seemed to limit their understanding of the divine image to just a spiritual aspect.[25] And it is a mistake that is still being made, with Machen, for example, writing: 'The "image of God" cannot well refer to man's body, because God is a spirit; it must, therefore, refer to man's soul.'[26] Actually, the human body is very important, though the extent to which human genetic and biological characteristics contribute to the specific aspects of the image of God in humankind cannot be defined.[27]

The correct biblical interpretation is that human beings, in their wholeness, soul and body, reflect the image of God. Of course, this does not mean that God has a physical body but simply stresses that it is only in the totality of the created nature of a human being that he or she can express his or her divine calling. Calvin emphasized this position by stating that, 'although the primary seat of the divine image was in the mind and heart, or in the soul and its powers, yet there was no part of man, not even the body itself, in which some sparks did not glow'.[28] In this, Calvin affirmed that even the fully restored image of God in humanity, in its heavenly state, will involve the human body.[29]

The original image was human and the final image of God's redeemed children in heaven will be human.

Substantive Aspects and Personhood

It has already been possible to explore briefly the idea that being a member of the *Homo sapiens* species automatically and inevitably implies personhood. Indeed, by agreeing to the concept of 'natural kinds' it is possible to affirm that to be a human being is to be a person.[30] However, a number of contemporary philosophers disagree with such a view, arguing instead that to be a person one must possess a certain number of characteristics and not just be a member of a particular species.

For example, the ethicist Michael Lockwood distinguishes strongly between a member of the species *Homo sapiens* and the concept of a human person, suggesting that personhood could also apply to chimpanzees or dolphins. Thus, he defines a person as:

A being that is conscious, in the sense of having the capacity for conscious thought and experiences, but not only that, it must have the capacity for reflective consciousness and self-consciousness. It must have, or at any rate have the ability to acquire, a concept of itself as a being with a past and a future.[31]

Another example of this line of reasoning comes from Michael Tooley. In a famous essay entitled 'Abortion and Infanticide' he insists that a distinction exists between the 'human being' as a biological fact and 'personhood' as a moral value judgement. For Tooley, a person is to be correlated with 'a moral right to life': 'An organism possesses a serious right to life only when it possesses the concept of a self as a continuing subject of experiences and other mental states and believes that it is itself such a continuing entity.'[32] This led Tooley to propose that infanticide may sometimes be justifiable.[33] It is also a position that supports a functional perspective, which will be examined later.

From a Christian perspective, it is a holistic anthropology that is the witness of the Bible. Even though some Cartesian influences remain[34] and some writers argue for a body–soul dualism,[35] Christian theology stresses the unitary nature of human beings. The Genesis 2.7 creation account clearly emphasizes that God 'breathed into his nostrils the breath of life, and the man became a living being' (*nephesh* in Hebrew; and *psyche*, soul, in the Septuagint). In other words, the human being is a living soul, meaning that the soul is not an independent constituent part of the human being but is a way of considering the human being in his or her entirety. For example, Barth stresses that the human being is an 'embodied soul and ensouled body'.[36]

The focus of the New Testament complements and emphasizes the thrust of the creation account with the same unitary perspective, but this is done through the incarnation where the 'Word became flesh' with the Son of God taking on physical humanity in perfect unity. Moreover, it was not just in the earthly life of Christ that the unity of Christ's being was manifested but in his death, resurrection and ascension. Although the resurrected and ascended Christ was transformed and glorified, he remains embodied as a human being.[37]

Thus, in the same way as the body–soul unity is celebrated in the ascension of Jesus Christ, it is also recognized in Christ's pre-natal life since it was at conception, and not at any later time, that Christ's embryonic human body came into being through the incarnation. As Rollinson notes: 'The Incarnation is the theological datum, which lays to rest all Cartesian dualism, and Aristotelian delayed animation.'[38]

At the incarnation, Jesus Christ was as fully body and fully soul as he was fully God and fully human.

Speciesism and the Moral Status of the Human Being

As already noted, Singer, in his influential essay 'Animals and the Value of Life', strongly resists the concept that human life, as such, has any special value. Valuing human life simply because it belongs to the *Homo sapiens* species is, he suggests, discriminatory in that it is speciesist. However, he does accept that arguments proposing that human beings are special in some particular way, for example that they possess self-consciousness, may be valid. But in the end, Singer maintains that not all human beings should be considered as persons or have the same dignity. For instance, he states that some human beings affected by a serious mental disorder may be considered of less moral value and worth than some of the healthy, more developed, non-human primates. A similar position is taken by Tooley who asks: 'Why should it be seriously wrong to kill an unborn member of the species *Homo sapiens*, but not seriously wrong to kill an unborn kitten? Difference in species is not, per se, a morally relevant difference.'[39]

In seeking to address these arguments, Warnock responds with the weak claim that 'speciesism' should not be considered as a form of prejudice since it is quite reasonable for a living being to seek to favour the survival of its own species or to take a prime interest in its survival.[40] Similarly, the English philosopher Peter Millican seeks to contest the argument of speciesism but without using the notion of the intrinsic moral worth of humans.[41] In this, he introduces two principles.

The first is one of special obligation: there is a greater obligation to one's own children than to those of the neighbour or other families. This does not mean, of course, that the intrinsic moral worth of others is any less but, because of these special obligations, it is possible to justify human beings giving more respect to a human embryo than to an adult non-human mammal.

His second principle is one of sympathetic respect. This arises when human individuals feel obliged towards someone because they respect his or her relationship with others. In other words, human beings give respect to those whom others consider important. The regard that prospective parents and the wider community have towards an unborn child should be honoured and respected. It is a level of reverence that would not be given to beings, at whatever stage of development, of other species.

Another response to the accusation of speciesism is the bold and unashamedly species-specific Christian emphasis that every human being is made in the image of God (Gen. 1.26–27). The very special and important nature of the human species is therefore a status conferred by God. It is blatant positive discrimination, originating in God, to be gratefully received by human beings and to be used responsibly. Moreover, the incarnation, whereby the Son of God chose to become a human being in the very image of God, is the most wonderful expression of this special status of humanity.

Though the image of God has been interpreted in many different manners,[42] it does reflect humanity's very being in the eyes of God. Of course, being created in the image of God does not license human beings to abuse nonhuman animals but it purposely sets humanity apart from all the other animals.

Singer, however, rejects any spiritual or religious dimension to human beings as lacking rational justification[43] and is thus limited, unfortunately, by the inability of science to seek value and meaning in biological life.

It should also be emphasized that the very definition of being a person cannot be limited or reduced to the context of humanity in itself. Indeed, if God's very being is inseparable from the three persons of the Triunity, then there must be a difference between being a person and being human.[44] The American Reformed theologian Lewis Smedes (1921–2002) summarized this understanding: 'No matter how we finally describe the essential ingredients which lift a life into personhood, we must distinguish living person from bodily life.'[45]

This section has demonstrated that it is very difficult to determine precisely what the substance of humanity actually is from the perspective of the image of God and what it means to be a person. But this does not mean that it is unimportant; just that there remains a mystery at the very heart of humanity as such. Taking this into account, it is now possible to discuss the manner in which substantive aspects can be considered with respect to the moral status of the embryo.

Substantive Aspects and the Moral Status of the Embryo

From a secular perspective, though it is agreed that a human embryo or foetus is a member of the species *Homo sapiens*, many questions remain concerning its status as a human person because of a lack of agreed definitions of personhood. As O'Donovan writes relating to the humanity of the foetus:

> There would be no difficulty in deciding that the fetus was 'human' if the only relevant criterion for humanity was that of species. Certainly it would then be 'human stuff' simply because it was not bovine, canine, fungoid, arboreal or any other kind of stuff ... Traditionally, then, the question about the humanity of the fetus has been interpreted as a question about the individual humanity of the fetus. But there is no obvious criterion for assessing what is and what is not 'individual'.[46]

Because of this ambiguity, many secular bioethicists believe that membership of the human species is secondary, from a moral perspective, and that human embryos cannot be considered as persons, for reasons that will be examined in subsequent chapters.[47] Nevertheless, because of the simple fact that early embryos are human and the continued uncertainty as to their moral status, they do still have some protection in most jurisdictions around the world.

From a Christian perspective, however, the concept of human personhood is understood to be inseparable from human nature. Indeed, if the Cartesian dualism between the body and the soul is rejected, then it is important to take human nature seriously. This suggests, for example, that if a living being is to attain self-consciousness at some stage (even after death), then it must be the kind of being that has an intrinsic capability of attaining such a consciousness. Hence, what makes the human being special is precisely what constitutes his or her humanness. Cameron comments:

> [W]hatever presents itself to us as *Homo sapiens*, man rather than some other species, is a bearer of the image of God. No-one would dispute that, from the moment of fertilization, the human embryo is a member of the species, a 'human being' rather than any other kind of being.[48]

The difficulty of recognizing moral status in embryos just because they are human from a substantive perspective, however, can lead to some very difficult situations. This happened, for example, in the British Parliament when human–nonhuman interspecies embryos were being discussed in the light of the Human Fertilisation and Embryology Act 2008 (HFE Act 2008). This sought to regulate through the UK Human Fertilisation and Embryology Authority (HFEA) human admixed embryos, which are embryos at the human end of the human–nonhuman spectrum. These included (in a catch-all category) any embryo containing genetic material (DNA) of a human and genetic material (DNA) of a nonhuman animal but in which the animal DNA is not predominant.[49]

At the time when the legislation was being drafted there was deep uncertainty about whether certain kinds of human–nonhuman inter-species embryos, and especially chimeras formed of both early human and nonhuman cells, should come under human or nonhuman legislation. In order to try to address these concerns, the Health Minister in the House of Lords, Lord Darzi of Denham, explained in 2008 that:

> If it were considered that an embryo was to be created in which the human DNA would ultimately predominate, an application for an admixed research licence would have to be made to the HFEA at the outset. This is because a licence is required to bring about the creation of a human admixed embryo. If a researcher was intending to create an embryo that would at some stage be predominantly human, for however short that time might be, they would need a licence to do so.[50]

This means that the word 'predominant' covers the whole period of an embryo's existence. Any chimeric embryos in which the nonhuman cells first predominate but where the human cells eventually develop into a majority – for however brief a time – would be covered by the catch-all category of the HFE Act 2008[51] and would need a licence from the Human Fertilisation and Embryology Authority.[52] This includes embryos that have predominantly nonhuman animal DNA in the first 14 days of development, but which would change if allowed to develop further, to become predominantly human, even if only for a short time.[53] Lord Darzi also indicated, on the same day, that human admixed embryos include those embryos in which human 'functionality' may predominate:

> In the case of an embryo in which the brain might be predominantly animal, it is worth reminding ourselves what we mean by 'predominant'. We refer not only to the percentage of the DNA but also to its location and functionality. If that entity had a human brain, that could clearly have a predominant function so, by definition, it would be at the human end of the spectrum of human admixed embryos and would require an HFEA licence.[54]

In reply to a question in the House of Lords asking whether this meant that, when the human cells of an interspecies embryo ended up being a minority in the brain of a nonhuman animal, they could still be considered to predominate in certain circumstances, Lord Darzi replied: '[T]he answer is yes. If that functionality predominates being human, that embryo will be classified as being at the human end of the spectrum of human admixed embryos.'[55]

However, this then raises the question of the definition of 'functionality', to which the House of Commons Minister of Health responded, in a 2009 letter:

> The point that Lord Darzi was making is that it is not necessarily the amount of DNA that would determine predominance, but what the DNA actually does ... Each case would have to be considered separately. It will be for the Human Fertilisation and Embryology Authority to apply the test in practice, and ultimately for the courts to determine in law what this test should be in any particular case.[56]

This means that if all the different parts of an embryo had a majority of animal DNA but that some parts, such as the brain, began to function as predominantly human (even though the majority of the DNA in the brain was animal), then this embryo would still be considered as a human admixed embryo and would come under the remit of the HFE Act 2008 instead of animal legislation. However, this determination is not mentioned in the HFE Act 2008 and so, according to the letter just quoted from the Health Minister, would be reliant on an initial decision by the Human Fertilisation and Embryology Authority, a decision which might well be open to legal challenge.[57]

This example demonstrates, once again, how difficult it is to determine what humanity actually represents and the challenges that exist in using the concept of the substance of humanity to confer moral status upon embryos. It also reflects how the arguments quickly turned into ones based on functionality, which Parliament seemed to suggest can better define what humanity actually represents. But this brings with it its own problems, as subsequent chapters of the book will show.

Notes

1 Judy Pearsall and Bill Trumble (eds), 1996, *The Oxford English Reference Dictionary*, second edition, Oxford: Oxford University Press, p. 1439.

2 David A. Jones et al., 2003, 'A Theologian's Brief on the Place of the Human Embryo within the Christian Tradition, and the Theological Principles for Evaluating its Moral Status', in B. Waters and R. Cole-Turner (eds), *God and the Embryo*, Washington, DC: Georgetown University Press, p. 194.

3 Richard Cross, 1998, *The Physics of Duns Scotus*, Oxford: Oxford University Press, p. 34.

4 Robert N. Wennberg, 1985, *Life in the Balance*, Grand Rapids: Eerdmans, pp. 36, 38.

5 Wennberg, *Life in the Balance*, pp. 40, 38.

6 Akin, Daniel L., 2007, *A Theology for the Church*, Nashville: B & H Publishing Group, p. 387.

7 Claus Westermann, 1984, *Genesis 1–11*, London: SPCK, pp. 202, 206.

8 Nigel M. de S. Cameron, 'Image in Embryo', in David C. Watts (ed.), *Creation and the Christian Response to Warnock*, Rugby: The Biblical Creation Society, pp. 9, 12.

9 Human–nonhuman interspecies persons will also, if they become self-aware and Christians, take the bread and wine at Communion representing the human body of Jesus Christ.

10 Reports to the General Assembly of the Church of Scotland, 1987, p. 309.

11 Jean-Claude Larchet, 1998, *Pour une éthique de la procréation: Éléments d'anthropologie patristique*, Paris: Les Éditions du Cerf, pp. 152–3.

12 David Atkinson, 1987, 'Some Theological Perspectives on the Human Embryo', in Nigel M. de S. Cameron (ed.), *Embryos and Ethics*, Edinburgh: Rutherford House Books, pp. 47–8.

13 Peter Singer, 1980, 'Animals and the Value of Life', in Tom Regan (ed.), *Matters of Life and Death*, Philadelphia: Temple University Press.

14 In Calvin's treatment concerning the divine image, he suggests that it is all creation which reflects the divine image in that it 'declares the glory of God' (Ps. 19). But he does, however, emphasize that it is in a very unique way that humankind reflects the image of God: 'It is certain that in every part of the world some lineaments of divine glory are beheld, and hence we may infer that when this image is placed in man, there is a kind of tacit antithesis, as it were, setting man apart from the crowd, and exalting him above all the other creatures.' John Calvin, *Commentary on Psalm 19*.

15 An enthusiastic exponent of this view is G. Wenham, 1987, *Genesis Chapters 1–15*, Word Bible Commentary, Waco: Word, p. 30.

16 Gerhard van Rad, quoted in Westermann, *Genesis 1–11*, p. 151.

17 Wenham, *Genesis Chapters 1–15*, p. 31.

18 A. McFadyen also stated: 'I take the image to be an ontological structure of freedom in response. As ontological, it is a permanent and indestructible structure, establishing homo sapiens as a being-in-relationship. Yet, as a structure of freedom, it has to be understood in terms of potential.' Alistair McFadyen, 1990, *The Call to Personhood*, Cambridge: Cambridge University Press, pp. 18, 41.

19 David Cairns, 1953, *The Image of God in Man*, first edition, London: SCM Press, p. 52.

20 Some, such as Gerrit C. Berkouwer, would argue that this verse (Gen. 9.6) looks back to what humans *were*, and forward to what they *could be*, but is not a statement of the *present*. This seems a strange way of speaking. Gerrit C. Berkouwer, 1962, *Man: The Image of God*, Grand Rapids: Eerdmans, pp. 56–9.

21 Anthony A. Hoekema, 1992, *Created in God's Image*, Grand Rapids: Eerdmans, p. 32.

22 Cairns, 1953, *Image of God*, first edition, p. 124.

23 Thomas F. Torrance, 1949, *Calvin's Doctrine of Man*, Edinburgh: T&T Clark, p. 36.

24 Emil Brunner, 1939, *Man in Revolt*, London: Lutterworth Press, p. 86.

25 Brunner, *Man in Revolt*, p. 401.

26 J. Gresham Machen, 'The Christian View of Man', quoted in Hoekema, *Created in God's Image*, p. 68.

27 Chris Darnbrough, 'Genetic Engineering: Monster or Miracle?', in Watts, *Creation and the Christian Response*, p. 26.

28 John Calvin, *Institutes* 1.15.3.

29 John Calvin, *Commentary on 1 Corinthians 15.49*.

30 Some, such as Baruch Brody, would argue that 'natural kind' needs itself to be defined. Thus for him it is the natural kind of human being which has a capacity for experience – in other words, a psychological life. Baruch Brody, 1988, 'On the Humanity of the Foetus', in Michael Goodman (ed.), *What Is a Person?*, Clifton: Humana Press.

31 Michael Lockwood (ed.), 1985, *Moral Dilemmas in Modern Medicine*, Oxford: Oxford University Press, pp. 11, 10.

32 Michael Tooley, 1974, 'Abortion and Infanticide', in M. Cohen, T. Nagel and T. Scanlon (eds), *The Rights and Wrongs of Abortion*, Princeton: Princeton University Press, p. 59.

33 Michael Tooley, 1988, 'In Defense of Abortion and Infanticide', in Goodman, *What Is a Person?*, pp. 83–114.

34 'It has, of course, become almost customary in these days to proclaim emancipation from a "Cartesian" body–soul dualism. For the most part, however, the emancipation has proved to be an empty boast.' O'Donovan makes this claim by way of comment on how bodily manifestations of humanity, such as our genetic structure, are often disregarded as important data in defining personhood. Oliver O'Donovan, 1985, 'Again, Who Is a Person?', in J. H. Channer (ed.), *Abortion and the Sanctity of Human Life*, Carlisle: Paternoster Press, p. 136.

35 Richard Swinburne, 1987, 'The Structure of the Soul', in A. R. Peacocke and G. Gillett (eds), *Persons and Personality: A Contemporary Inquiry*, Oxford: Blackwell, pp. 33–55.

36 Karl Barth, 1957–75, *Church Dogmatics*, Edinburgh: T&T Clark, Vol. III.2, p. 325.

37 Adrian Thatcher, 1987, 'Christian Theism and the Concept of a Person', in Peacocke and Gillett, *Persons and Personality*, p. 184; Chandra Sethurajan and Nigel M. de S. Cameron, 1989, *Sexuality and Fertility*, Edinburgh: Rutherford House, p. 24.

38 Andrew R. Rollinson, 'The Incarnation and the Status of the Human Embryo', a thesis submitted for the degree of M.Litt. with the Religious Studies Department of Newcastle University, p. 174.

39 Tooley, 'Abortion and Infanticide', p. 66.

40 Mary Warnock, '*In vitro* fertilisation: The ethical issues II', *Philosophical Quarterly* 33:132 (1983), p. 242.

41 Peter Millican, 1992, 'The Complex Problem of Abortion', in D. R. Bromham, M. E. Dalton, J. C. Jackson and P. J. R. Millican (eds), *Ethics in Reproductive Medicine*, New York: Springer, p. 178.

42 Henri Blocher, 1984, *In the Beginning*, Leicester: InterVarsity Press; see the chapter 'The Image of God'.

43 Singer, 'Animals', p. 227.

44 Wennberg, *Life in the Balance*, p. 33.

45 Lewis Smedes, 1983, *Mere Morality*, Grand Rapids: Eerdmans, p. 107.

46 Oliver O'Donovan, 1973, *The Christian and the Unborn Child*, Bramcote, Nottinghamshire: Grove Books, p. 10.

47 Pia Matthews, 2010, 'Discerning Persons: How the early theology can illuminate contemporary bioethical approaches to the concept of person', doctoral thesis, Saint Mary's University College, p. 31.

48 Nigel M. de S. Cameron, 1986, *Abortion: The Crisis in Morals and Medicine*, Leicester: InterVarsity Press, p. 16.

49 Human Fertilisation and Embryology Act 2008, Section 4A(6)(e).

50 Lords Hansard, 29 October 2008, Column 1624.

51 Human Fertilisation and Embryology Act 2008, Section 4A(6)(e).

52 Or the HFEA's successor body.

53 Lords Hansard, 29 October 2008, Columns 1619–26.

54 Lords Hansard, 29 October 2008, Column 1625.

55 Lords Hansard, 29 October 2008, Column 1626.

56 Letter from the Health Minister to Calum MacKellar's Member of Parliament, 22 May 2009.

57 It would be useful to clarify that the Home Office would, presumably, still have regulatory and inspection roles.

7

Relational Aspects and the Embryo

The concept of relationships between persons has been one of the most important notions to be used down throughout history to help determine both the image of God and what it means to be a person.

Relationships between persons are indeed crucial in theology because they enable interactions of love to exist – a love that confers value and meaning while bringing joy into the relationship. This is as true between human persons as between God and his human children.

But a relationship also emphasizes the mutual, holistic existence of two beings. This was one of the main conclusions of the Austrian-born Israeli Jewish philosopher Martin Buber (1878–1965), in his influential 1923 book *Ich und Du* (I and Thou).[1] For him, in order to experience this I–Thou relationship, a person must also be open to the idea of such a relationship with another personal being.

Relational Aspects and the Image of God

From the beginning of Genesis, there is a strong reflection of who God is in the relational character of creation. 'Let us make mankind in our image ...' (Gen. 1.26) expresses, in some way, the creational relationship in love of a Godhead-in-community – a love existing from all eternity in personal relationship between the persons of the Trinity.

Thus, when God says in Genesis, 'Let us make mankind in our image', the 'us' represents the relational aspect in God which expands onto his children. It means that God creates persons using images or templates (from himself and his image) so that his creatures can also express the love from which his creation originates. Each time the image of God is mentioned in Genesis, it is always associated with relationships. In other words, to be created in the image of God is to be created as a person in a community of relationships with God and with others.

The first epistle of John declares: 'No one has ever seen God; but if we love one another, God lives in us and his love is made complete in us' (1 John 4.12). John, in this way, indicates that something of the image of God can be seen when persons love God and each other. In fact, in Trinitarian theology, the very definition and meaning of being a person is based on the existence of a loving relationship with others.[2]

Indeed, any appropriate understanding of the image of God involves a relationship between the origin of this image (God) and the image itself in human persons. God always intended to have a loving relationship with human persons who reflect something of himself in his image. As the British physician and ethicist John Wyatt explains, 'God's creation of humans in his image is also a call to relationship with him. God creates us as relational beings and calls us to enter into communion with him.'[3]

In this context, and using Calvin's exposition of the divine image, both Brunner and Barth, in two different ways, developed a relational understanding of the image of God.

For Brunner, the very nature of humankind is based on the reality that human beings stand before God in a relationship which exists even if they reject God. Moreover, this relationship is a 'living', dynamic and existential one whereby each and every human being is constantly standing, as a morally responsible agent, before the Word of God. By examining the whole of creation, Brunner then distinguishes between two perspectives when considering created human beings. The first considers human beings as having a human nature stamped upon them as an image is stamped upon a coin. The second perspective considers human creatures as incomplete and unfinished items who are, nevertheless, constantly being held in God's hands as well as constantly being sustained, confronted and loved. Such an I–God (vertical) relationship, moreover, is complemented by I–Thou (horizontal) relationships. In other words, the universal image in humankind, though primarily consisting in the inalienable confrontation of human beings with the Word of God, also involves relationships with fellow humans. The International Theological Commission of the Holy See states that 'human persons are created in the image of God in order to enjoy personal communion with the Father, Son and Holy Spirit and with one another in them'.[4]

As already indicated, for Brunner, the image of God includes the creaturely nature of bodily existence. But the most important concept, for him, is one of relationship. Human beings, as sinners in their guilty existence, still stand confronted by God. This is the 'formal image'. Faith in Christ brings a renewal of that image, a restoration of the 'material image'.[5]

With Barth, an even stronger statement of this emphasis is presented whereby he recognizes a special meaning in the last words of Genesis 1.27, 'in the image of God he created them; male and female he created them'. Barth asserts that the loving face-to-face confrontation of man and woman reflects the loving 'face-to-face relationships' of the persons of the triune God, and it is this very relational existence which is at the heart of humanity being made in the divine image.[6]

The very fact that God speaks in the plural – 'Let us make mankind in our image' – may be taken as a confirmation of this understanding of 'face-to-face relationships'. This relational existence again involves a relationship between human beings and God as well as between a man and a woman. Thus, Barth emphasizes that the image does not consist in a particular characteristic that human beings can do or have but is constituted by their very relational existence. It is the orientation of human beings that is determinative and not their capabilities.[7]

Barth's understanding of the image of God is also strongly Christological in that humankind stands and is represented before God in the person of the incarnate Word of God, Jesus Christ. In addition, human beings have not lost their divine image through the Fall; rather, sin obscures or hides their true nature from themselves and others. It is only through a grateful acceptance of God's good news in Christ that the real human being can begin to be revealed.

Thus, the divine image in humanity has both vertical and horizontal dimensions.[8]

The 'vertical image' can be expressed by Barth's vivid definition of the human being as 'a being-in-gratitude'[9] through his or her creaturely relationship with God. It is a relationship in which a dialogue exists, which was initiated by God and which enables human beings to become beings-in-partnership with God. As McFadyen comments: 'God's creative and sustaining activity elicits, enables and deserves a free and thankful response.'[10] This relationship, he suggests, is the very basis of what it means to be made in the image of God.

But it is also a vertical relationship supported by love. As Kilner writes: 'Complete conformation to Christ's image in Romans 8:29 entails not only experiencing God's love but also loving God in return (v.28).' This means that one of the most important ways in which the relational aspect of humanity's renewal, according to God's image, is expressed in Scripture is in terms of loving (*agape*) relationship with God.[11] This also means that Jesus Christ is the perfect reflection of the image of God because he perfectly reflects the love coming from the Father while returning this love to him. Fallen humanity, on the other hand, does not reflect the perfect image of God because it reflects only partially the love coming from God.

The horizontal aspect of the image is the reality that persons are persons-in-community. In other words, personal identity cannot be found only in a human being's unique individuality but in the relationships he or she has with others. For McFadyen, such a notion of beings-in-relationship originates from the model found in the Trinity, 'a community of persons in which person and relation are interdependent moments in a process of mutuality'. It follows that Father, Son and Spirit are not simply constituted of relationships, nor are they absolute, discrete and independent individuals but 'Persons in relation and Persons only through relation'.[12]

In the biblical text, this horizontal dimension is best described in Genesis 1.27 where the image of God is clearly related to the face-to-face relationship of man and woman: 'So God created mankind in his own image, in the image of God he created them; male and female he created them.' Though there is no direct equation of the image of God in humanity with human existence as male and female, the close proximity of the concepts certainly suggests that it is a significant dimension. Adam was not complete without his human companion (Gen. 2.18). This forms a paradigm, a typical example or pattern, emphasizing the importance of social relationships as well as a relationship with God for any appropriate understanding of what it means to be a human person.

It may also be useful to note that the Apostle Paul experienced a glimpse of the mystery of the relationship of love between two persons of different sex when he studied the relationship of love between Christ and his 'bride' the Church, as indicated in Ephesians 5.23: 'For the husband is the head of the wife as Christ is the head of the church, his body, of which he is the Saviour.'

In a way, the relationship between a man and a woman is an *eikon* of the relationship between Jesus Christ and his human children. Moreover, as already noted, in ancient thought the *eikon* was not considered only a copy of the reality being portrayed, but was thought somehow to participate in the very substance of the reality it symbolized. It is not just a reflection of reality, but is that same reality.[13] Hence, the image of God is clearly related to the face-to-face relationship between God and his human children which is expressed in the man–woman relationship.

In this way, McFadyen understands the divine image as being related to a permanent and indestructible structural dimension defining who human beings are as *Homo sapiens*. But there is also a dimension of freedom, where there is a moral direction. He writes: 'The assertion that we are created in the divine image operates both as an assertion of the way things are – an ontological given – and as an ideal regulating personal and social conduct. It is both an "is" and an "ought".'[14]

It is worth noting that Barth's powerful emphasis on the I–Thou relationship may still have its limitations. His argument gives the impression that there is something not quite real about those who do not love God. There may be some uncertainty between the 'real man' (the universal image of humanity) and the 'true man' (the redeemed image). This means that creatureliness as well as relationships needs to be emphasized,[15] while remembering that there is a structural, as well as a functional, dimension to the image of God.[16]

Interestingly, Barth's understanding of the image of God was criticized by Brunner who suggested that it portrayed human destiny rather than defining humanity's very being.[17] However, it is difficult to condense Barth's colossal and intricate description of the image of God and it can only stand as a radical Christological and relational understanding of the divine image.

A further insight of the nature of the image of God can be examined in that, unlike all the other animals, humankind has been made God's counterpart. As Westermann affirms: 'The relationship to God is not something which is added to human existence; humans are created in such a way that their very existence is intended to be their relationship to God.'[18]

This understanding of relationships with respect to the image of God is also reflected in the fundamental self-transcendence which is present in all human persons who are searching for fulfilment and meaning in their existence: a search that is brought to an end only when they find their genuine identity in Jesus Christ, the fulfilment of the image of God.[19]

This insight is also taken up by T. F. Torrance who argues that human persons can be seen as transcendentally determined in their very existence as soul and body. This enables them to understand themselves as personal beings before God. For Torrance this is also where the concept of the spirit of a person becomes important:

> By spirit is not meant that man was created as body, soul, and spirit, but rather that as spirit, man as body of his soul and soul of his body, is given a transcendental determination of his human condition before God. As Holy Spirit God is here to be thought of as transcendent personalising Being, and the human creature as spirit is to be thought of as personalised being. Through the creative power and personal presence of his Spirit God realises the relation of the creature to himself, constituting him a spiritual being capable of meeting God and of enjoying personal relation with him.[20]

The spirit of a human person, therefore, is his or her openness to the Spirit of God through a relationship. However, it is not a matter of a human being's addressability but rather the reality that human beings are constantly being addressed as 'thou' by the divine 'I'. In the same way, Gunton comments that to be addressed by God is one of the notions that is sometimes used to characterize the image of God. He adds: 'To be human is to be addressed by God, to be called to be in particular forms of relationship with him, with one another and with the rest of the created world.'[21]

In ending this section, it should be noted that many who believe that being in God's image somehow involves relationship are also aware of the insufficiency of the concept of relationship alone as the essence of what creation in God's image entails.[22] Other factors must come into play, and relationships are only an element of the overall picture.

Relational Aspects and Personhood

The previous understanding of the image of God implies that it is only through a relationship of love with God that any meaning in existence can be expressed. Human persons were created from and for a relationship with their creator.

As already mentioned, from a Trinitarian perspective, classical theology does not consider three completely separate persons in the Godhead but three persons defined by one another and who cohere consubstantially in one another. This is characterized by T. F. Torrance in the expression of 'onto-relations', which means that personhood is intrinsically defined by relationships with other persons.

Interestingly, this notion of relationship is what Torrance compares to Einstein's relativity theory by explaining that human persons, on their creaturely level, only exist in such a way that the relations between them belong to what persons essentially are. They bear, in this way, a created reflection of the transcendent relatedness or 'community-ness' inherent in God. It is in the light of this personal and interpersonal nature of human beings that one may rightly think of man and woman as imaging or reflecting God the creator.[23]

Gunton expands Torrance when he states:

The one [God] who is known by virtue of His free and personal relatedness to the world is one who is a relational being in Himself. God, that is to say, is a communion: one who exists in the communion of the Father, Son and Spirit: each with His own distinctive and particular being, yet all are only what they are as a result of their relations in perichoresis[24] with one another. It follows that God is personal, for to be a person is to exist in relations of free mutuality with other persons. Equally, it follows that God is love, for it is of the essence of love to exist through reciprocal giving and receiving.[25]

Similarly, Wyatt suggests:

This is the ultimate meaning behind the biblical statement, 'God is love', a continual self-giving of the persons of the Trinity. It seems that the persons of the Godhead do not, even cannot, exist in isolation. God's being is defined as being in relationship. To be a person is both to be a unique 'other' and to be in relationship with others.[26]

This means that who and what persons are is derived not only from their relations to the creator God but to those others who have made and continue to make persons what they are. Just as the Father, Son and Holy Spirit constitute the being of God, so created persons are those who, insofar as they are authentically personal, exist in mutually constitutive relations of love with one another.[27]

This exchange of love is also what should be expressed in the personal relation of complementarity between men and women. Indeed, the division of sexes enables human beings to know one of the most intimate I–thou relationships through love.[28]

From a more secular perspective, John Harris also considers the relational element of personhood though this is done in a self-reflective manner. He suggests that a person should only be defined as 'a creature capable of valuing its own existence' in such a way that he or she can give himself or herself inherent dignity in a kind of relationship with one's self. But in so doing, he rejects the personhood of embryos, foetuses, newborn children and individuals who do not have the capacity to value their own existence.[29] On the other hand, in selecting this definition Harris acknowledges that persons 'may include animals, machines, extra-terrestrials, gods, angels and devils'.[30]

Unfortunately, this understanding of personhood based on an individual's own capacity to have a relationship with, while giving personhood and value to, himself or herself, is limited to the physical capacities and creaturely perspectives of humanity. As such, it begs the question whether any real worth and meaning can arise from physical science since it cannot give any answer to the ultimate value of humankind. As T. F. Torrance notes:

[F]ailure to develop understanding of the different levels of human existence in their relation to higher levels, and so to cut short their meaningful reference beyond themselves, beyond what we can determine merely by physical, neurological, and psychiatric analyses, would be to truncate what we learn in those ways, and limit the value of what we have already determined. The human being is characterised by an indefinite openness to what is beyond, and is properly to be understood in that open-structured way.[31]

In other words, real value and meaning can only come from God and cannot be found without transcending the physical cosmos.

Theological Anthropology and Relationships

There is a general agreement in all aspects of contemporary anthropology that human beings are relational beings. But what is so special to theological anthropology is the affirmation that the relationship of God to humanity is crucial to any appropriate understanding of all the relationships in which human beings exist. What is more, a human person's 'relational being' is rooted in humanity's relationship to a God who is triune and who is himself relational.[32]

As already indicated, this is an important emphasis and T. F. Torrance argues that the three persons of the Godhead must be understood in relational terms: 'The Persons are who they are in their mutual and perichoretic relations with one another in one and the same divine Being.'[33]

The French Catholic theologian Jean Galot SJ (1919–2008) argued in a similar fashion[34] using the doctrine of the Trinity as interpreted by Augustine. In this way, Galot comes to understand the concept of a 'person' as a 'relational being' (*être relationnel*), from which he emphasizes that the notion of human personhood cannot be defined by a nature of identifiable characteristics which then enable relations. Instead, personhood should be seen as being constituted by these very relations. 'Human persons approximate to the divine Persons by the fact that, while each has an individual nature, they are nevertheless essentially constituted by a relation, a hypostatic relation.'[35] Human beings' relationships with one another and their relationship with God are the necessary constitutive elements for them to be defined as persons.

O'Donovan further argues that, by definition, it is impossible to 'examine' a person in a purely disconnected and observational manner since it is possible to discern a person only if one commits oneself to interacting and having a relationship with this person.[36]

As already mentioned, in the Christological debates of the early Church, Christ's two natures in one person implies that no living human nature can exist without being a person. The notion of personhood, therefore, must come before the concept of properties (or nature). In other words, properties do not give rise to personhood but personhood to properties. This means that, from a Trinitarian and Christological perspective, an important progression seems to take place which implies that personal characteristics arise out of being a person which, itself, requires relationships.

As already noted, MacQuarrie asserts that a person cannot exist without a relationship to another person, indicating that persons are 'beings-with-others'.[37] This has been described very sensitively by the Canadian philosopher Jean Vanier, who used his knowledge of working with disabled adults to emphasize the joy of communion with another person, a communion which is crucial to experiencing a fuller and more meaningful life.[38] The emphasis here is not on a human being's capacity to form human relationships. Neither do personal relationships all by themselves simply create personhood. What matters is being considered, valued and loved by another in a relationship.

For example, many societies consider babies as persons from the moment of birth and even before. Through the process of imitation, a baby seems to replicate the words and behaviour of the persons who consider him or her as a person and thereby learns to treat others as persons. By learning this behaviour the baby may even be acquiring a concept of self.[39]

In summary, it is not only the existence of a being that matters, but also the relationship(s) that are made possible because of this existence, which enables this being to be a person.

But it is important to emphasize, yet again, that the very basis and foundation of personhood is God's relationship of love with human beings as his creatures. Human beings are persons in relationship with God who is himself a mutual indwelling and communion of the Father, Son and Holy Spirit.[40] Moreover, persons are created by, and living in dialogue with, a creator God. The grace of God is freely given to sustain humanity's creaturely personhood and the incarnation is the supreme basis and guarantee of such a relationship.

Relational Aspects and the Moral Status of the Embryo

The position that an embryo may be considered as having a moral status if another person gives this status through a relationship is a valid one. But it is important to define who this other person is.

In this respect, one argument often presented is that it is the mother who is this important other person. For example, some bioethical commentators do not believe that pre-implantation embryos can be regarded as human persons. This is because, for them, the crucial stage from a biological perspective is implantation, enabling a relationship between the embryo and the mother to be established and allowing this embryo to develop further.[41]

But this still has its problems since, to be able to give moral status to the embryo, the mother must have moral status herself. Furthermore, from a purely scientific perspective, the mother is as much a 'pile of cells' as the implanted embryo and any 'pile of cells' is incapable of giving any moral status to anything. Indeed, without God, 'Man is like a mere breath; his days are like a passing shadow' (Ps. 144.4).

It is thus only when God, the source of all real value and worth, loves a being that any real meaning for this being exists. As already noted it is God who is the original source of all personhood and not anyone else. As T. F. Torrance puts it:

> Certainly it is God himself who is the Creative Source of all personal being and inter-personal relations – he is the personalising Person, who brings us into personal life and being through the inter-personal activity of a father and mother, which begins with our conception, develops in our pre-natal life, reaches fruition in birth and childhood, and blossoms within the inter-personal life and love of a human family.[42]

Thus, in the most fundamental manner, a being only becomes a true person through a relationship with God, the personalizing Person, and this is independent of anything an individual can be or do. This perspective on relationships is interesting because it enables human beings who are not rational, such as embryos and foetuses (but also infants, the profoundly mentally disabled, and the hopelessly comatose) to be considered as persons. Indeed, God will always have a personalizing relationship of love for them since he created them in a special way out of his love. As Psalm 139 declares, what is crucial is not whether an embryo is aware of God but that God is aware of and committed by grace and love to the embryo.[43]

Gunton supports this view by recognizing the personhood of those so incapacitated as to be incapable of any human response, such as the foetus: 'We must say at least that those whose physical shape is ... not yet fully formed retain the intrinsic dignity conferred by virtue of their inextinguishable relation to God the Father through Christ and the Spirit.'[44]

But even on a human level, an embryo is never just brought into existence from absolutely nothing. A relationship always exists between his or her parents. In other words, he or she was procreated by them with the same moral value and nature as they possess. As a result, society must reconsider what it means to be a person, recognizing that each child is already personal from the very beginning of his or her life, in the oneness of body and soul, and grows as a personal being with a body and a soul.[45]

This is also considered by McCarthy, who cites the manner in which persons are called before birth in the following passages of the Bible:

> Listen to me, you islands;
> hear this, you distant nations:
> Before I was born the LORD called me;
> from my mother's womb he has spoken my name.

And now the LORD says –
he who formed me in the womb to be his servant
to bring Jacob back to him
and gather Israel to himself ... (Isaiah 49.1,5)

Before I formed you in the womb I knew you,
before you were born I set you apart;
I appointed you as a prophet to the nations. (Jeremiah 1.5)

But when God, who set me apart from my mother's womb and called me by his grace, was pleased to reveal his Son in me so that I might preach him among the Gentiles ... (Galatians 1.15–16)

McCarthy explains that to 'know' or to 'call' a person before he or she was even conceived means that the person already exists in a relationship from God's perspective who is outside of time and physics. Hence, anyone 'known' or 'called' by God must exist in all eternity but also at some stage in time on this physical earth. It is therefore the existence of this person that matters to God and not whether he or she exists in this physical universe as an embryo or as adult human being. This is because only persons can be 'known' or 'called' by God. McCarthy notes:

To state that the individual existed 'only in the mind of God' is not to deny the individual's existence. To exist 'in God's mind' is surely to exist even if that existence is not experienced by anyone (including the individual concerned) other than God. God's thoughts are reality in the fullest sense. We cannot speak of God 'imagining' something, for his thoughts are inherently creative, since whatever is in the 'mind of God' must exist. There is no other ultimate reality to any existence other than its being in the mind of God.[46]

McCarthy continues by explaining that it is impossible to consider God calling his children in any other way than in a personal way, or that there is a time in the history of humankind when any person was not part of God's call. If God calls a person from all the eternity of time to have a relationship of fellowship with him there is never a moment in time when this calling into relationship is not taking place. Thus, there cannot be a meaningful discontinuity between any stage in the existence of the person being called by God, whether before or after birth.

We may therefore argue that everyone 'called' by God enjoys the status of a human person even at the moment of conception, even though they may not at that time experience the attributes normally associated with a person. This has the important effect of making the ground for assessing the status of the human embryo the purposes of God rather than any functional attribute of the embryo.[47]

He does admit, however, that this understanding does not demonstrate that every embryo is always a person as it is impossible to know whether every human embryo is called by God. But McCarthy recognizes that it is very unlikely that two kinds of embryo exist depending on whether or not they are called, and that such a concept is not supported, in any way, by the scriptural message.[48]

It should further be emphasized that God's calling of his child from all eternity cannot be separated from his love. This then strengthens the case, made previously, that there is never a moment in time when God does not have a personalizing relationship of love for the early embryo since, at this stage (as indeed at all the subsequent stages of its personal existence until old age, death and even after death), this human being exists in his mind.

Notes

1 Martin Buber, 1923, *Ich und Du*, Leipzig: Insel Verlag.

2 Denis R Alexander, 'Cloning humans – distorting the image of God?' *Cambridge Papers, Jubilee Centre* 10:2 (2001); John Wyatt, 1998, *Matters of Life and Death: Today's Healthcare Dilemmas in the Light of Christian Faith*, Leicester: InterVarsity Press, p. 54. The thought experiment of a completely isolated individual, where God as well as others do not exist and who refuses even to have a relationship with himself or herself, can never be a person.

3 Wyatt, *Matters of Life*, p. 54.

4 International Theological Commission, *Communion and Stewardship: Human Persons Created in the Image of God*, The Vatican, 2002, paragraph 4.

5 Emil Brunner, 1956, 'Nature and Grace', in Emil Brunner and Karl Barth, *Natural Theology*, London: Geoffrey Bles, pp. 10–11.

6 Karl Barth, 1957–75, *Church Dogmatics*, Edinburgh: T&T Clark, Vol. III.1, p. 183.

7 Barth writes that '[the image] ... is constituted by the very existence of man as such, and as a creature of God. He would not be man if he were not God's image. He is God's image inasmuch as he is man.' Barth, *Church Dogmatics*, Vol. III.1, pp. 206–7.

8 A full exposition of this theme is given in Alistair I. McFadyen, 1990, *The Call to Personhood*, Cambridge: Cambridge University Press.

9 Barth, *Church Dogmatics*, Vol. III.2, pp. 168 and 193.

10 McFadyen, *Call to Personhood*, p. 19.

11 John F. Kilner, 2015, *Dignity and Destiny: Humanity in the Image of God*, Grand Rapids: Eerdmans, pp. 298, 297.

12 McFadyen, *Call to Personhood*, p. 27.

13 The Greek word *charakter* (representation) in Hebrews 1.3, 'the exact representation of his being', is an even more categorical word than *eikon*, expressing the inherent correspondence and identity of the image to the nature of what is being represented.

F. F. Bruce, 1964, *The Epistle to the Hebrews*, New London Commentary on the New Testament, London: Marshall, Morgan & Scott, p. 6.

14 McFadyen, *Call to Personhood*, p. 18.

15 C. F. H. Henry explains: 'The image is not reducible simply to a relation in which man stands to God, but rather is the precondition of such a relationship.' C. F. H. Henry, 1984, 'Image of God', in W. A. Elwell (ed.), *Evangelical Dictionary of Theology*, Grand Rapids: Baker.

David Cairns writes: 'While man's mode of existence is his act of response to God's creative call, man's being is not reduced to act or relation. As endowment, man's being is a substance which exists in responsive act to God, and in personal confrontation with Him.' David Cairns, 1953, *The Image of God in Man*, first edition, London: SCM Press, p. 190.

16 This is how Anthony A. Hoekema refers to it in Anthony A. Hoekema, 1992, *Created in God's Image*, Grand Rapids: Eerdmans, pp. 68–73.

17 Quoted in Cairns, 1953, *Image of God*, first edition, p. 173, fn. 2.

18 Claus Westermann, 1984, *Genesis 1–11*, London: SPCK, p. 158.

19 R. J. Berry and M. Jeeves, 'The Nature of Human Nature', *Science & Christian Belief* 20:1 (2008), p. 26.

20 Thomas F. Torrance, 1999, *The Soul and Person of the Unborn Child*, Edinburgh: Scottish Order of Christian Unity/Handsel Press, pp. 18–19.

21 Colin Gunton, 1998, *The Triune Creator: A Historical and Systematic Study*, Grand Rapids: Eerdmans, p. 206.

22 Kilner, *Dignity and Destiny*, p. 219.

23 Torrance, *Soul and Person*, p. 18.

24 The 'interpenetration' of the three persons of the Trinity.

25 Colin Gunton, 1992, *Christ and Creation*, Carlisle: Paternoster Press, p. 74.

26 Wyatt, *Matters of Life*, p. 54.

27 Colin Gunton, *Triune Creator*, p. 208.

28 Al Truesdale, 'Preface to Bioethics: Some Foundations for a Christian Approach to Bioethics', *Perspectives on Science and Christian Faith* 48:4 (1996), p. 227.

29 This may also include individuals with potentially suicidal depression.

30 John Harris, 'The concept of the person and the value of life', *Kennedy Institute of Ethics Journal* 9:4 (1999), pp. 293–308.

31 Torrance, *Soul and Person*, p. 6.

32 Christoph Schwobel, 1991, 'Human Beings as Relational Beings', in Christoph Schwobel and Colin Gunton (eds), *Persons, Divine and Human*, Edinburgh: T&T Clark, p. 142.

33 Thomas F. Torrance, 1989, 'The Soul and Person in Theological Perspective in Religion, Reason and Self', in S. R. Sutherland and T. A. Roberts (eds), *Essays in Honour of Hywel D. Lewis*, Cardiff: University of Wales Press.

34 Jean Galot, *La Personne du Christ*, quoted in Eric L. Mascall, 1977, *Theology and the Gospel of Christ*, London: SPCK, Appendix I.

35 Galot, *La Personne du Christ*, quoted in Mascall, *Theology and the Gospel*, p. 39.

36 Oliver O'Donovan, 1984, *Begotten or Made?*, Oxford: Oxford University Press, p. 60.

37 John MacQuarrie (ed.), 1967, *Dictionary of Christian Ethics*, London: SCM Press, p. 177. The South African Archbishop Desmond Tutu, interviewed in 2008 on the Canadian radio programme *One Hour*, said, 'A person is a person through other persons.'

38 Jean Vanier, 1985, *Man and Woman He Made Them*, London: Darton, Longman & Todd, p. 20.

39 Jean Vanier explains: 'We know that an intense dialogue, harmony, relationship already exist between the baby and mother – even before the child is born.' Vanier, *Man and Woman*, p. 13.

40 Colin E. Gunton, 1993, *The One, the Three and the Many*, 1992 Bampton Lectures, Cambridge: Cambridge University Press, p. 168.

41 John Bryant and John Searle, 2004, *Life in Our Hands: A Christian Perspective on Genetics and Cloning*, Leicester: InterVarsity Press, p. 58.

42 Torrance, *Soul and Person*, pp. 15–16.

43 Thomas F. Torrance, 1974, *Test-tube Babies: Morals – Science – and the Law*, Edinburgh: Scottish Academic Press, p. 11.

44 Gunton, *Triune Creator*, p. 203.

45 Torrance, *Soul and Person*, p. 17.

46 Brendan McCarthy, 1997, *Fertility & Faith*, Leicester: InterVarsity Press, p. 74.

47 McCarthy, *Fertility & Faith*, pp. 122, 74–75.

48 McCarthy, *Fertility & Faith*, pp. 74–5.

8

Functional Aspects and the Embryo

The *Oxford English Reference Dictionary* defines functional as 'serving a function' and function as 'an activity proper to a person'.[1] This means that functional aspects are reflected in a capacity to do or be something. Because a capacity to do something is often seen as enabling an individual to be something, these two notions will be examined together in this chapter.

This, as will be discussed, has also become the crucial factor for a number of modern secular thinkers who would ascribe personhood to a being only if it can demonstrate a number of capacities to do certain things, accomplish certain functionalities or fulfil certain characteristics.

Thus the following section on the functional aspects of the image of God will include a discussion on the capacities a being may have to do certain things or attain specific characteristics while also examining what this may then mean for the status and function of this being.

But, as already noted, this is not to say that some of these capacities cannot also be included under the previous chapters on the substantive and relational aspects of the image of God. Indeed, the boundaries between these different aspects are in no way immutable.

Functional Aspects and the Image of God

Before examining the function or status an individual may have in reflecting the image of God, it may be useful and even necessary to study the different capacities or functionalities that have been seen as important in past Christian discussions to reach such a function or status. Indeed, ever since the early Christian Church was formed, some writers have suggested that the image of God must lie with certain spiritual qualities or capacities such as reason (or intellect), free will and self-consciousness.

For example, one dominant and highly influential interpretation of the image of God in the Christian tradition came from Augustine who argued that, since God is a Trinity, some derivative trinitarian structure may be found in humankind. In his *De Trinitate* he reviews a number of possible suggestions, in particular 'the memory, understanding and will'[2] which enable human beings to have rationality. This was actually the most favoured interpretation by writers on the divine image up to Aquinas, including dominant figures such as Irenaeus, Clement of Alexandria and Athanasius of Alexandria,[3] who were also influenced by pre-Christian Greek philosophers.[4]

But the ability to reason, mentioned by commentators such as Irenaeus, had a relatively broad meaning and included a person's freedom and responsibility. Often, a distinction was also made between the rationality that cannot be lost, such as thoughts and accountability for actions, and a higher rationality that can be and has been lost.[5] This second rationality reflects not only a person's ability to reason but his or her capacity to be reasonable while recognizing and responding to the gifts of God.[6]

More modern writers are similarly very much influenced by the ability to reason. For example, the German Protestant theologian Walther Eichrodt (1890–1978) suggested that a human being's likeness to God is principally 'in his capacity for self-consciousness and self-determination; in short, in those capacities which we are accustomed to regard as typical of personality'.[7]

But rationality was not the only human function to be considered; many other capacities were used to interpret the divine image. For example, Stott writes:

Some think [the image of God] means that human beings are God's representatives, exercising dominion over the rest of creation in his place. Others conclude that God's image alludes to the special relationship that he has established between himself and us. But if we see the expression both in its immediate context in Genesis and in the broader perspective of Scripture, it seems to refer to all those human qualities or capacities that render us unlike the animals and like God.

Stott goes on to enumerate some of these human qualities, including:

1 rationality and self-consciousness,
2 a capacity to discern what is moral and having a conscience to do what is perceived to be right;
3 creativity which reflects a similar capacity in the creator to make beautiful things;
4 sociability and the ability to establish authentic relationships of love reflecting the reality that God is love; and
5 spirituality which makes humanity hunger for God.[8]

All this makes human beings unique in being able to decide, to create, and to celebrate their love for God and others.

In the end, however, all these interpretations may eventually prove insufficient since they are unable to emphasize the more important defining elements in humankind's being. As the American theologian Noreen L. Herzfeld explains: 'Identifying a quality or set of qualities as the image of God implies a hierarchy of traits within the human person, a hierarchy that has generally been detrimental to the Christian view of the body.'[9] Gunton refers to this process as 'a substantialising of the divine image, a tendency to conceive it to consist in the possession of certain fixed characteristics, characteristics moreover which tend to preclude relationality'.[10] Barth simply calls them 'symptoms of humanity' or, more specifically, observations which can only be understood once one is in possession of the full text.[11] In addition, Cairns argues that the emphasis given by the early Church writers on the capacity to reason may in fact only reflect their own preferences and values as to what is important.[12]

Perhaps all that can really be deduced from human beings' functionalities or capacities is the observation, by the British theologian John Sawyer, that '[God] chose to reveal some of his transcendent nature in man, the crowning glory of his creation'.[13] This reflects the very important transcendent and open nature of humanity which is similar to the teachings of some of the Greek Fathers. For example, Gregory of Nyssa maintained: 'One of the characteristics of the Godhead is to be in its essence beyond our understanding, and so the image should also express this.'[14] Interestingly, these early writers also considered human persons as small gods (*microtheos*) because of their ability to communicate with the transcendent God; or, as Gregory of Nazianzus suggested, human beings are *megalocosmos*, 'a great universe within a little one'.[15]

In short, the biblical text ascertains that human persons reflect the image of God by emphasizing that there is something of God in all of them without exception, although human beings are entirely different from God in nature and essence and are not gods. Although the faculties of reason, freedom and discernment are undoubtedly qualities that many human beings possess, and manifestations of the divine image, understanding the image of God cannot be reduced to these characteristics.[16] As Wyatt puts it:

> [I]n Christian thought, the dignity of a human being resides not in what you can do, but in what you are, by creation. Human beings do not need to earn the right to be treated as Godlike beings. Our dignity is *intrinsic*, in the way we have been made.[17]

The image of God reflects a divinely bestowed status, which is equal to all and is independent of any functionality or capacity.

The Function of Stewardship

Because all human beings are created in the image of God in order to experience and receive the communion of the Trinitarian love, they have a special status and place in the created world. It follows that, not only do they all possess a common and equal position, but they also share a special God-given responsibility for overseeing his creation (Gen. 1.26). However, this privileged position of ruler, under God, is also one of steward since human beings remain accountable to him for what they do.[18]

The Holy See's 1965 Pastoral Constitution on the Church in the World *Gaudium et Spes* states:

> For man, created to God's image, received a mandate to subject to himself the earth and all it contains, and to govern the world with justice and holiness; a mandate to relate himself and the totality of things to Him Who was to be acknowledged as the Lord and Creator of all. Thus, by the subjection of all things to man, the name of God would be wonderful in all the earth.[19]

In Christian theology this special role is expressed using the image of a sovereign since human beings are called by God to have the exalted royal position over the visible creation. But this dominion, as so well exemplified by Jesus Christ, is also that of a servant king who is prepared to give of himself completely in service and care for his dominion.

Functional Aspects and Personhood

From a secular perspective, a number of philosophers have proposed that a person is any being that shows a certain capacity to exhibit specific functionalities. This view is sometimes described as the performance theory and is generally associated with having a brain since consciousness is often considered to be necessary. Singer speaks for many when he explains that life without consciousness does not have any value.[20] He defines a human person as 'a being possessing at least at a minimal level, the capacities distinctive of our species, which include consciousness, the ability to relate to others, perhaps even rationality and self-consciousness'.[21]

The capacities or functionalities generally suggested for a being to be a person include:[22]

1 the ability to feel pleasure and pain;
2 the use of language;

3 consciousness and rationality;
4 the possibility of forming rich and meaningful relationships;
5 the potential to have complex emotions;
6 an unparalleled ability to imagine a future and remember the past;
7 a capacity for moral behaviour and moral or altruistic agency;
8 a capacity for free will, responsibility and sacrificial love;
9 a capacity to recognize human dignity in, and confer it to, other persons;
10 a capacity to have faith and believe in a god.[23]

One of the greatest proponents of the association of personhood with the capacity to make autonomous rational decisions was Kant, who noted:

> Beings whose existence depends not on our will but on nature have, nevertheless, if they are not rational beings, only a relative value as means and are therefore called 'things' [*Sachen*]. On the other hand, rational beings are called 'persons' inasmuch as their nature already marks them out as ends in themselves, i.e., a something which is not to be used merely as means and hence there is imposed thereby a limit on all arbitrary use of such beings, which are thus objects of respect.[24]

Interestingly, according to this definition, personhood is not dependent on being a member of the species *Homo sapiens*. Just as some nonhumans may be considered persons, other humans may not be considered persons because they do not exemplify the relevant capacities. Suggested examples include human foetuses, anencephalic children and irreversibly comatose patients. Insofar as performance theorists define the boundaries of a person's existence according to the manifestation of self-conscious rationality, the criterion for determining such boundaries is, at a minimum, the presence of a fully formed and functioning brain.[25]

Such a position, in which personhood is defined by a set of characteristics originating from within the being, is also influenced by Locke's empiricism.[26] In his (1690) *Essay Concerning Human Understanding* he wrote:

> We must consider what person stands for; which I think is a thinking intelligent being, that has reason and reflection, and can consider itself the same thinking thing, in different times and places; which it does only by that consciousness which is inseparable from thinking and seems to me essential to it; it being impossible for anyone to perceive without perceiving that he does perceive.[27]

Being able to perceive that one perceives then includes, for Locke, characteristics such as intelligence, self-consciousness, memory and foresight.

These have also become the main necessary characteristics for person-hood in many contemporary secular positions.[28]

An interesting point to consider here is the moment when human personhood is actually lost through death, though it may continue in an after-life. Indeed, an important question is whether brain death (and the different criteria associated with such a death) suggests that a living being may no longer be a person. This is because the living brain supports important characteristics, such as consciousness, the control of bodily integration, reasoning and feelings, and whatever else is considered essential to be a living person with a personal identity, at least before death.[29]

In seeking to bring together these disparate positions, it is possible to propose the essential property of personhood as either the capacity to actually exhibit self-conscious rational thought (performance theory), or the capacity to exhibit self-conscious rational thought, given time and proper development, both before and/or after death (in an after-life); the latter would be more in line with Christian beliefs.[30]

Functional Aspects and the Moral Status of the Embryo

As already discussed, personhood has been defined by many commentators as being associated with certain characteristics and abilities. For example, Aquinas adopted Boethius's definition of personhood which concurs with performance theory insofar as 'rationality' is taken as its definitive feature. But Aquinas differed from performance theorists because he held that every human being is a person.[31] It is possible to interpret his position by suggesting that all the relevant future capacities of the individual are important at every stage of his or her existence, whether before or even after death (in an after-life). At the embryonic stage, these future capacities are present because the embryo has the complete and whole human body of an embryonic person. It also means that an embryo can be considered as a person because it can develop into a self-conscious rational being even if this may happen only after the death of the embryo in an after-life.

But, as already mentioned, for many secular philosophers person-hood is reduced to those capacities found in this present 'earthly' life. It is, then, these characteristics that define the existence of a person. This means that 'ability criteria' precede 'being'.

From this perspective, personhood can only be considered in the developing foetus (or neonate) if it reaches a stage when it can be demonstrated that certain characteristics are present which enable, for example, conscious activity since they make possible the existence of relationship.[32]

In this way, the bioethical philosopher Walter Glannon, in Canada, writes:

> A person begins to exist when the fetal stage of the organism develops the structure and function of the brain necessary to generate and support consciousness and mental life. This is when the fetus becomes sentient, at around 23–24 weeks of gestation.[33]

In a similar fashion, but in a manner that is less dependent on brain characteristics, Dunstan considered the developmental stage when the foetus awakens a maternal response in, and interaction with, the mother to be crucial:

> If we could know at what point a mother, as a human being, as a source of specifically human relationship, becomes irreplaceably necessary to the development of the human embryo into a human child, then we should see a threshold at which experiment must cease, a step which must not be crossed. For beyond it lies the life of a man, the image and glory of God; and this is holy ground.[34]

However, O'Donovan rejects any notion that a functional brain or any other observable function is necessary for a person to exist:

> The scientific evidence about the development of the unborn child does not prove that the unborn child is a person because that cannot in principle be proved. We cannot accept any equation of personhood with brain activity, genotype, implantation, or whatever for that is to reduce personhood, which is known only in personal engagement, to a function of some observable criteria.[35]

He then asserts that science can only explain and identify with greater accuracy the objective boundaries of an existence, including the 'beginning' of an individual human biological existence. O'Donovan argues that the biological beginning of a human being is sufficiently important for this existence to be respected through personal commitment, adding: 'The only ground we have for risking commitment in the first encounters with the new human being is biological appearance.'[36]

In summary, functions by themselves are not sufficient to determine whether or not an embryonic being is a person. This is because the definition of a person cannot be reduced to science or any observable characteristics. Personhood has a far deeper, more wonderful and more profound meaning than what can be observed by embryonic or other functionalities.

Nonetheless a number of arguments have been attempted to demonstrate that human embryos cannot be considered as persons worthy of protection based on functional characteristics; these will now be addressed.

Functional Aspects and Arguments Pertaining to the Moral Status of the Embryo

In coming near the end of this study concerning the moral status of the human embryo and the manner in which it relates to the image of God, it is now necessary to give a brief overview of the different ways in which the embryo is considered among secular but also Christian writers. This will be undertaken especially in the light of the functional arguments which, as already indicated, have become central to many discussions. In doing so, it will be important to develop the different arguments both carefully and clearly in order to expose their substance while avoiding any bias.

Each of the central arguments raises important moral questions which cannot be answered by one single discipline since a simplistic reduction to one single authority such as biology, philosophy or theology would become meaningless. Moreover, it must be recognized that the 'givenness' of the moral order is not ready to hand but has to be painfully brought together out of the interplay of these disciplines.[37]

To begin with, it is important to clarify the concept of the 'potential' of a human embryo to develop into a human person since this has already led to a lot of misunderstanding.

The Potentiality Argument

The concept of potentiality has proved particularly slippery in the debate relating to the moral status of the human embryo. For some, it has been crucial to their moral stance,[38] although for others the concept does not have any bearing on their understanding of the value and worth of the embryo. As already indicated, the concept of 'potential' may be used in different ways, leading to significant confusion.[39] T. F. Torrance talks of 'a serious ambiguity'.[40]

For example, sperm and egg cells have potential since they assist in bringing a person into existence, but they are not given any moral value as such. The concept of 'potential' can, therefore, relate to completely different notions. As Harris points out: 'We are all potentially dead, but no one supposes that this fact constitutes a reason for treating us as if we were already dead.'[41]

The bioethicist John Mahoney emphasizes the concept of 'promise' in preference to 'potential', while also noting: 'What appears very elusive to grasp is the moral purchasing power simply of promise as such.'[42]

Another way of understanding the concept of potentiality is to carefully distinguish its meaning from the concept of *opportunity*. Thus, if an appropriate environment is denied to the embryo, it will certainly not develop, though this would not demonstrate a lack of potential. But this is exactly the sort of argument that is used by some commentators. For example, Singer maintains that IVF emphasizes the requirement of an external intervention for both fertilization and subsequent implantation of the embryo.[43] This suggests that through external interventions both (1) the moral status of gametes is very different from that of the resulting embryo and (2) the moral status of the embryo in the laboratory is very different from when it is implanted in a woman. In the same manner, Warnock asserts:

> To say that eggs and sperm cannot by themselves become human but only if bound together, does not seem to me to differentiate them from the early embryo which by itself will not become human either, but will die unless it is implanted.[44]

This implies that because IVF embryos in the laboratory have no potential if they are not implanted into a woman, they cannot have the same moral status as those that are implanted, and thus may be used for destructive research. But this is a circular argument since it suggests that there is no potential *if* opportunity is denied and, because there is no potentiality, opportunity *is* denied.[45] In order to address such empty rhetoric there is a need to distinguish between what ability a being has within itself and what it receives from its environment. For instance, Rollinson gives as an example: 'If oxygen is withdrawn from a room full of law students they will die, but it does not imply they are not potential lawyers!'[46]

Here, however, the definition of 'potential' needs to be clarified since there are generally three ways of considering this concept.

Full Moral Status of the Embryo Who Has a Potential to Develop

First, it is possible to consider an embryo as having a full moral status with the potential to continue in its development for a certain amount of time (be it short or long). This would mean accepting the moral imperative to fully respect and protect the embryo from the moment of its creation, thus prohibiting destructive embryo experimentation.

For example, T. F. Torrance recognizes that the potential of a human embryo is not the potential to become something else, but of becoming what it essentially is. This can be described as the difference between the potential *to produce* (something else) and the potential *to become*.[47] It mirrors Tertullian when he affirmed, 'that is a man which is going to be one; you have the fruit already in its seed'.[48] In a similar fashion Ramsey stated: 'The human individual comes into existence as a minute informational speck ... his subsequent pre-natal and post-natal development may be described as a process of becoming what he already is from the moment he was conceived.'[49]

In other words, a living healthy embryo already has within it the potential for full development into an infant.[50] Iglesias summarizes this position:

> The actual power to achieve a particular type of development must always have been present prior to the development, and is therefore significant in determining what kind of being we are dealing with, even in the earliest stages of its existence.[51]

This means that an early embryo has built into it a complete, intrinsic and inherent potential which allows a new individual to unfold. The ability to develop as a person, given the right environment, is already there. Such an understanding implies that full respect and protection must be given to the human embryo from the moment of its creation.

The Embryo Has the Potential to Develop into a Being with Greater Moral Status

The second way of understanding the concept of 'potential' represents the situation whereby the embryo has a partial moral status, at most, but could develop into a being with a greater or full moral status. In other words, the embryo may have some kind of limited moral value, depending on the stage of development and because it could grow into a being with greater or full moral status.

In this case, the embryo may either (1) be left to develop in such a way that it does attain greater or full moral status or (2) be destroyed before it attains such a status.

For some commentators, such as D. Gareth Jones, it follows that the potentiality principle leads to a gradualist approach to the moral status of the embryo. He argues that equating the potential to become a human person with being an actual human being overlooks biological and human development,[52] though he still maintains that the potentiality principle gives the foetus some claim to life. This also reflects the position of Millican, who argues that, if it is true that the moral status of 'potential personhood' is less than that of 'actual personhood', then at each growing developmental stage the potential to become the next stage has less moral status than the actual next stage.[53] Such an argument repeated for each stage of the growing foetus results in a developmental approach.

From this perspective, an early embryo does not have any, or has only a partial, moral status, and it is only because the embryo has a potential to become something else, with more moral value, that its present status is given in a kind of projected anticipation.

However, a number of difficulties arise with such an approach. To begin with, it is difficult to give an entity only some moral status and a certain number of rights just because it can eventually become something else. This is especially the case if it is remembered that all human persons eventually die and become corpses. There is also the possibility that some embryos, for a number of reasons, may never eventually attain the anticipated full moral status of a person who has been born. Questions can then be asked as to why they should be considered morally different from embryos who do eventually develop into a child.[54]

Thus, on the grounds of coherence, such an understanding of 'potential' is difficult to accept.

The Moral Status of the Embryo is Uncertain

The third way in which to understand the concept of 'potential' reflects uncertainty regarding the exact moral status of an embryo. In other words, while it may 'potentially' already be entitled to full moral status, it is impossible to determine this with any certainty.

Most of the time, such a usage of the term 'potential' reflects sincere agnosticism relating to the moral status of a created being. This happens, for example, when those who would normally give full moral status to an early fully human embryo have to consider the moral status of an embryo obtained through the fertilization of a chimpanzee egg with human sperm.

This survey of the concept of potentiality makes it now possible to discuss some of the extensive arguments of the gradualist position.

The Gradualist Position

One of the most common positions in contemporary society relating to the moral status of the human embryo is the gradualist approach. This maintains that as the embryo or foetus develops, and its body differentiates into different parts, its moral status also increases and is entitled to a greater claim of protection. Certain specific stages have to be determined for legislative reasons (such as the UK Warnock Report's recommendation to prohibit experimentation on human embryos after 14 days from fertilization), but gradualists do not have any robust, reasoned approach as to the moral status of the embryo or foetus. This means that bound-aries are set because they are necessary but these are, to some extent, arbitrary with no specific defining point being established. For example, the previous Anglican Archbishop of York, John Habgood, rhetorically asks: '[B]irth may be the equivalent of full dawn. But when was first light?'[55] The gradualist position of Edwards is also typical, as in this comment on the prohibition of human embryonic research in the UK after the fourteenth day from fertilization:

> In my opinion rules like that cannot be made about embryology which is a gradual process of steady change, for there are no specific days here or there which can be used to justify a belief that something new and fundamental has occurred, and which indicates without any doubt that research should then end.[56]

This basic premise is also accepted by Warnock herself who stated that 'there is no particular point in the process that is more important than another'.[57] It is interesting, however, that for many commentators this rather weak approach is the only perspective being considered.[58]

From a Christian perspective, some of the greatest proponents of the gradualist viewpoint were Mahoney, who comes from a Roman Catholic background, and Dunstan.[59] Mahoney applies the French philosopher and Jesuit priest Pierre Teilhard de Chardin's (1881–1955) evolutionary term 'hominization' to human embryological development in arguing for a gradual and delayed, rather than an instantaneous, *hominization*.[60]

The German Jesuit priest Karl Rahner (1904–84) also borrowed from de Chardin the term 'hominization', which he uses for both the grad-ual evolution of the human species and the gradual development of the human embryo, seeing them as comparable processes of development: 'In both cases a not yet human biological organism develops towards a condition in which the coming into existence of a spiritual soul has its sufficient biological substratum.'[61]

In a similar fashion, the Dutch Christian ethicist Egbert Schroten main-tained that 'embryology ... pushes us into the direction of a "process anthropology". One is not immediately a person from the beginning, but one becomes a human being, a person.'[62] This gradualist perspective is also a contemporary Jewish view.[63]

The possibility of considering the moral status of the embryo as increasing either gradually or when it reaches a certain stage of develop-ment has proved to be very popular in society. But there has always been a difficulty in rigorously defining the process by which this actually happens.[64]

At the very basis of the gradualist understanding are certain philosophical suppositions. These include the view that factual decisions should, and can, be based on empirical observation but that, since the moral status of the human embryo cannot be determined by scientific observable data, it can only be considered from a subjective perspective based on moral judgement.

It is the position of Warnock who indicated that the moral status of the embryo is one of 'judgement and decision according to a particular moral standpoint. It is not a question of fact, but a question of value.'[65]

This is the basis for the gradualists' moral agnosticism which, in all honesty, must also extend to the moral status of the adult human being making the moral judgement about the embryo. Indeed, the moral status of neither the embryo nor the adult can be determined by science. In fact, biology or any other scientific discipline will never be able to demonstrate, logically, that a rational, autonomous, sensitive being has any moral worth. It can only show that the human being is a pile of biological cells of the species *Homo sapiens*.

What should be considered, therefore, is not human biological matter but human personhood which, as already indicated, transcends science and the cosmos. This means that defining the time and stage when a new human *individual person* (defined by Aquinas as 'that which is undivided in itself and distinct from others'[66]) begins his or her existence is the most important and critical question.

Another difficulty with the gradualist position is that the moral status or human rights of an embryonic or foetal entity is dependent on whether it attains a specific structure, function or capacity that characterizes human persons. These include, for example, whether it has a functioning nervous system, is viable outside the womb or is even conscious.[67] But this would then mean that infants, but also other individuals such as those affected by severe mental disabilities or suffering from dementia, may not be recognized as persons.[68] As O'Donovan explains:

> The perfect specimen of humanity, mentally, physically and spiritually developed, has become the mark to which any candidate for humanity must in some measure approximate. Higher and higher criteria of individuation have been assumed, so that more and more living creatures, whose bodies are organized in a human kind of way, are deemed by virtue of their failure to realise full human potential, 'not yet persons', and so not yet protected.[69]

One of the main problems with the gradualist position, however, is that it does not indicate whether moral status is acquired incrementally or at some specific stage after fertilization. If it is the former, then both the human body and the soul are acquired incrementally if the important principle of an ensouled body and an embodied soul is to be maintained. But no explanation is usually given about the manner in which this process can actually take place. Are some souls (living beings) more important, morally, than others?

If, on the other hand, moral status is acquired at a specific developmental stage after creation, then the gradualist position must accept that the soul and the biological body are brought into existence at different stages.

As already noted, this kind of philosophical dualism, whereby a distinction is made between the embryo or the early foetus and its soul, has its origins in the philosophy of Aristotle for whom the embryonic human body developed through different stages with different kinds of souls. For Aristotle, the real question was not, 'When does human life begin?' but 'When does individual personal life exist?'[70] This means that before full personal ensoulment takes place, the moral status of a biological entity remains limited. Reflecting this kind of thinking, the British philosopher Michael Coughlan writes:

> Before personhood is attained, the life of the embryo or fetus is not the bodily life of the person to be, but the life of the body of the person to be. That is to say, the life of the embryo from which I grew was not a stage of my life, but a stage in the life of my body ... The life of the embryo was a stage in the life of the body which came to be my body when I came to be. It cannot properly be described as 'my body' before then.[71]

But this kind of dualism, whereby a certain dissociation exists between the union of the body and the soul, has generally been rejected by many early and contemporary scholars.[72] For example, Tertullian argued that 'the flesh, being conceived, formed, and generated along with the soul from its earliest existence in the womb, is mixed up with it likewise in all its operations'.[73] For Tertullian, there is never a moment in the entire existence of a person where the body and the soul are not present together:

> We have already demonstrated the conjunction of the body and the soul, from the concretion of their very seminations to the complete formation of the *foetus*. We now maintain their conjunction likewise from the birth onwards; in the first place, because they both grow together, only each in a different manner suited to the diversity of their nature.[74]

Maximus the Confessor, for his part, did not only contest the pre-existence of the soul with respect to the body but rejected any suggestion that there was a pre-existence of the body in relation to the soul. He argued, instead, that there is always a simultaneous origin and coexistence of the soul and the body.

One of the arguments given by Maximus supporting this inherent union of the soul and the body was that they form harmoniously ordered parts of a whole human person. They exist as elements of this whole person and must, therefore, be everywhere and in every case perfectly simultaneous with respect to their coming into existence. This is because they form in their union an entire entity which is that of a human person. In other words, the soul and the body of the human person cannot exist separately one before the other from a chronological perspective.[75]

This reflects the Hebraic manner of understanding human beings in that a person does not *have* a soul but *is* a soul. Similarly, a person does not *have* a body but *is* a body.[76]

The human soul, moreover, cannot exist in degrees. A human person always consists of a whole body and a whole soul which give this individual the same worth and value as that of any other person. The body or the soul of a person cannot exist in degrees or have less value at different stages in time or in comparison with another person. This would otherwise undermine the very basis of the concept of personhood and civilized society.

The gradualist position and delayed animation, whereby a human living being may exist without a soul or with a lesser soul, giving this individual less moral status, is difficult therefore to accept from a rational perspective.

It is probably because of pressures arising from secular society to accept many forms of abortion and the use of embryos in destructive research that a lot of confused theology has resulted with respect to the gradualist position. Indeed, this required an uncoupling of the human soul from the body in order to deny the full moral status of early human embryos.

For example, Reginald Gardner, a Christian gynaecologist and Pentecostal minister, whose book *Abortion: The Personal Dilemma*, published in the early 1970s, was very influential in leading many Christians to a compromised view on abortion, argued that the soul only enters the body when the baby takes his or her first breath.[77]

But O'Donovan laments this confusion:

In a period when the most orthodox ... theological anthropology has been that the Bible teaches 'body-soul unity', it is ironical that Christians should have allowed their view of the fetal soul to drift upon a sea of speculation without seeking anchorage in any account of the fetal body.[78]

This is a case of society influencing theology and not Christian theology witnessing to society.

A far more rational perspective which seeks to challenge this idea of delayed animation is given by Breck, who explains that, from an Orthodox perspective, even for embryos: 'Personhood, then, depends neither on an "infused soul" nor on one's conscious relationship with others. It depends rather on the love of God that embraces the bearer of his divine image from conception, through death and beyond.' He continues:

> Language such as 'ensoulment,' 'infusion of an immaterial rational soul,' or simply 'a principle of immaterial individuality or selfhood,' sounds dualistic to Orthodox ears ... From an Eastern patristic (and biblical) perspective, the soul or *nephesh* constitutes the very personhood of the individual (Gen 1:26–27; 2:7). Accordingly, one may properly affirm 'I am a soul' rather than 'I have a soul.'[79]

The suggestion, therefore, that the material body is animated by a rational soul which is created separately and is then infused into this body at fertilization, at implantation, or at some subsequent stage in its development, is based on a mistaken understanding of Christian anthropology.[80]

The Concept of Full Moral Status May Be Undermined by the Gradualist Position

In the cases where full moral status of the embryo is held to be acquired either (1) incrementally or (2) at some other specific stage after the embryo is brought into existence, there is a risk that the very manner of conferring moral status in this way may undermine the concept. This is because the bestowing of full moral status becomes arbitrary and dependent on human decisions. For example, because of utilitarian pressures, there is a risk that the stages in which moral status is recognized in the human embryo or foetus are pushed back to ever later development periods. Eventually, the 'special status' of the embryo or foetus may be completely undermined or even become non-existent.

In 1984, for instance, Warnock (one of the main architects of the embryology legislation in the UK) commented, in her report that led to the Human Fertilisation and Embryology Act of 1990, that the embryo 'ought to have a special status' under British law.[81] But in December 2002 her position had changed significantly: 'I regret that in the original report that led up to the 1990 legislation we used words such as "respect for the embryo" ... I think that what we meant by the rather foolish expression "respect" was that the early embryo should never be used frivolously for research purposes'. She added:

[Y]ou cannot respectfully pour something down the sink – which is the fate of the embryo after it has been used for research, or if it is not going to be used for research or for anything else.[82]

This example demonstrates how an entity which should have been considered as having a special status in the 1980s no longer has such a status and, in fact, has lost all moral status. From this perspective, it is apparently only the biomedical research (and not the embryo) that should now be respected in the UK.

It is also unfortunate that the general public is, generally, unaware that embryos are, at present, simply being considered as useful 'piles of cells' in biomedical research. Indeed, since the concept of a 'special status' for the embryo was always completely subjective it was inevitable that this ambiguous gradualist position would eventually become ethically meaningless.

The Scottish ethicist Kenneth Boyd, seeking to defend a gradualist position on the moral status of the human embryo, commented that, however much Christian thinkers try to be 'objective', 'the moral question could only be finally settled if we knew, "how God sees early embryos". But this is precisely what we do not know'.[83]

But maybe this is exactly what is known if the argument about the image of God in embryos is taken seriously. This is because there is never a moment when these embryos are not loved by God, the creator, as was confirmed when the Word of God became an incarnate embryonic person in Christ. Even though some commentators may disparagingly present this as an extreme position,[84] it should be noted that the incarnation, itself, is extreme in its wonderful workings of redemption and grace.

Who Decides Whether Embryos Should Have Full Moral Status with the Gradualist Position?

Concerns also exist as to the organizations or persons who would be given responsibility to decide whether an embryo should be recognized as having full moral status, and whether the decision should even be taken by other human beings. This is because human decision making is dangerous and unreliable. For example, before the slave trade was abolished, or during the Second World War, many persons and governments believed that specific categories of individuals did not have full moral status and considered them second-class citizens. Indeed, when moral status is decided by others, there is always the danger that this status may be taken away by others.

Another question is the manner in which this moral status is recognized. Should this simply take place by a majority vote in an assembly, such as a parliament, which may be swayed either way for a number of reasons and could even reverse its decision in a subsequent vote by different representatives? Making a decision in this way on the crucially important matter of the moral status of an entity may seem completely inappropriate.

For example, when deciding whether human embryos should be created for destructive research, the influential Warnock Committee in the 1980s agreed only by a very small majority of nine votes to seven in favour of creating such embryos.[85] This decision then went on to influence the UK and many other foreign parliaments to take a similar stance.[86]

How Should Full Moral Status Be Ascribed to the Embryo in the Gradualist Position?

There are also misgivings as to the stage in which full moral status is recognized for the embryo or foetus within the gradualist position since this can be considered arbitrary or subjective. Indeed, a number of different stages have been suggested at which an embryo or foetus can be considered to deserve partial or full protection. These include:

- implantation and the apparition of the primitive streak, corresponding to the end of individuation and the beginning of neurological development (about 14 days after fertilization);
- the legal limit for abortions in many continental European countries (12 weeks after fertilization);
- the present stage at which a human foetus may be viable (21–22 weeks after fertilization);
- the legal limit of a termination in the UK (24 weeks after fertilization);
- the birth of the infant, at which stage most legislations confer full protection;
- after birth, as suggested by some professional ethicists who believe that infanticide should be legalized in the UK under certain circumstances.[87]

Such a list implies that no universally accepted stage has yet been determined by those who support the gradualist position. As a result, there is a lot that remains unclear, speculative and uncertain in this position where an ill-defined 'intermediate' or 'special' moral status of the human embryo or foetus exists – an ambiguity open to serious rational questioning on a matter that is not inconsequential.

The Full Protective Position

The full protective position argues that the embryo should be considered as a new, complete and whole person as soon as it comes into existence as an organism and at no later stage. In other words, an embryonic person exists as soon as an integrated, self-developing and self-maintaining, organized unity exists which retains both in space and in time a wholeness which precedes and produces its organic elements.

In contrast to an ordinary somatic cell, an early human embryo is a new whole being of the human species. A central qualitative change has occurred which is different from any other point in the developmental process. The leading French geneticist who discovered Trisomy 21, Jérome Lejeune (1926–94), commented: 'Life has a very, very long history, but each individual has a very neat beginning, the moment of its conception.'[88]

The full protective position, which argues that a human embryo should be respected and protected as a human person from the moment of embryonic creation, is based on the premise that only at this stage is a new member of the species *Homo sapiens* in existence. This is because at no other point in embryonic development is there any further, significant, qualitative change.

In contrast to building a house out of different bricks which do not express a plan of what the completed house will be like, the very early embryo is already a whole and complete being reflecting a human biological person. As explained by the American biologist Maureen Condic, the cells, tissues and organs produced during embryonic development 'do not somehow "generate" the embryo (as if there were some unseen, mysterious "manufacturer" directing this process), they are produced *by the embryo* as it directs its own development to more mature stages of human life'.[89] This is unlike the builder who cannot just lay his first brick and leave it to build a house. A human embryo does not develop into a human person. It is a full human person.[90]

In this sense there is no discontinuity between the fellowship of God and the parents towards the child who brought it into existence as an early embryo. There is no moment, in the existence of the embryo, when it is not a person in fellowship with God and his or her parents.

This position also reflects the idea that human life should not be considered as having different values at different stages in time. From God's eternal perspective (outside of time which was created with the universe) a human life can be seen in a sense as being 'complete' even as it occurs. In this case, the term 'human life' could be replaced with 'human personal existence' both before and after death.[91] Indeed, any appropriate study of humanity may only be possible from the perspective of a resurrected body. In this regard, earthly humanity is maybe far too preoccupied with only earthly aspects.

Finally, it should be noted that, for those who accept that human embryos do indeed have the same moral status as children who have been born, the use of human embryos for destructive experimentation would, unfortunately, be similar to some kind of human sacrifice of children (the wording may, sadly, be apposite) to the benefit of biomedical research. Such a blunt conclusion may be difficult to accept in a modern society but this truth is, unfortunately, impossible to avoid.

Moreover, the number of lives saved through such research cannot have any bearing on the way a human embryonic being is considered. This is because the moral status of a being cannot be reduced to his or her usefulness in research.[92]

Arguments Opposing the Full Moral Status of the Human Embryo and their Responses

In the debate concerning the moral status of the human embryo a number of influential arguments have been employed which generally come from the functionalist perspective. In other words, the aim is to demonstrate that early embryos cannot be considered as having the same moral status as adult human beings because they do not have certain characteristics.

The following section will present some of the most influential of these arguments, which deny full moral status to early human embryos, while opening them up to more considered analysis and thereby questioning the conclusions which they tend to make.

Viability Outside the Womb

As mentioned previously, for many in secular society a specific structure, function or capacity is seen as necessary in an embryonic entity before it can be recognized as being a human person with full moral status. In this regard, one of the most important properties often mentioned is that of viability outside the womb – a capacity which has generally been recognized as being reached earlier in the gestation of the foetus over the past decades. Indeed, with the introduction of new technology, a 22–23-week foetus can now survive birth in many modern neonatal intensive care clinics. In the future, it is likely that even younger foetuses may survive.

This means that linking the recognition of full moral status to the viability of the foetus outside the womb reduces the argument to technological improvements, which is not very consistent.[93]

A more reasonable position is to suggest that it is not the length of time that a person exists, before or after birth, that matters but the fact that they actually exist (even just for a few seconds), are alive and 'complete' and 'whole'. Thus, the question of whether an embryo is 'viable' is not morally important, since all embryos are alive and all biological life in this universe is ultimately non-viable (all biological life eventually dies).

Small Number of Undifferentiated Cells

One of the more common arguments against recognizing full moral status for early embryos is based on the fact that they are composed of a very small number of undifferentiated cells. As the British biologist Sir Ian Wilmut (the creator of Dolly the sheep) observed when defending destructive embryo research: 'A critical element in this [view] is to recognise we would only be working at a very early stage with a maximum of 200 cells', adding, 'I wouldn't think of a human embryo at that stage as being a person.'[94]

From a theological perspective, however, it is useful to remember that from God's standpoint, which is the true basis of all value and worth, the number of cells or their state of differentiation in a person may not really matter. Instead, as already indicated, it is whether the embryo exists, is complete and is whole that is important.

Small Size

Another argument related to the small number of cells that are present in an early embryo is the somewhat strange suggestion that it should not be recognized as having full moral status because it has a very small size. As the American biologist and Nobel Laureate David Baltimore commented: 'To me, a tiny mass of cells that has never been in a uterus is hardly a human being – even if it has the potential to become human.'[95]

But, in this regard, it may be appropriate to remember that, from God's perspective and from beyond the galaxies and the universe, size is of course of no consequence. Considered from this divine viewpoint, the size of every adult human being would be even smaller than that of embryos seen from the scale of human individuals. As the American political scientist Hadley Arkes pointed out:

> The question, however, is not what the organism 'looks' like, but what it is. The embryo may not look like the average undergraduate – some people may even think that it looks like a tadpole – but it is never the equivalent of a tadpole even when it 'looks' like one. That apparently formless mass is already 'programmed' with the instructions that will make its tissues the source of specialized functions and aptitudes discriminably different from the organs and talents of tadpoles. This

'tadpole' is likely to come out with hands and feet and with a capacity to conjugate verbs.[96]

In the end, however, it should be remembered that, without God, the whole universe, including galaxies, embryos and adult individuals, has no worth and is in fact a 'pile of dust'. The human embryo or adult can only receive incredible meaning, worth and value through the love of God. This is wonderfully manifested in the birth, death and resurrection of Jesus Christ whereby God demonstrated that he values and loves his children to such an extent that he was prepared to go to the cross for them out of love.

Twinning and Recombination

A more substantial challenge to the position stating that very early embryos can be considered as persons relates to their biological capacity and characteristics *before* the stage of segmentation which, though not clearly defined in biology,[97] is considered to take place at about the thirteenth or fourteenth day after fertilization.[98] Indeed, this is the last stage in which (1) the twinning of one embryo into two distinct embryos may take place or (2) two or more early embryos (which would normally develop to give two or more non-identical twins or individuals) may combine to form one single individual embryo. These two possibilities will now be examined in turn.

Twinning

Interestingly, an early embryo up to the 14-day stage following fertilization is sometimes able to give rise to two (or more) identical daughter cell-clusters, which may develop separately, and eventually be born, as identical twins (or multiples). It means that a single embryo is capable of giving rise to two genetically identical but distinct individual persons.[99]

As a result, it is suggested that individual personhood cannot exist for the early embryo. In other words, since it is uncertain whether the original embryo will become one or more persons, it is argued that the original embryo cannot then be considered as a person.[100]

This is the argument of a number of influential scholars such as the Australian Roman Catholic priest Norman Ford, in his book *When Did I Begin?* He states:

The first cleavage produces two identical cells of about equal size, each with 46 chromosomes. Each cell is an individual living being that is distinct and totipotent. Each is able to give rise to an adult human being. Whatever potential is possessed by the original fertilized egg is also possessed by each of its daughter cells. The existence of monozygotic or identical twins from the two-cell stage suggests in a convincing way ... that the fertilized ovum is far from being actually organized into a single continuing ontological human individual.

Thus, according to Ford: 'An individual that was capable of becoming one or more persons could only be a potential person, not a distinct actual person ... The same would apply for a cluster of individual cells with the same capacity.'[101]

He then goes on to question what actually happens to the one-cell embryo when it splits in two, suggesting that one human individual cannot give rise to two distinct human individuals without the original embryo ceasing to exist. In this regard, rather than arguing that the original human individual ceased to exist in the twinning process, he believes that it would be more credible to accept that the original individual never really existed as a person in the first place. Thus, for Ford, the evidence is not convincing that an individual continuity can exist from the one-cell embryo (zygote) to the foetus, infant, child and adult.[102]

As already indicated, the 14-day segmentation stage after the formation of the human embryo is also about the stage when the primitive streak begins to appear from which the first rudiment of the nervous system is developed. The British biologist Anne McLaren (1927–2007) wrote:

If we are talking not about the origin of life ... but about the origin of an individual life, one can trace back directly from the newborn baby to the foetus, and back further to the origin of the individual embryo at the primitive streak stage in the embryonic plate at sixteen or seventeen days. If one tries to trace back further than that there is no longer a coherent entity. Instead there is a larger collection of cells, some of which are going to take part in the subsequent development of the embryo and some of which aren't.[103]

Similarly, Warnock, who chaired the committee that was prominent in shaping human fertilization and embryology legislation in the UK, which had such a significant influence on the rest of the world, explained why this group believed the primitive streak stage to be very important:

We, the majority of the Inquiry, recommend that research on the human embryo should be brought to an end on the fourteenth day because of the development then of the primitive streak. Up to that time, it is difficult to think of the embryo as an individual, because it might still become two individuals ... The collection of cells though loosely strung together, is hardly yet one thing, nor is it several. It is not yet determined to be either one or several.

It means that up to this time, Warnock suggests that the whole collection of cells cannot be thought of as an individual embryo.[104]

Thus, one of the more common positions which questions whether embryos less than two weeks old should be fully protected is that they have not yet developed into indivisible human beings. Indeed, a number of commentators maintain that biological stability in an organism is required before its individuality can be firmly established.[105] It is for this reason that the Warnock Committee recommended that research on human embryos must stop at the 14-day stage.[106]

This position was also taken up by Ramsey, who had earlier favoured fertilization as the decisive step, when he wrote:

It might be asserted that it is at the time of segmentation, and not earlier, that life comes to be the individual human being it is ever thereafter to be ... If there is a moment in the development of these nascent lives of ours, subsequent to fertilisation and prior to birth (or graduation from college), at which it would be reasonable to believe that an individual human life begins and therefore to be inviolate, that moment is at the stage when segmentation may or may not take place.[107]

In order to try to address the argument stating that an individual cannot exist before the 14-day stage, Iglesias suggests that the original organism may not cease to exist when it divides in two. In other words, an embryonic division may only represent one part splitting off from the original whole. The part fragmented off has the capacity to become a new whole but the 'parent' continues to remain a whole, though at first somewhat depleted. There is, therefore, no division of living beings which cease to exist as total wholes.[108]

In response, however, Ford considers this argument to be insufficient. He compares Iglesias' proposal to the horticultural equivalent of taking a cutting from a plant for it to grow into a new plant while the original continues its individual existence. But he questions whether what happens with plants is an appropriate analogy. For example, an early embryo containing four cells can divide into two genetically identical but distinct individuals. Moreover, because the cells in the four-cell embryo are totipotent they could also all be separated from one another to give rise to four distinct entities which, if they were developed in the right environment, would give rise to quadruplets. In the light of this, Ford concludes that individuation can have meaning only if there is some shape and stability in the embryo preventing it from dividing into new individuals.[109]

Nevertheless, the scientific possibility of Iglesias' argument may have been shown when a pair of identical (monozygotic) twins was discovered, one of which was affected by Down's syndrome (having three chromosome 21s in its cells) while the other was normal (with the expected two chromosome 21s in its cells). In this case, it was suggested that the trisomic twin was the original individual created through fertilization, while the second (unaffected) embryo was created through the separation of one or a number of cells from the trisomic embryo; a procedure which apparently enabled the cell(s) of the second embryo to lose one chromosome 21 resulting in an embryo with the normal two chromosome 21s.[110]

Moreover, it is difficult to understand why the argument based on the cloning of plants in horticulture, whereby a branch of a shrub is cut off and planted to form another shrub next to the original one, is dismissed. Indeed, it would resemble the cloning of an adult person using his or her cells if this ever became possible. A new person would have been split off from the original individual, but this does not mean that the initial individual was not a person.

It is interesting how influential the twinning argument has become over the years, which suggests that, because a living entity may give rise to two distinct new individuals (by whatever means), then the original living entity cannot be an individual. This is surprising because strong counter-arguments have been presented, and none more so than that of the simple flatworm. As the American philosopher Patrick Lee and the jurist Robert George write:

> Viewed biologically, the occurrence of monozygotic twinning and the possibility of fusion fail to show that in the first fourteen days the cells within the embryo constituted only an incidental mass. Just as the division of a single, whole flatworm into two whole flatworms does not show that prior to that division the flatworm was not a unitary individual, just so with the human embryo that twins.

Thus, in a similar manner to when a flatworm is cut in two giving rise to two new parts which can both become new whole flatworms, when an early human embryo splits in two it is also possible for the two parts to become new embryos. But this does not mean that, prior to division, either the original flatworm or the embryo did not exist as single, complex, actively developing, living organisms.[111]

In the splitting of a two-cell embryo it may be impossible to say whether the original embryo remains or two new ones are created. Some commentators, such as D. A. Jones,[112] suggest that the process of twinning may be considered as (1) the ending of existence of one embryonic individual (a form of death) to give rise to two new individuals, or (2) the continuation of the original individual in its development from which a number of cells separate giving rise to a new individual.[113] What is certain is that, as with the original flatworm, the original embryo did exist as a whole individual.

The Australian Jesuit priest and philosopher Thomas Daly (1924–2014) summarizes this argument:

> There is nothing philosophically troublesome about one organized whole developing within it another circle of organization which eventually breaks off from it while the original individual retains its identity. One living thing has given rise to another and this can happen in a wide variety of ways, most of which are quite familiar, though so many writers on the embryo assume that this would destroy all previous individuality. The twinning that they see as an unsuperable [sic] obstacle to previous establishment of identity is no more difficult to explain than is the vegetative propagation of a plant by removing a bulb, or by taking a cutting. An amoeba is no less of a real concrete individual living thing if later on it reproduces and initiates a new amoeba by fission.[114]

Accordingly, individuality is compatible with divisibility. To accept that an early embryo is a human person is dependent not on whether or not it can divide but, instead, on whether a dynamic unity and organic system exists. When an embryo splits in two, what matters is that both before and after the separation of the embryo into two new embryos all the entities are distinct whole organisms, embryos and thus persons.[115]

Recombination

Arguments relating to individuation have also focused on the possibility, already mentioned, of two or more early embryos in the womb of a woman (which would normally develop to give two or more siblings) combining to form one single individual embryo. Again questions are asked as to the moral status of these two or more early embryos since, apparently, they can fuse to become one single individual.[116]

This took place, for example, for a woman who discovered that her sons were in fact only half-brothers even though she had conceived naturally with her husband.[117] In this case, researchers suggested that the most likely explanation was that her body, including her ovaries, was the result of two non-identical early embryonic twin girls who had fused.

Again, it can be suggested that the combination could be considered as either (1) the ending of biological existence (a form of death) of two embryonic individuals to give rise to one new individual, or (2) the fusion of one of the embryos into the second one (a form of death for this first embryo), after which the second embryo continues its original individual existence.[118] But, once more, it may never be possible to know for certain which one of these alternatives is true.

Coughlan comments: 'It looks as though there has been a death without a body! Apart from any other considerations, this would give rise to theological difficulties in connection with the doctrine of the resurrection of the body.'[119] But would it? Does a human body actually have to remain in existence for it to be resurrected? There is indeed no basis for this in theology.

More interestingly from a biological perspective, the possibility of two individual early embryos combining to form only one single new embryo is similar to what is already happening in normal human reproduction. In this case, two persons eventually give rise to one person (their child), the parents eventually die and the child survives.[120]

The capacity for a whole living organism to split or to combine with others to form new living wholes is something that should also come as no surprise to Christians. Indeed, these kinds of possibilities are similar to what may already happen in living Christian churches whereby one single, whole church may eventually divide to become two (or more) whole churches. Or two (or more) whole churches may combine to eventually become one whole, single church. Each time, however, it would be impossible to suggest that the original churches, as living, whole entities, did not exist.

To summarize, in all these different cases, the troublesome questions of whether one, two or more whole individuals are contained in an early embryo and whether it has full moral status become unimportant if each embryonic entity is considered to be a whole person in the sense of 'being' a soul rather than 'possessing' a soul.[121] In other words, the manner in which an embryo was created or ceases to exist is actually irrelevant to its existence, its life and whether it should be ascribed full moral status. Instead, what matters is that the entity exists, is complete and is whole in space, throughout the time of its life on earth (even if this means only a few seconds or minutes) and beyond death.

Totipotent Cells May also Be Embryos

As already indicated, totipotent cells are cells which should also be considered as embryos in their own right, if they are on their own, since they can then behave as mature whole organisms. As Condic explains:

> Producing a mature organism requires the ability to both generate all the cells of the body and to organize them in a specific temporal and spatial sequence; i.e. to undergo a coordinated process of development.

Totipotency in this strict sense is demonstrated by the ability of an isolated cell to produce a fertile, adult individual. Consequently, a cell that is totipotent is also a one-cell embryo; i.e., a cell that is capable of generating a globally coordinated developmental sequence.[122]

Studies with a number of mammals have demonstrated that if a single cell from an early embryo up to the eight-cell stage is taken and implanted into the corresponding female animal, then a pregnancy and even the birth of a new animal is sometimes achievable. This happens even though a declining success rate is noticed with ever older cells from the one- to the eight-cell stages of the embryos.[123]

A successful pregnancy has not yet been obtained from cells isolated from a 16-cell mammalian embryo. As a result, it is believed that cells in a 16-cell embryo are no longer totipotent; and even before this stage it is likely that only some of them may be totipotent.[124] It should also be noted that a grouping of early embryonic cells in a cell-cluster may be totipotent even though some cells, by themselves, in this cluster have lost such a property.

Because of these totipotent cell characteristics, the Embryo Protection Act (12.13.1990) in Germany defines an embryo as 'the fertilised egg from the moment of the fusion of the cell nuclei of egg and spermium, and every totipotent cell taken from an embryo since these cells have the potential to develop into a human individual'.[125] Moreover, this Act states that it is forbidden 'to dispose of an embryo, or to deliver, acquire, or use an embryo for purposes not serving its preservation';[126] this means that embryos are protected from the one-cell stage until their complete implantation in the uterus. As a result, according to German legislation, every cell up to the eight-cell stage of the embryo (reached on the third or fourth day of embryonic development) which is separated from the original embryo is also under the strongest possible protection. This is because it is probable (subject to confirmation) that some of these cells are totipotent and may legally qualify as embryos in their own right.[127]

Consequently, under German law, all biopsies of totipotent cells for research or analytical purposes are similarly protected even if the original embryo, from which the cells were taken, is not harmed. But if the cells are not totipotent then the removal of cells for genetic testing (in which the removed cells would be destroyed) becomes possible.[128] This means that only cells taken from an embryo later than the fourth day after fertilization can be used in Germany for testing since, by then, all the early cells making up the original embryo have lost totipotency.[129]

In the light of these properties of totipotent cells, another argument that is sometimes used to question the full moral status of very early human embryos is that it would be impossible to know whether just one or several embryos are present, all at the same time, in the early embryonic cluster of totipotent cells.[130] For example, it may be possible to separate an eight-cell embryo into eight separate cells which could all be considered as embryos, in their own right, and then recombine all of them again to form one single embryo (or any other number of embryos depending on the number of cells used).[131] As Ford writes:

> [I]t appears that at least up to the eight-cell stage in the human embryo there are eight distinct individuals rather than one multicellular individual. It is the zona pellucida that gives the appearance of a single organism or unity by holding the eight distinct individual cells together.

He goes on to argue:

> If the natural active potentiality of the zygote and cluster of cells to develop into an adult person were enough to constitute an actual person, we would have to claim that the zygote and cluster of cells at the same time, was both one person and more than one person. We cannot accept this at all, so it would be reasonable to deny that the zygote and cluster of cells are persons on the simple grounds of their potentiality or inherent capacity to develop into one or more than one adult person.

This led Ford to argue that it is difficult to consider embryos, up to the eight-cell stage, as single whole individuals since they contain parts that are potential individuals in their own right. As a result he suggests that it is challenging to consider such early embryos as individual human beings instead of just clusters of cells.[132]

For example, if an embryo reaches the three-cell stage (about 24 hours after fertilization), it is possible to indicate that it forms all at the same time:

1   one embryo made up of three totipotent cells;
2   three embryos, each made up of one totipotent cell;
3   two embryos, the first made up of two, and the second of one, totipotent cells.

The argument then suggests that because of this multiplicity of individuals existing all at the same time, questions can be asked about the moral status of the original one, then two, then four cells which slowly divide to become the eight totipotent cells of an embryo. How can a single embryo exist as a person while also existing as a cluster of eight embryonic persons all at the same time?

In response, it may be noted that a very different picture appears if an organism (a living whole expressing an integrated coordination of parts) is examined while not being restricted by the manner in which it is constituted. In this respect it may first be observed that very early totipotent cells in the two-cell stage of a primitive embryo may already be communicating with each other and, as a result, may already be considered as a single, whole, living, interdependent organism.

For example, in the case of the fertilization of frog and toad eggs, the symmetry of the two-cell embryo which is formed on division of the original one-cell zygote depends on the exact position of the penetration by the sperm cell of the egg. This means that the point of penetration of the sperm defines the body plan of the future multi-cellular embryo and which parts will become, for instance, the dorsal side of the amphibian.[133]

With many mammals, on the other hand, there is still some uncertainty as to whether the body plan of an embryo depends on the position of the sperm when it fertilizes the egg. But scientists believe that, with mice, the sperm entry position does predict the plane of initial cleavage of the mouse egg and can define the different parts of the future early embryo.[134] In addition, the cell inheriting the sperm entry position seems to acquire a division advantage and tends to cleave ahead of its sister cell.[135] Furthermore, the cells resulting from the first cell to divide from a two-cell mouse embryo generally develop in a specific manner since they contribute a greater number of cells to the inner cell mass than to the outer cells of the embryo.[136] This means that the cell in a two-cell mouse embryo which divides first is the one that generally produces the cells that make up the embryonic body. The other cell generally gives rise to the placenta and other supporting tissue.[137] It is also noticed that the cells divide asynchronously from the two-cell stage.[138] Consequently, with other mammals (such as humans), it is believed that the first cell to further divide in two-cell embryos is very likely to have a significant influence on the subsequent development of these embryos.[139]

All this means that interactions seem to be taking place right from the beginning of embryonic development, enabling the cluster of all the very early cells to be considered as a single, whole organism whereby each cell behaves as part of this organism, a living organism that would only be divided into new organisms if the cells ceased to communicate in any way. From this perspective, what matters is whether a whole organism exists, not whether some cells in this organism are totipotent. In a similar manner, if two completely distinct early embryos fuse with one another enabling their cells to communicate, they would then be unified into one single embryo – a single whole organism.[140]

Second, it is accepted that when cells in an eight-cell human embryo begin gradually to lose their totipotency, one after the other, they still only form one integrated whole organism even if, for example, it is at a stage when only half of them remain totipotent. Again, it is the very fact that they form one single organism that matters, not whether some of the cells in the embryo can still become other individual organisms if separated from the original organism.

Finally, it should be noted that, when different possibilities of whole individuals exist inside a group such as a cluster of cells in an early embryo, the concept of something being characterized as a 'whole' means that it is the greatest number of constituents of this single 'whole' that should be considered.

Again this is similar to what happens with Christian churches. If, for example, a church with ten members is examined, it is possible to consider this church as being formed of many different numbers of possible sub-churches with different numbers of parishioners. For instance, it would be possible to suggest that the church is made up of three sub-churches containing three, four and three members respectively. Or it could be considered as being formed of two sub-churches containing four and six members.

However, when they all come together, the 'whole' church is made up of ten members representing the greatest number of constituents of this whole, making it impossible to deny that this ten-member church is a real, single and whole, living church.

This kind of reasoning is reflected in German legislation which indicates that it is only when a totipotent cell is separated from the early embryo for testing that it becomes an embryo in its own right and on its own. Before this stage, it was part of the original whole embryo made up of several totipotent cells.

In summary, the arguments based on totipotency put forward by some commentators cannot rationally demonstrate that an early embryo before the 14-day stage of its existence is not a person in whom the image of God is reflected and whom he loves. Early embryos may possess certain biological abilities that are lost in later life but this does not mean that they have to conform to the 'usual' manner in which many believe personhood should be conferred.

Implantation and Relational Arguments

It is sometimes suggested that it is on the basis of the existence of a possible relationship with others and with God that it is reasonable to conclude that early embryos have a special moral status.

For instance, it is argued that it is only when an embryo is implanted within the uterus of its mother that it can have a biophysical contact with her and that it can then be considered as being a relational person. The British Christian clinical geneticist Caroline Berry states, for example:

God seems to have arranged the natural order so that the mother only becomes aware of her fetus and [is] able to value it *after* implantation has taken place. Is there any suggestion here that God himself values the embryo more after implantation?

Similarly, the British physician David Millar, discussing embryos created by *in vitro* fertilization, writes that they can be defined as potential human beings only if they are transferred into a woman's womb, since otherwise they would die.[141]

It is further argued from a Christian perspective that a being can only be considered as having full moral status if it can relate to God with a wider self-awareness and consciousness.

In response, and as already shown, it should be emphasized that a capacity to relate to God cannot be the central argument for personhood since it would also mean that infants and the severely mentally disabled would not be persons, which is difficult to accept. Moreover, such arguments limit an understanding of personhood and the moral status of human embryos to the perspective of physical development and the relationship that they can have with their mothers, humanity or God. The Church of Scotland 1996 Report was right when it stated that 'attempts to determine whether or not the embryo at any given stage in its development is a person or manifests God's image, in order that we might know how to behave towards it, can only end in sterile argument'.[142]

What is important is how God considers this existence which he created. God can of course have a relationship of love and grace with any individual (either adult or embryonic) even if this person is not implanted into a womb, is not self-aware or cannot consciously respond to this love.

The Church of Scotland 1996 Report further stated: 'The use of various criteria to define personhood and establish the point at which an embryo or fetus becomes a person is arbitrary and subjective.'[143] This means that, since the process of human development is continuous, any demarcation can only be arbitrary and merely conventional, as exemplified by the different upper time limits for abortion and destructive research on embryos across Europe and the world. Within the development process it is indeed impossible to indicate a non-arbitrary point of transition from human non-person to human person.

High Incidence of Spontaneous Abortions

A further objection to the full protective position is the very high incidence of spontaneous abortions,[144] with the majority of human embryos (up to 50–60 per cent) failing to implant and develop into infants.[145] This means that most human embryos are spontaneously aborted and die in the womb of their mother who may not even be aware of their existence.

FUNCTIONAL ASPECTS AND THE EMBRYO

This high level of deaths is then used to suggest that such embryos cannot have the same moral status as infants who have in fact been born. Schroten represents many commentators when he objects:

[I]t is logically possible that God has a special relationship with each human (pre)embryo in particular. But then we would be facing the absurd situation that in reality God allows more than 50 per cent of these beloved (pre)embryos to perish.[146]

It has further been argued that those supporting a full protection of embryos should be actively involved in the prevention of such spontaneous miscarriages if they are to be consistent.[147]

In response, however, a distinction should be made between natural processes, for which human individuals cannot be held morally accountable, and deliberate actions on embryonic life which certainly are the responsibility of the perpetrators.

In addition, if the high rate of miscarriages is an issue, then it is little different from the high infant mortality rates which remain in many parts of the world, and the 50 per cent rate which generally existed throughout most of human history.[148] Of course, such high rates of death are deeply distressing but they cannot ultimately be determinative in any assessment of the moral status of embryonic life.

As the British Christian philosopher Michael Banner comments:

It is difficult to see what, if any, significance should be attached to the natural wastage of early embryos or to the fact that many so lost are genetically impaired. The fact that infant mortality has often stood at very high levels, especially so in the case of the handicapped, does not cause us to doubt our duty to respect the sanctity of the life of the handicapped in particular.[149]

Furthermore, it should be remembered that 100 per cent of all living beings in the cosmos will eventually die, which means that the viability argument of a biological being cannot readily be used as a basis for its moral status, especially if the length of a life is morally irrelevant. A similar view is expressed by the Church of Scotland 1996 Report: '[L]arge numbers of people lose their lives as a result of natural occurrences like floods, drought, and earthquakes, but such loss does not tell us anything about the nature of the individuals lost.' Again, the moral status of a person, made in the image of God, is only dependent on the love of God that embraces the bearer from creation, through death and beyond. As the Church of Scotland 1996 Report states, 'each person, irrespective of who he or she is, enjoys equality of dignity and status with every other person before God and must be treated with appropriate respect.'[150]

A final and somewhat odd argument sometimes presented against the moral status of embryos who died through spontaneous abortion is that, were these embryos to be considered as persons, heaven would be over-populated by individuals who were never born. But to this, O'Donovan responds by suggesting that Christians should not be concerned by such matters since they will eventually discover how God has prepared a full and meaningful place for them. In the meantime, O'Donovan adds that, with respect to human embryos, 'we know that they make a human claim upon us which we evade only at the cost of our own full realization of humanity'.[151]

Brain Activity and Self-awareness

For many in secular society, recognizing the full moral status of an entity is dependent on finding specific human structural or functional capacities such as those associated with the human nervous system. Brain functions such as self-awareness, memory and reason are, in this regard, consid-ered to be some of the most important characteristics for the attainment of human rights and dignity. But this would then mean that some kind of relationship could exist between well-functioning brains or intelligence and human rights, which would be extremely dangerous for a civilized society to accept.[152]

In this context, the specific developmental stage at which the nerv-ous system is considered to confer special moral status can vary quite considerably between commentators. This begins, as already discussed, at 14 days with the beginning of the primitive streak, with initial neural functioning being observed at around 10 weeks. The development of a 'coordinated neural function' takes place at about 23 weeks with a rudi-mentary complete brain being recognized at between 30 and 35 weeks.[153]

From this perspective, Lockwood asserts that an established human identity is a continuity of identity, and can arise only with functional brain activity. Because of this, he argues: 'It is morally permissible to do whatever one likes with a human embryo or foetus before brain develop-ment' (and as long as the embryo is not allowed to develop further),[154] including destructive experimentation.

An extreme example of the manner in which this kind of argument based on decisive brain activity can be taken is given by Tooley, who argues that a human being can only be entitled to a serious right to life 'if it possesses the concept of a self as a continuing subject of experiences and other mental states, and believes that it is itself such a continuing entity'.[155] In this he also acknowledges that such a definition may make some forms of infanticide, as already mentioned, morally permissible.

A more religious angle to this argument was given by the Belgian Catholic theologian Joseph Donceel (1924–94), who stressed that for

Aristotle and Aquinas the essence of all substance in the natural or physical world can be explained by the 'hylomorphic' (literally 'matter–form') theory of substance. He then states: 'If form and matter are strictly complementary, as hylomorphism holds, there can be an actual human soul only in a body endowed with the organs required for the spiritual activities of man.' Because of this, Donceel believed that a soul can be present in a human body only if it has the capacity for spiritual activity which implies the existence of a developed functioning brain.[156]

Another supporter of a similar approach was the Scottish neuro-scientist Donald MacKay (1922–87) who suggested that a foetus cannot be considered to have 'personal significance of the self-conscious kind' until it has the ability to relate to other persons through the development of a brain.

By way of supporting his argument he emphasized that a person ceases to exist when he or she dies, which is often defined by 'brain death'. In other words, it is argued that if a person ceases to exist with his or her neural activity, then a person should only be seen to begin existence with brain activity.[157] Similar arguments were also held by Dunstan[158] and the Catholic ethicist Bernard Häring (1912–98).[159]

At this stage, however, it is important to note that a brain-dead person is neither a complete nor a whole living entity. Though not identical with the 'organism as a whole', the brain is a vital element in the integration of a developed whole person and, if it stops working, the integrity of the whole is lost. This is in contrast to an early human embryo which is a living organic whole with a unified, harmonious and dynamic constitution. The unity of a living whole is brought to life as a whole, develops and sustains itself as a whole and ends its life as a whole. As Iglesias argued:

> The unity of the living whole does not reside in any of its parts, because, that unity is not caused by any of its parts … The true primacy is that of the whole, of the living unit and its organisation; it is an ontological primacy over all the parts either considered singly or as a totality.[160]

A related argument to the brain activity argument suggests that destructive experimentation on human embryos may be acceptable if they are not sentient, though it recognizes that it is very difficult to determine at what stage these embryos can begin to feel pain.[161] But the absence of certain neural configurations does not necessarily mean that organisms in general, and embryos or foetuses in particular, are totally incapable of feeling physical suffering.

Moreover, if the risk of sentience is the only reason for avoiding the use of more developed embryos or foetuses in experiments, this could be addressed by using pain-killing drugs. Hence, the argument using the development of sentience as a final limit for experimentation may just be an attempt to bypass the more central questions relating to the moral status of the embryo.[162]

To summarize, the capacity for self-awareness and rational thought cannot be the sole basis of the image of God in humankind and its associated inherent human dignity. From a biblical perspective it is the whole being of the person, in his or her entirety, who reflects the image of God, and not just certain functions such as rationality. Moreover, this unity exists from the moment of creation of the being and gives an identity which can continue over time.[163]

The Moral Status of the Embryo and the Relief of Suffering

One of the main challenges in recognizing full moral status in the early human embryos is that many in society believe that they are necessary for research in the development of therapies. In fact, it is very likely that human embryos would have retained a far greater level of protection in legislation if they could not be used for biomedical research or destroyed after an unwanted pregnancy. There is, therefore, a tension between recognizing moral status in embryos and the relief of suffering that might be possible if they were not considered as having any value or worth. For example, one of the most controversial issues in medical ethics is whether the life of a foetal child should be destroyed in order to show compassion to the mother and reduce the burden that this child may represent.

From this perspective, a number of points may be examined. First, it is very important to express genuine sympathy and compassion to those who find themselves in a very difficult situation which is the source of profound suffering – a situation which may lead them to believe that an embryo or foetus may not have a similar value and worth to that of any other human being who has been born.

Second, the inherent value and worth of human life and the relief of suffering are not competing moral principles and are very different in nature. The inherent worth of human life exists because, at its very basis, this life is created in the image of God. This human worth is the reason why human beings behave in a respectful manner with each other.

Third, the very notion of inherent human dignity is undermined if a human life is taken to relieve suffering. This is because human dignity would be negated in order to relieve suffering, with the result that there would eventually be no reason to alleviate suffering since human dignity would no longer have any real worth.[164]

Thus, both the relief of suffering and the inherent worth of human life are only compatible if the taking of life is not a solution to the relief of suffering. As the 1987 Report to the General Assembly of the Church of Scotland states:

> [T]he sanctity of human life can never be qualified ... The sanctity imparted to human life by its bearing the image of God is absolute. It cannot be set aside even in the interests of relieving the suffering of the person who is suffering ..., still less in order to relieve the suffering of someone other than the person whose life is at stake.[165]

From a Christian perspective, though the virtue of compassion is central, the very purpose of life cannot simply be happiness and the avoidance of suffering. Instead, the meaning of the Christian message is to come ever closer to God and walk in the paths of sacrificial love – a path that was exemplified by Jesus Christ.

The Russian novelist Aleksandr Solzhenitsyn (1918–2008) supported the same idea in philosophical terms:

> If Humanism were right in declaring that man is born to be happy, he would not be born to die. Since his body is doomed to die, his task on earth evidently must be of a spiritual nature. It cannot be unrestrained enjoyment of everyday life. It has to be the fulfilment of a permanent, earnest duty so that one's life journey may become an experience of moral growth, so that one may leave life a better human being than one started it.[166]

Of course, a Christian response to suffering cannot be a fatalistic acceptance of suffering but neither is it an avoidance of suffering by undermining the inherent dignity of human life which gives this life its very meaning.

The Lord's words to the Apostle Paul are relevant: 'My grace is sufficient for you, for my power is made perfect in weakness' (2 Cor. 12.9). Paul was later able to assert, 'I have learned the secret of being content in any and every situation' (Phil. 4.12); and, 'For to me, to live is Christ and to die is gain' (Phil. 1.21).

Notes

1 Judy Pearsall and Bill Trumble (eds), 1996, *The Oxford English Reference Dictionary*, second edition, Oxford: Oxford University Press, p. 561.

2 St Augustine, *De Trinitate* X.12.

3 David Cairns, 1953, *The Image of God in Man*, first edition, London: SCM Press, pp. 110–13.

4 Both Plato and Aristotle called the human intellect divine, 'the spark of divinity in us'. Plato, *The Timaeus* 90C, Aristotle, *De Anima*, Book 1, 408b, both quoted in Anthony A. Hoekema, 1992, *Created in God's Image*, Grand Rapids: Eerdmans, p. 39.

5 Colin Gunton, 1998, *The Triune Creator: A Historical and Systematic Study*, Grand Rapids: Eerdmans, p. 194.

6 David Cairns, 1973, *Image of God*, second edition, London: Fontana Library of Theology and Philosophy, p. 116.

7 Walther Eichrodt, 1961, *The Theology of the Old Testament II*, London: SCM Press, p. 60.

8 John Stott, 2006, *Through the Bible Through the Year*, Oxford: Lion Hudson, p. 18.

9 Noreen L. Herzfeld, 2002, *In Our Image: Artificial Intelligence and the Human Spirit*, Minneapolis: Fortress Press, p. 19.

10 Colin E. Gunton, 1993, *The One, the Three and the Many*, 1992 Bampton Lectures, Cambridge: Cambridge University Press, p. 52.

11 Karl Barth, 1957–75, *Church Dogmatics*, Edinburgh: T&T Clark, Vol. III.2, pp. 83–157.

12 Cairns, 1973, *Image of God*, second edition, pp. 116–19.

13 John F. A. Sawyer, 'The meaning of "In the Image of God" in Genesis I–VI', *Journal of Theological Studies*, 25/2 (1974), p. 426.

14 St Gregory of Nyssa, 'On the creation of man' II, *Patrologia Series Graeca*, J. P. Migne, 44, 153D, 156B.

15 Quoted in Kallistos Ware, 1987, 'The Unity of the Human Person According to the Greek Fathers', in A. R. Peacocke and G. Gillett (eds), *Persons and Personality*, Oxford: Blackwell, p. 203.

16 Pia Matthews, 2010, 'Discerning Persons: How the early theology can illuminate contemporary bioethical approaches to the concept of person', doctoral thesis, Saint Mary's University College, pp. 143, 160.

17 John Wyatt, 2001, *Matters of Life and Death: Today's Healthcare Dilemmas in the Light of Christian Faith*, Leicester: InterVarsity Press, p. 55.

18 International Theological Commission, Communion and Stewardship: *Human Persons Created in the Image of God*, The Vatican, 2002, paragraph 57,

19 *Gaudium et Spes*, paragraph 34.

20 Peter Singer, 1994, *Rethinking Life and Death: The Collapse of Our Traditional Ethics*, New York: St Martin's Griffon, p. 190.

21 Peter Singer and D. Wells, 1984, *The Reproductive Revolution*, Oxford: Oxford University Press, p. 90.

22 Jamie Shreeve, 'The Other Stem-Cell Debate', *New York Times*, 10 April 2005.

23 Julian Savulescu, 'Human–Animal Transgenesis and Chimeras Might Be an Expression of Our Humanity', *American Journal of Bioethics* 3:3 (2003), pp. 22–5.

24 Immanuel Kant, *Grounding for the Metaphysics of Morals* (1785), trans. James W. Ellington, second edition, Indianapolis, IN: Hackett Publishing Company, 1981, pp. 35–6.

25 J. T. Eberl, 'Creating Non-Human Persons: Might it be worth the risk?' *American Journal of Bioethics* 7:5 (2007), pp. 52–4.

26 John Locke defines a person as 'a thinking, intelligent being, that has reason and reflection, and can consider itself, the same thinking thing in different places and times'. *Essay Concerning Human Understanding*, Book II, ch. XXVII. Quoted in Norman Ford, 1988, *When Did I Begin?*, Cambridge: Cambridge University Press, p. 69.

27 John Locke, *An Essay Concerning Human Understanding* (1690), Oxford: Clarendon Press, 1975, p. 335.

28 Peter Singer defines 'person' as 'a rational, self-conscious being': Singer and Wells, *The Reproductive Revolution*, p. 90; Robert N. Wennberg states: 'A person is, in a strict sense, a being which possesses the developed capacity to engage in acts of intellect, acts of emotion and acts of will.' Robert N. Wennberg, 1985, *Life in the Balance: Exploring the Abortion Controversy*, Grand Rapids: Eerdmans, p. 33.

29 Matthews, 'Discerning Persons', pp. 38–9.

30 Eberl, 'Creating Non-Human Persons', pp. 52–4.

31 Thomas Aquinas, *Summa Theologica*, Ia, q. 29. a. 1; IIIa, q. 16. a. 12, *ad* 1.

32 Donald Mackay, 1977, *Human Science and Human Dignity*, London: Hodder & Stoughton.

33 Walter Glannon, 'Genes, Embryos, and Future People', *Bioethics* 12 (1998), p. 190.

34 Gordon R. Dunstan, 1974, *The Artifice of Ethics*, London: SCM Press, p. 71.

35 Oliver O'Donovan, 1985, 'Again: Who Is a Person?', in J. H. Channer (ed.), *Abortion and the Sanctity of Human Life*, Exeter: Paternoster Press, p. 136.

36 O'Donovan, 'Again: Who Is a Person?', p. 136.

37 Anthony Dyson, 1990, 'At Heaven's Command', in Anthony Dyson and John Harris (eds), *Experiments on Embryos*, London: Routledge, p. 102.

38 M. Carriline, J. Marshall and J. Walker state: 'It is in our view wrong to create something with the potential for becoming a human person, and then deliberately destroy it.' M. Carriline, J. Marshall and J. Walker in Mary Warnock, 1985, *A Question of Life: The Warnock Report on Human Fertilisation and Embryology*, Oxford: Blackwell, p. 90.

39 S. Buckle comments: 'I think it not unfair to say that both advocates and critics of the potentiality argument are frequently not clear about what they understand potentiality to be, and that discussion of the argument has suffered from not distinguishing causes from their effects.' S. Buckle, 1990, 'Arguing from Potential', in P. Singer and H. Kuhse (eds), *Embryo Experimentation*, Cambridge: Cambridge University Press, p. 95.

40 T. F. Torrance, 1984, *Test-tube Babies: Morals – Science – and the Law*, Edinburgh: Scottish Academic Press, p. 3.

41 John Harris, 1985, *The Value of Life*, London: Routledge & Kegan Paul, p. 70.

42 John Mahoney, 1984, *Bioethics and Belief*, London: Sheed and Ward, pp. 84, 97.

43 Peter Singer and Karen Dawson, 1990, 'I.V.F. Technology and the Argument from Potential', in Singer and Kuhse, *Embryo Experimentation*, p. 78.

44 Mary Warnock, 'Do Human Cells Have Rights?', *Bioethics* 1:1 (1987), pp. 2–3.

45 This is exactly the argument of D. R. Millar who states: 'This creation of man [i.e. an IVF embryo] could not be called a potential human being, unless it is transferred to a receptive womb, for it inevitably dies in a few days.' D. R. Millar, 1984, *Respect for Life*, London: Christian Medical Fellowship, p. 27.

46 Andrew R. Rollinson, 'The Incarnation and the Status of the Human Embryo', thesis submitted for the degree of M.Litt. with the Religious Studies Department of Newcastle University, p. 39.

47 Buckle, 'Arguing from Potential', p. 95.

48 Tertullian, *Apologia* 9.8, Ante-Nicene Christian Library, Vol. XI, 72.

49 Paul Ramsey, 1970, *Fabricated Man: The Ethics of Genetic Control*, New Haven: Yale University Press, p. 11.

50 J. Foster, 1985, 'Personhood and the Ethics of Abortion', in Channer, *Abortion and Sanctity*, p. 37.

51 Teresa Iglesias, 1990, *I.V.F. and Justice*, London: Linacre Centre for Health Care Ethics, p. 67.

52 Gareth Jones, 1987, *Manufacturing Humans: The Challenge of the New Reproductive Technologies*, Leicester: InterVarsity Press, pp. 134–63.

53 Peter Millican, 1992, 'The Complex Problem of Abortion', in D. R. Bromham, M. E. Dalton, J. C. Jackson and P. J. R. Millican (eds), *Ethics in Reproductive Medicine*, New York: Springer, p. 180.

54 N. Poplawski and G. Gillett, 'Ethics and embryos', *Journal of Medical Ethics* 17:2 (1991), pp. 62–9.

55 Archbishop of York, diocesan leaflet, December 1989.

56 R. Edwards, 1990, 'Ethics and Embryology: The Case for Experimentation', in Dyson and Harris, *Experiments on Embryos*, p. 41.

57 Warnock, *A Question of Life*, p. 65.

58 P. Millican writes: 'It is ... so overwhelmingly natural to see a massive moral distinction between the microscopic blob which is the early pre-embryo and the fully formed sentient and active individual which is the nine-month foetus, that only the spurious demands of religious dogma or of simplistic theoretical systematisation could ever lead anyone to deny it.' Millican, 'Complex Problem', p. 183.

59 G. R. Dunstan, '*In vitro* fertilisation: The ethics', *Human Reproduction* 1:1 (1986), pp. 41–4.

60 Mahoney, *Bioethics and Belief*, p. 78; J. Donceel, 'Immediate animation and delayed hominisation', *Theological Studies* 31 (1970), pp. 76–105. For a similar, but Protestant, viewpoint, see Wennberg, *Life in the Balance*.

61 Karl Rahner, 1965, *Hominisation: The Evolutionary Origin of Man as a Theological Problem*, London: Burns & Oates, p. 94. In the nineteenth century Ernst Haeckel suggested that the stages of development of the embryo repeat the stages of evolution (from simple organism, to fish, to amphibian, to simple mammal, to primate, etc.). For an excellent historical overview of this topic see S. J. Gould, 1977, *Ontogeny and Phylogeny*, Cambridge, MS: The Belknap Press of Harvard University Press.

Haeckel's ideas have long since been abandoned by scientists. Moreover, it should be noted that an embryo does not become a person in the same way as humans may eventually have become persons through the theory of evolution. Human evolution would suggest that before some specific moment in time hominid bodies existed that were not persons but after which some were persons. But these two sets of beings would have been very different individuals with separate bodies. In the case of the developing embryo, however, it is the same body that must be considered. In other words, the whole existence of this body in time can only be, or not be, a person if a body–soul dualistic approach is rejected.

62 Egbert Schroten, 'What Makes a Person', *Theology* 97:776 (March–April 1994), pp. 98–105 (p. 102).

63 Lord Jakobovits, 1992, 'Respect for Life: Embryonic Considerations', in Bromham et al., *Ethics in Reproductive Medicine*, pp. 47–8.

64 Gilbert Meilaender and Robert P. George, 'That Thing in a Petri Dish', *National Review Online*, 21 February 2006.

65 Warnock, 'Do Human Cells Have Rights?', pp. 2–3.

66 Aquinas, *Summa Theologica* 1. Ia, q. 29. a. 4.

67 Maureen L. Condic, 2001, 'Preimplantation Stages of Human Development: The Biological and Moral Status of Early Embryos', in Antoine Suarez and Joachim Huarte (eds), *Is This Cell a Human Being?*, Berlin/Heidelberg: Springer, pp. 37–8.

68 Meilaender and George, 'That Thing'.

69 Oliver O'Donovan, 1973, *The Christian and the Unborn Child*, Bramcote, Nottinghamshire: Grove Books, p. 11.

70 The concept of a delayed animation is also accepted by Judaism and Islam. According to the Talmud, which refers back to Exodus 21.22, animation takes place 40 days after conception. For some in the Muslim tradition, who refer back to sura 23.12–14 of the Qur'an, there are four distinct stages of 30 days and it is only in the 120th day that the spirit is breathed into the embryo. Others in the Muslim tradition refer to a hadith (a word from the prophet Muhammad) indicating that this breathing of the spirit into the embryo already happens on the 40th day.

71 Michael J. Coughlan, 1990, *The Vatican, the Law and the Human Embryo*, London: Macmillan, p. 110.

72 Wyatt, *Matters of Life*, p. 152.

73 Tertullian, *On the Resurrection of the Flesh*, ch. 16

74 Tertullian, *A Treatise on the Soul*, ch. 37.

75 *Ambigua à Jean*, 42, Patrologia, Series Graeca, J. P. Migne, 91, 1325D; 7, 91, 1100CD; trans. E. Ponsoye in *Maxime Le Confesseur, Ambigua*, Paris: Suresnes, 1994.

76 David Atkinson, 1987, 'Some Theological Perspectives on the Human Embryo', in Nigel M. de S. Cameron (ed.), *Embryos and Ethics*, Edinburgh: Rutherford House Books, p. 56.

77 Reginald Frank Robert Gardner, 1972, *Abortion: The Personal Dilemma*, Carlisle: Paternoster Press.

78 O'Donovan, *Christian and the Unborn Child*, p. 11.

79 John Breck, 2000, *The Sacred Gift of Life: Orthodox Christianity and Bioethics*, New York: St. Vladimir's Seminary Press, pp. 141 fn., 140.

80 Breck, *Sacred Gift*, p. 140.

81 *Report of the Committee of Inquiry into Human Fertilisation and Embryology* (The Warnock Report), London: Her Majesty's Stationery Office, 1984, p. 63.

82 House of Lords Hansard, Volume 641, Part 14, Column 1327, 5 December 2002.

83 Kenneth Boyd, 1987, 'Response to Richard Higginson', in Church of Scotland Board of Social Responsibility, *Abortion in Debate*, Edinburgh: Quorum Press, p. 63.

84 Millican, 'Complex Problem of Abortion', p. 167.

85 The Warnock Report, pp. 90–4.

86 'The challenge of the biotech century', *The Guardian*, 21 May 2005, https://www.theguardian.com/society/2005/may/21/health.research (accessed 21 July 2016).

87 'Adviser sparks infanticide debate', BBC News, 26 January 2004, http://news.bbc.co.uk/1/hi/health/3429269.stm (accessed 21 July 2016).

88 Jérome Lejeune, 1984, in *Test-tube Babies: A Christian View*, Oxford: Unity Press, p. 35. J. Lejeune criticizes the idea of 'hominization': 'I must say, very simply, as a geneticist, I have never heard any specialist in husbandry of animals thinking about the "cattlisation" of cattle. They know that the embryo of a cow would be a calf.' Senate Select Committee on the Human Experimentation Bill 1985, quoted in N. Ford, 1988, *When Did Life Begin?*, Cambridge: Cambridge University Press, p. 127.

89 Maureen Condic, 'A Scientific View of When Life Begins', *On Point – Charlotte Lozier Institute*, June 2014, p. 4.

90 Teresa Iglesias, '*In vitro* fertilisation: The Major Issues', *Journal of Medical Ethics* 10:1 (1984), pp. 32–7.

91 Calum MacKellar, 2001, *The Value of the Human Gene*, Edinburgh: Rutherford House, p. 20.

92 This means that destructive embryonic stem cell research – of the kind already taking place in the UK – may be regarded as inherently unethical and should be rejected.

This has already been prohibited in Austria, Ireland, Lithuania, Slovakia and Poland. In addition countries such as Malta and Portugal do not have specific legislation but have a national constitutional position which protects early human life. The production of any kind of human embryo for research is prohibited by the European Convention on Human Rights and Biomedicine which was signed (as of July 2016) by 35 out of the 47 Member States of the Council of Europe. The UK has not signed this Convention, which states in Article 18: 'The creation of human embryos for research purposes is prohibited.'

93 Condic, 'Preimplantation Stages', pp. 37–8.

94 Ian Johnston, 'Scientists set to create human–rabbit hybrid', *The Scotsman*, 13 January 2006.

95 David Baltimore, 'Don't Impede Medical Progress', *Wall Street Journal*, 30 July 2001.

96 Hadley Arkes, 1986, *First Things*, Princeton: Princeton University Press, p. 364.

97 Karen Dawson, 1990, 'Segmentation and the Moral Status: A Scientific Perspective', in Singer and Kuhse, *Embryo Experimentation*, Cambridge: Cambridge University Press, p. 53.

98 Ford, *When Did I Begin?*, p. 176.

99 Mahoney, *Bioethics and Belief*, London: Sheed and Ward, p. 64.

100 Berit Brogaard, 2007, 'The Moral Status of the Human Embryo: The Twinning Argument', in Paul Kurtz (ed.), *Science and Ethics*, Amherst, NY: Prometheus Books, pp. 87–94.

101 Ford, *When Did I Begin?*, pp. 133, 136.

102 Ford, *When Did I Begin?*, pp. xvi, xvii.

103 Anne McLaren, 1986, 'Prelude to Embryogenesis', in The Ciba Foundation, *Human Embryo Research: Yes or No?*, London: Tavistock Publications, p. 22.

104 Mary Warnock, 'Do Human Cells Have Rights?', pp. 11–12.

105 John Mahoney writes: 'Some biological stability in the organism is essential for its individuality to be firmly established, and that without this stable individuation of the organism one cannot begin to speak of a human individual.' Mahoney, *Bioethics and Belief*, p. 64.

106 Warnock, *A Question of Life*, p. 66.

107 Paul Ramsey, 1970, 'Reference Points in Deciding about Abortion', in J. T. Noonan (ed.), *The Morality of Abortion: Legal and Historical Perspectives*, Cambridge, MA: Harvard University Press, pp. 65–6.

108 Teresa Iglesias, 1987, 'What Kind of Being is the Human Embryo?', in Cameron, *Embryos and Ethics*, p. 71; Paul Ramsey, 'Abortion, a Review Article', *The Thomist* 37 (1973), p. 190.

109 'The appearance of one primitive streak signals that only one embryo proper and a human individual has been formed and begun to exist. Prior to this stage, it would be pointless to speak about the presence of a true human being in an ontological sense. A human individual could scarcely exist before a definitive human body is formed.' Ford, *When Did I Begin?*, p. 172.

110 Angelo Serra, 'Advances in Medical Genetics: Prospectives and Ethical Problems', *Melita Theologica* 48:1 (1997), p. xvi.

111 Patrick Lee and Robert P. George, 'The First Fourteen Days of Human Life', *New Atlantis* 13 (2006), pp. 61–7.

112 David A. Jones, 2004, *The Soul of the Embryo*, London: Continuum, pp. 226–7. See also Peter E. Bristow, 1997, *The Moral Dignity of Man*, Dublin: Four Courts Press, pp. 134–5.

113 Lee and George, 'The First Fourteen Days'. An embryo's potential for spontaneous twinning seems to be established at an early stage by factors determining the
thickness of the zona pellucida: Richard M. Doerflinger, 'The Ethics of Funding Embryonic Stem Cell Research: A Catholic Viewpoint', *Kennedy Institute of Ethics Journal*
9:2 (1999), p. 138.

114 T. V. Daly, SJ, 1985, 'The Status of Embryonic Human Life: A Crucial Issue
in Genetic Counselling', in N. Tonti-Filippini (ed.), *Health Care Priorities in Australia: Proceedings of the 1985 Annual Conference on Bioethics*, Melbourne: St Vincent's
Bioethics Centre, p. 52.

115 Elisa Garcia and Henk Jochemsen, 2005, 'Ethics of Stem Cell Research', in Henk
Jochemsen (ed.), *Human Stem Cells; Sources of Hope and of Controversy*, Amersfoort:
Prof. Dr G. A. Lindeboom Institute and Business Ethics Center of Jerusalem, p. 89.

116 Coughlan, *The Vatican, the Law*, pp. 70–1.

117 Roger Highfield, 'Sons I gave birth to are "unrelated" to me', *Daily Telegraph*,
13 November 2003.

118 Breck, *Sacred Gift*, p. 141.

119 Coughlan, *The Vatican, the Law*, p. 72.

120 This comparison was suggested by Mr David Moyes.

121 Breck, *Sacred Gift*, p. 141.

122 Maureen L. Condic, 'Totipotency: What It Is and What It Is Not', *Stem Cells
and Development* 23:8 (2014), pp. 796–812.

123 R. G. Edwards and H. K. Beard, 'Oocyte Polarity and cell determination in early
mammalian embryos'. *Molecular Human Reproduction* 3 (1997), pp. 863–905; Hilde
Van de Velde, Greet Cauffman, Herman Tournaye, Paul Devroey and Inge Liebaers,
'The four blastomeres of a 4-cell stage human embryo are able to develop individually
into blastocysts with inner cell mass and trophectoderm', *Human Reproduction* 23:8
(2008), pp. 1742–7.

124 Van de Velde et al., 'Four Blastomeres'.

125 R. Wolfrum and A. C. Zeller, 'Legal Aspects of Research with Human Pluripotent Stem Cells in Germany', *Biomedical Ethics* 4:3 (1999), p. 102.

126 Embryo Protection Act (12.13.1990), translated and quoted in Wolfrum and
Zeller, 'Legal Aspects', p. 103.

127 Wolfrum and Zeller, 'Legal Aspects', pp. 102–07. By the eight-cell stage, only
a very few number of blastomeres are totipotent. In experiments in various mammals,
only one or two blastomeres remain totipotent at this stage. See Deutsche Akademie der
Naturforscher Leopoldina – Nationale Akademie der Wissenschaften, 2011, *Ad-hoc
statement Preimplantation genetic diagnosis (PGD) The effects of limited approval in
Germany*, Deutsche Akademie der Naturforscher Leopoldina – Nationale Akademie
der Wissenschaften, January 2011. E. Hildt, 'Preimplantation Diagnosis in Germany',
Biomedical Ethics 1:2 (1996), pp. 28–9.

128 The position on Preimplantation Embryonic Selection in Germany has developed
since 2010, when Germany's Federal Supreme Court decided to acquit a gynaecologist
of an illegal abortion after he chose to carry out Preimplantation Genetic Diagnosis
on several human embryos and discard those with a genetic disorder. A. Tuffs, 'Court
Allows Preimplantation Genetic Diagnosis in Germany', *British Medical Journal* 341
(2010), pp. 120–1; in July 2011, the German parliament also voted to allow Preimplantation Genetic Diagnosis in certain circumstances. These are if the parents are
at high risk of passing on a genetic disorder to their children or if there is a high risk of
miscarriage or stillbirth because of a genetic dysfunction. A. Tuffs, 'Germany Relaxes
Law on Preimplantation Genetic Diagnosis', *British Medical Journal* 343 (2011), p. 119.

129 The German Ethics Council, 2012, *Preimplantation Genetic Diagnosis: Opinion*, Berlin: The German Ethics Council, p. 14.

130 Brogaard, 'Moral Status'; Coughlan, *The Vatican, the Law*, pp. 72–3.

131 In this regard, it should be noted that results from experiments in a number of mammals indicate that only one or two cells at the eight-cell stage remain totipotent.

132 Ford, *When Did I Begin?*, pp. 137, 136, 145.

133 Jonathan M. W. Slack, 1983, *From Egg to Embryo: Determinative Events in Early Development*, Cambridge: Cambridge University Press, pp. 32–4.

134 Helen Pearson, 'Developmental biology: Your destiny, from day one', *Nature* 418 (2002), pp. 14–15.

135 Karolina Piotrowska and Magdalena Zernicka-Goetz, 'Role for sperm in spatial patterning of the early mouse embryo', *Nature* 409 (2001), pp. 517–21.

136 Anne McLaren, 1982, 'The Embryo', in C. R. Austin and R. V. Short (eds), *Embryonic and Fetal Development, Reproduction in Mammals*, Book 2, Cambridge: Cambridge University Press, p. 3.

137 Karolina Piotrowska, Florence Wianny, Roger A. Pedersen and Magdalena Zernicka-Goetz, 'Blastomeres arising from the first cleavage division have distinguishable fates in normal mouse development', *Development* 128:19 (2001), pp. 3739–48.

138 Ford, *When Did I Begin?*, p. 147.

139 Ford, *When Did I Begin?*, p. 146.

140 Lee and George, 'First Fourteen'.

141 Caroline Berry, 1993, *Beginnings: Christian Views of the Early Embryo*, London: Christian Medical Fellowship, p. 28; Millar, *Respect for Life*.

142 Church of Scotland Board of Social Responsibility, 1996, *Pre-Conceived Ideas: A Christian Perspective of IVF and Embryology*, Edinburgh: Saint Andrew Press, p. 60.

143 Church of Scotland Board of Social Responsibility, *Pre-Conceived Ideas*, p. 56.

144 One-third of all fertilized human ova never implant in the uterine wall. Some estimates are significantly higher, but there is considerable debate on this issue. See Pamela Sims, 'Test-tube babies in debate', *Ethics and Medicine* 4:3 (1988), p. 4.

145 K. Moore, 1982, *The Developing Human: Clinically Oriented Embryology*, third edition, Philadelphia: W. B. Saunders, pp. 36, 49.

146 Schroten, 'What Makes a Person', *Theology* 97:776 (1994), p. 103.

147 T. F. Murphy, 'The moral significance of spontaneous abortion', *Journal of Medical Ethics* 11 (1985), pp. 79–83; Giuseppe Benagiano, Maurizio Mori, Norman Ford and Gedis Grudzinskas, 'Early pregnancy wastage: Ethical considerations', *Reproductive BioMedicine Online* 22 (2011), pp. 692–700.

148 Benedict M. Ashley and Kevin D. O'Rourke, 1982, *Health Care Ethics: A Theological Analysis*, St Louis: The Catholic Health Association of the USA, p. 223.

149 Michael Banner, 1999, *Christian Ethics and Contemporary Moral Problems*, Cambridge: Cambridge University Press, p. 112.

150 Church of Scotland Board of Social Responsibility, *Pre-Conceived Ideas*, pp. 55, 9.

151 O'Donovan, *Christian and Unborn Child*, p. 16.

152 Condic, 'Preimplantation Stages', p. 39.

153 Condic, 'Preimplantation Stages', pp. 37–8.

154 Michael Lockwood (ed.), 1985, *Moral Dilemmas in Modern Medicine*, Oxford: Oxford University Press, p. 24. He also states: 'We must conclude that before the brain comes into being, there is no human being there to worry about', p. 19.

155 Michael Tooley, 1974, 'Abortion and Infanticide', in M. Cohen, T. Nagel and T. Scanlon (eds), *The Rights and Wrongs of Abortion*, Princeton: Princeton University Press, p. 59.

156 Joseph F. Donceel, 'Immediate Animation and Delayed Hominization', *Theological Studies* 31:1 (1970), pp. 76–105 (p. 83).

157 Donald Mackay, 1977, *Human Science and Human Dignity*, London: Hodder & Stoughton. See also D. Mackay, 'The Beginning of Personal Life', *In the Service of Medicine*, 30:2 (1984), pp. 9–13 and D. G. Jones, 'Brain birth and personal identity', *Journal of Medical Ethics* 15 (1989), pp. 173–8.

158 Gordon R. Dunstan, 1974, *The Artifice of Ethics*, London: SCM Press, p. 71.

159 'I think it can be said that at least before the twenty-fifth to fortieth day, the embryo cannot yet (with certainty) be considered as a human person.' Häring adds that if 'the theory of hominisation as dependent on the development of the cerebral cortex ... gains general acceptance by those competent in this field, it could then contribute greatly to the resolution of those difficult cases involving conflict of conscience or conflict of duties'. Bernard Häring, 1973, *Medical Ethics*, Notre Dame, IN: Fides Publishers, pp. 84–5.

160 Iglesias, 'What Kind of Being?', pp. 65–6.

161 John Marshall, 1988, 'Experiment on Human Rmbryos: Sentience as the Cut-off Point?', in G. R. Dunstan and Mary J. Seller (eds), *The Status of the Human Embryo: Perspectives from the Moral Tradition*, London: King Edward's Hospital Fund for London, p. 58.

162 Marshall, 'Experiment on Human Embryos', p. 60.

163 Reports to the General Assembly of the Church of Scotland, 1987, p. 311.

164 Reports to the General Assembly, pp. 285–6.

165 Reports to the General Assembly, p. 312. The Church of Scotland went on to say that 'the child created by an act of rape is, despite the circumstances of his or her origins, still a child with the right to life. Christians must believe that all children are precious to God. The conceived child is an innocent party and has done nothing to deserve destruction.'

166 Aleksandr Solzhenitsyn at Harvard Class Day Afternoon Exercises, 8 June 1978.

Conclusion

This book has never been about proving that the image of God is reflected in the human embryo. This will never be possible. Indeed, it is only because of the Christian faith in God that a belief in the image of God in persons is possible which then enables a belief in the image of God in embryonic persons.

But by examining the central Christian concept of the image of God, it has been possible to see how central doctrines, such as the creation by God of humanity and the incarnation of the Word of God, can be used to bring into focus a rich variety of themes which may otherwise have remained out of sight. These are of crucial importance to the manner in which the very understanding of science is considered. As Gunton comments:

> The chief basis of human science, technology, craft and art is ... christological. The teaching that the one through whom the world was made became part of that world, even in its fullness, affirms the readiness of that world for human knowledge, action and shaping.[1]

One of the more specific responsibilities of those created in the divine image is to exercise dominion over the whole of creation. This was also reflected in the way Jesus Christ, the perfect divine image, demonstrated his total control over creation through, for example, his nature miracles. It is because of this that T. F. Torrance described science as 'a religious duty' and characterized the scientist as 'the priest of creation'.[2]

Even though clear answers to many ethical dilemmas cannot easily be derived from biblical analysis, it is still useful to study theological ethics from the basis of Christian doctrinal principles because they may eventually enable specific moral conclusions to be recognized.[3]

Of course, questions remain as to how far such an ethical approach may command general, let alone universal, appeal in the present pluralist societies. Is this approach just another example of one understanding among many others in today's fragmented ethical scene? Or does this perspective have within it themes that engage the more widespread debate?

It is hoped that this study will have, in some way, demonstrated the latter. In any event, an examination of the image of God through the rich and far-reaching implications of creation, incarnation and other aspects can only be seen as a useful addition to a Christian understanding of the moral status of the human embryo.

Admittedly, this book has not been able to fully answer the question, 'What is the image of God in the embryo?' As already mentioned, this image, by its very nature in reflecting God, will never be completely understood or defined. A certain amount of humility is, therefore, required in recognizing that it will never be possible to completely characterize the moral status of an embryo – or for that matter, that of any adult human being – which is dependent on this image. They are both based on a belief – a belief in God and that human beings are created in his image which give them immeasurable worth, value and meaning.

Of course, a lot more may be said about the image of God from a theological perspective. But this is not a book about the theology of this image. Instead, it has argued that the image of God can rationally be accepted as being reflected in the very earliest of human embryos which deserve, as a result, to be loved, respected, celebrated and protected.

Creation, Incarnation, the Nature of Existence and Ethics

The conclusion of this book argues that the image of God is fundamental in trying to understand the moral status of the human embryo and foetus – an image which may be expressed from many different angles including functional, substantive and relational perspectives. But probably the most useful expression of this image of God, as it relates to the human embryo, may be obtained by studying the way God creates persons and how the Word of God became a human person in Jesus Christ.

Because humankind is created 'in the image of God, after his likeness' it has a unique position in creation which enables human persons to experience a unique relationship with their creator. It also enables human beings to take responsibility for looking after the created world with, and on behalf of, the creator God.

At the same time, because the image of God comes from God and is created by him, it is not dependent on anything humankind can do. This is further confirmed through the incarnation in that God, in Christ, does not only emphasize the importance and uniqueness of humankind, but gives value and worth to all human beings independently of any capacities, functions or abilities. As the 1985 Church of Scotland Report to the General Assembly states:

> The value of human life and the dignity of life, derive from how God regards and treats us, and not on any status which legal or moral codes and conventions may confer at particular ages and stages of development. Thus, human beings may never treat each other as means to ends, but only as ends, and as ends backed by ultimate sanction of God's own being and love incarnate in Jesus Christ.[4]

The reality that the eternal Son of God became incarnate in Jesus, and took on humanity, is the ultimate and transcendent origin of the immeasurable order of rational love which is behind the creation of each human being.[5] That the living Word of God has come into creation is the crucial witness to the truth that God has established a wonderful relationship with his created children. As already emphasized by T. F. Torrance, the incarnation focuses and even radicalizes the manner in which God's relationship with his creation, and humankind within it, is perceived.

God, who first created humankind in his image, has presented the 'original' in his incarnate Son. Furthermore, Jesus Christ, as the 'image of the invisible God' (Col. 1.15), certifies the inherent dignity and immeasurable moral worth of that image not only by sharing it, but by revealing its very origins and foundations. This original image in the incarnate Son entered the whole of creation at the moment when his embryonic human body came into being. In the same way, it is possible to recognize the image of God in human beings at their earliest embryonic stages.[6]

Moreover, because the union of Christ's humanity and divinity in one hypostasis (or individual existence) implies personhood from the moment of his conception, a model or paradigm now exists of God's relationship with all human beings, stretching back to their own embryonic beginnings:[7] a relationship of love with his human children which has a personalizing effect.

The broad themes of creation and incarnation are all about God's love uniquely expressed in human form. In Jesus Christ, it is possible to see what it really means to 'love one's neighbour as one's self' (Lev. 19.18; Matt. 22.39). O'Donovan has suggested that persons can only be discerned existentially through love: 'We discern persons only by love, by discovering through interaction and commitment that this human being is irreplaceable.'[8]

But, unfortunately, this is not happening with the various forms of destructive human embryonic experiments that now exist in certain countries, reflecting the reality that human beings no longer know what is precious in humanity and are deliberately alienating themselves from themselves. The crime, O'Donovan suggests, is not 'the old crime of killing babies, but the new and subtle crime of making babies to be ambiguously human'.[9] In a way, this is the complete opposite to what happened in the incarnation. Indeed, no ambiguity was present when Jesus Christ, the Word of God, became existentially involved in humanity while treating all those he encountered, including the weakest and most vulnerable, with an immeasurable love and dignity.

This also means that the concept of personhood is intrinsically defined by relationships with other persons, uniquely expressed and manifested in the very Being of the Trinity, and also reflected in the creator–creature relationship. The supreme biblical witness to this is Psalm 139.13–17:

> For you created my inmost being; you knit me together in my mother's womb.
> I praise you because I am fearfully and wonderfully made; your works are wonderful, I know that full well.
> My frame was not hidden from you when I was made in the secret place.
> When I was woven together in the depths of the earth, your eyes saw my unformed body.
> All the days ordained for me were written in your book before one of them came to be.
> How precious to me are your thoughts, O God! How vast is the sum of them!

Stott commented that this was 'perhaps the most radically personal statement in the Old Testament of God's relationship to the individual … The Psalmist is aware of no discontinuity between his antenatal and postnatal being.'[10] This is what the psalm expresses and what the incarnation reveals.

God, who became a human being in Jesus Christ at the point of human conception, loves and 'personalizes' all human beings right down to their embryonic origins. Greek patristic anthropology emphasized such a relationship by describing the human person as 'indivisible; body of his soul and soul of his body' while being related to God through the creating and sustaining work of the Holy Spirit and thereby having a human 'spirit'. As such, this human 'spirit' was not seen as a third part of a human person but as a dynamic correlate of the divine Spirit.[11] It is through the Holy Spirit that God's relationship with human beings personalizes them.

Another important conclusion of this book is that the very basis for the focus and priority of human personhood is given expression in the 'image of God'. Indeed, the concept of personhood expresses, in a fundamental manner, the 'I–Thou' relationship between God and each human being, unique in his creation. As T. F. Torrance argued, God is the 'personalising Person' and human beings are personalized persons. This also means that the image of God cannot be characterized in any qualitative manner.

Another outcome of this study is that 'being' has priority over 'attributes'. This implies that human beings, including human embryos, reflect the image of God because God created them in a special way. As Rollinson observed, '"Being" then has priority over "behaving", just as in the christological paradigm "person" has priority over "nature".' What is fundamental to human personhood is this continuing creaturely relatedness to God since his relationship of grace and love to his human children is prior to, and independent of, any possibility of returning this relationship in any appropriate way. The stone from which the concept of being a person was hewn in the patristic Trinitarian debates is the stone that supports the very understanding of being a person as such.[12]

This implies that it is only through the wonderful love of God that human embryos (and adults) can be recognized as persons – persons who can only be defined through Jesus Christ. It is no coincidence that, just as the incarnate Word of God was present before, in and through the conception of Jesus Christ, so the love of God is present before, in and through the creation of all human embryonic persons.

Practical Implications

Since it is possible to believe, rationally, that early human embryos do indeed reflect the image of God, a number of practical implications arise of importance for those who either hold such a view or do not share this view but respect it in others.

Giving the Embryo the Benefit of the Doubt

It will never be possible to determine the exact moment, at the embryonic stage, when a human person begins to exist. Fertilization is itself a process taking up to 24 hours to complete.[13] As the British Christian ethicist Helen Oppenheimer emphasizes: 'It is ironical that the "moment of conception" doctrine should be gaining ground just now, when increased knowledge of human beginnings has indicated that there is no such moment.'[14] Or more exactly, it is not that such a moment does not exist but rather that it is impossible to specifically determine it. It is a kind of mystery point to which one may come ever closer but which is never finally attained.[15]

In this context of uncertainty, where no final conclusions may ever exist as to the exact moment when early embryonic entities become persons, caution is required. This means that the only acceptable alternative may be to give them the benefit of the doubt as soon as they come into existence.

For example, Norman Ford writes:

> I am not alone in finding the argument that the zygote is an ongoing human individual unconvincing. But I admit it is plausible both on account of its intrinsic merit and by reason of the number of eminent scientists and philosophers who support it. So long as there are good reasons to believe the zygote is already a human individual and a person, prudence required that any reasonable doubt should be ethically resolved in favor of treating the zygote as a person.[16]

Wyatt further commented:

> [I]f we recognize a deep uncertainty and ambiguity about the moral significance of the embryo or early fetus, we have to ask: 'What is an authentically Christian response to this deep ontological uncertainty?' Surely an appropriate response is to vote in favour of protection and against intentional destruction.[17]

This is all the more relevant since, as already mentioned, science will never be able to demonstrate whether an early embryo, or for that matter a fully formed child or adult, has full moral value since this concept is based on beliefs and is an ethical rather than, solely, a scientific concept.

This argument based on caution is also reflected in the use which is sometimes made of the concept of a 'potential person'. Because uncertainty exists about the exact status of the embryo and the fact that it may be a person, it is meaningful to be cautious and consider the embryo as having the same moral status as an adult.

Of course, only God will know the correct manner in which to consider certain kinds of embryo or foetus. But until this is made clear, this side of eternity, the decision should be in favour of protection.[18]

Giving the embryo the benefit of the doubt is also the official position of the Roman Catholic Church. The Holy See's 1974 *Declaration on Procured Abortion* in paragraph 13 stated:

> [I]t is not up to biological sciences to make a definitive judgment on questions which are properly philosophical and moral, such as the moment when a human person is constituted or the legitimacy of abortion. From a moral point of view this is certain: even if a doubt existed

concerning whether the fruit of conception is already a human person, it is objectively a grave sin to dare to risk murder. 'The one who will be a man is already one.'[19]

Later on, in 1995, John Paul II wrote in *Evangelium vitae*:

> Furthermore, what is at stake is so important that, from the stand-point of moral obligation, the mere probability that a human person is involved would suffice to justify an absolutely clear prohibition of any intervention aimed at killing a human embryo. Precisely for this reason, over and above all scientific debates and those philosophical affirmations to which the Magisterium has not expressly committed itself, the Church has always taught and continues to teach that the result of human procreation, from the first moment of its existence, must be guaranteed that unconditional respect which is morally due to the human being in his or her totality and unity as body and spirit: 'The human being is to be respected and treated as a person from the moment of conception; and therefore from that same moment his rights as a person must be recognized, among which in the first place is the inviolable right of every innocent human being to life'.[20]

In other words, because a fully personal human life may be present, there is a moral imperative to resolve any doubts on the side of protect-ing life.[21] As D. A. Jones and others emphasize: 'The Christian churches teach not that the early embryo is certainly a person, but that the embryo should always be treated as if it were a person.'[22]

Giving the embryo the benefit of the doubt would also be appropriate when scientists are unsure whether or not it even exists. This would be the case, for example, for certain kinds of human–nonhuman embry-onic combinations or entities resulting from parthenogenesis whereby an egg is tricked into replicating its own set of chromosomes instead of being fertilized by sperm. In these instances, scientists do not even know whether embryos are actually created or if they are just a sort of cluster of disorganized cells. But until further biological information is forthcoming as to whether they are actually embryos, many believe that such entities should be considered as persons under the precautionary principle. O'Donovan even goes so far as to argue:

> [U]nless we approach new human beings, including those whose humanity is ambiguous and uncertain to us, with the expectancy and hope that we shall discern how God has called them out of nothing into personal being, then I do not see how we shall ever learn to love another human being at all.[23]

The principle of giving the benefit of the doubt is also the position taken in a court of law when a judge is unsure whether or not an accused is guilty of a crime. The magistrate cannot simply condemn the accused because this may be beneficial to society (this principle is called *in dubio pro reo*). The accused has rights which have priority over the possible consequences for society. In the same way, the full protective position for the embryo indicates that it has a right to life which has priority over the possible positive consequences for society through its destruction, such as in biomedical research.

The British Christian ethicist Robert Song states that 'it is my conviction that the arguments in favour of the personhood of the early embryo certainly are strong enough to sustain a reasonable doubt whether embryos may ever be subjected to lethal research'.[24] Again the ends do not justify the means.

With respect to the moral status of the early embryo developing inside its mother, O'Donovan further argues with respect to the foetus (though the argument is similar for embryos):

> To encourage or allow abortion because one does not know for certain that the fetus is a human being, is to engage in moral thought in a rare spirit of frivolity. In just such a spirit a rescue team might decide not to go out on a cold night if there was at least an even chance that the lost mountaineers were already dead.[25]

In a similar vein, Banner argues:

> In the present state of scientific knowledge we do not know what the outcome of the development of a particular embryo will be. It is, however, odd to argue from our uncertainty about whether something is true (i.e., whether the early embryo will finally become an individual human being) to its being false (i.e., that the early embryo is not an individual human being) or to its being permissible for us to act as if it were false.[26]

In this context, the act of killing an embryo does not only point to an action that may transgress a very serious moral imperative to protect human life, but may also reflect the character of the person who is prepared to undertake such an act.[27] As the German Roman Catholic theologian Bernhard Häring (1912–98) argued, 'every mortal attack upon a life which is at least probably an actual human life manifests the spirit and disposition of a murderer'.[28] Similarly, the Catholic philosopher and theologian Germain Grisez wrote that 'to be willing to kill what for all one knows is a person is to be willing to kill a person'.[29]

The Embryo and the God of Love

In the end, the only real value the human embryo can have is the same as that of any adult human person. It is a wonderful value, worth and meaning that can only come from the love of God whose existence will never be logically demonstrated. This means that it will never be possible to prove, scientifically, that an embryo or an adult human person has any value or worth. Without God, the whole universe is but a 'pile of dust', be it embryonic, post-natal or galactic. As Genesis 3.19 puts it, 'for dust you are and to dust you will return'.

In other words, in the same manner as it is a love for, and belief in, God, the Father, Son and Holy Spirit that gives meaning in life from a Christian perspective, it is also a belief in the inherent worth and value given by God to all his pre-natal and post-natal children that gives them meaning. It is because human beings are believed to be created in the image of God and out of his love that each member of humanity, including each embryo, has full inherent dignity and should be protected from destruction.

As Pope John Paul II said, 'when God turns his gaze on man, the first thing he sees and loves in him is not the deeds he succeeds in doing, but his own image'.[30] This affirms the supernatural and transcendent origins of genuine human dignity. As the British Christian scientist and bioethicist John Ling states:

> God made man as the pinnacle of His creation. We have extrinsic dignity – derived from the intrinsic dignity of the one whose image we bear. That is why each of us is unique and each of us is special – we are the bearers of the *imago Dei*.[31]

This is amazingly manifested in the birth and death of Jesus Christ whereby God demonstrated that he values and loves his children to such an extent that he was prepared to go to the cross for them.

Christ, as the perfect human being, was also the perfect image of God – an image that Adam had concealed through sin. Tertullian maintains, in his treatise on the resurrection of the body, that 'in whatever way the clay was pressed out, He [God] was thinking of Christ, the man who was one day to be: because the Word, too, was to be both clay and flesh'.[32]

As the Vatican's *Gaudium et Spes* further comments, 'human nature, by the very fact that it was assumed, not absorbed, in him has been raised in us also to a dignity beyond compare'. Through the incarnation, the Second Person of the Trinity has entered into solidarity with human beings so that 'he, the Son of God, has in a certain way united himself with each man'.[33] Though human beings gave themselves over to sin, they have been redeemed through the passion, death and resurrection of Jesus Christ. As Matthews explains, being 'destined to share eternal life in friendship with God, human beings journey towards this communion with Christ who is the perfect image of the Father'. And she adds: 'The solidarity of Christ with humanity sharpens, as it were, the image of God in human beings such that each person is called to see the other as another Christ.'[34]

This also means that the concepts both of inherent human dignity and of personhood do not rest on a human being's ability to do anything such as to reason, to practise autonomy or to communicate. Instead, they depend on and originate in God, who embraces the bearer of his divine image during all the stages of his or her existence on earth, through death and beyond.

Consequentially, it is not so much the value that other people or society give to the pre- and post-natal person that really matters, but the value that God gives to this individual through his relationship of love. McCarthy writes:

> Because of the continuity between the adult and the embryo, there is no reason for assuming that, even from the earliest moments of human existence, we are dealing with anything other than an embryonic person who, given the right environment, will become the adult human person whom all will acknowledge as fully and personally human. God's call to fellowship, rooted in eternity, must extend to every moment of this individual's life; even to the earliest moments following conception. For this reason, even though the embryo is not a person in the same way as is an adult, he or she is still a person as an embryo and is deserving of the same respect, dignity and sanctity as any other member of the human race.[35]

This means that the embryo is a person because God created this person to have a relationship of fellowship and love with him or her.

The act of creation by God of humanity and the incarnation implies that the human embryo is fully loved by God and has sacred, inviolable moral status from the very beginning of his or her creaturely embryonic existence.[36] Indeed, the crucial focus on humanity's creaturely relatedness to God has very important implications since all other aspects become secondary. This means that Schroten, for example, is misguided when he prioritizes other relationships, explaining: 'I propose not to treat a (pre) embryo in a test-tube as a future person, because one of the necessary conditions, namely the relationship with the future mother, has not yet been satisfied.'[37]

This is precisely the wrong conclusion relating to the moral status of the human embryo. Personal status cannot be determined by science or any biological development. As Wyatt argued:

> I therefore find myself driven by the thrust of the biblical material, by theological arguments and by the undeniable reality of widespread human intuitions about abortion, to the conclusion that we owe a duty of protection and care to the embryo and the early fetus as much as to the mature fetus and newborn baby. Even the earliest stages of human development deserve respect and protection. There is no point from fertilization onwards at which we can reliably conclude that a human being is not a member of the human family, one who is known and called by God, one with whom we are locked in community.[38]

In other words, no human being, even at the very early stages of embryonic development, should be treated in a manner that would violate the respect and protection due to his or her nature as a human person made in the image of God. This is because, from the moment of its creation, the human embryo is an organized, living unity. It has the right to be protected as any other human being and not used for the sole benefit of others in their quest, for example, of improved health and greater happiness.[39] As T. F. Torrance argued:

> The human embryo is fully *human being, personal being* in the sight and love of his or her Creator, and must be recognised, accepted, and cherished as such, not only by his or her mother and father, but by science and medicine.[40]

Theology has often struggled to understand the nature of the human person but it does recognize that persons are a unity of the transcendent: embodied souls and ensouled bodies. As such, seeking to understand or determine what makes human beings so special in a reductionist manner from both a scientific or spiritual perspective is impossible.[41] Human beings will always remain a mystery because they are created in the image of God whose very nature will always remain a mystery.

But although the very basis of the moral status of an embryo will never be completely determined, this does not mean that deliberately destroying an embryo with this mysterious image of God is an unimportant matter. This is because, as Kilner explains: 'Destroying someone in God's image, in light of God's connection with humanity, is tantamount to attacking God personally.'[42]

Moreover, because of the deep commitment of love that God has given to his image, he has also opened himself up to being vulnerable with this image. This also means that because God's throne in heaven is indestructible and totally secure, the only war against God that is open to rebellious human beings is a war against his image.[43] This may be one of the reasons why this image has come under so much attack in both history and modern society. In addition, if human embryos may be considered to reflect the image of God, as this study suggests, and they are deliberately being destroyed by society, then this may be just another front of the war against God personally. But it is also a front with which Christians should engage with God's help, love, compassion and wisdom.

This implies that the Christian Church should be profoundly challenged by the millions of human embryos which are being destroyed in countries such as the UK and the USA without the expression of any significant protest or compassion. As one member of the House of Lords, Lord Alton, said in 2012, the destruction of human embryos, human persons made in the image of God, has reached an 'industrial' scale in 'casual indifference'.[44] One of the moral measures of a Christian church is how it considers the smallest, weakest and most helpless individuals with the most vulnerable claims of personhood reflecting the image of God.

Notes

1 Colin E. Gunton, 1992, *Christ and Creation*, 1990 Didsbury Lectures, Carlisle: Paternoster Press, p. 123.

2 Thomas F. Torrance, 1984, *Transformation and Convergence in the Frame of Knowledge: Explorations in the Interrelations of Scientific and Theological Enterprise*, Belfast: Christian Journals, p. 263.

3 Peter Sedgwick, 1991, 'Theological Reflection', in Daniel Hardy and P. H. Sedgwick (eds), *The Weight of Glory, A Vision and Practice for Christian Faith: The Future of Liberal Theology*, Edinburgh: T&T Clark, p. 124.

4 Reports to the General Assembly of the Church of Scotland, 1985, p. 288.

5 Thomas F. Torrance, 2000, *The Being and Nature of the Unborn Child*, Edinburgh: Scottish Order of Christian Unity/Handsel Press, p. 4.

6 Andrew R. Rollinson, 'The Incarnation and the Status of the Human Embryo', thesis submitted for the degree of the M.Litt. with the Religious Studies Department of Newcastle University, November 1994, pp. 220-1.

7 Rollinson, 'Incarnation and Status', p. 219.

8 Oliver O'Donovan, 1984, *Begotten or Made?*, Oxford: Clarendon Press, p. 59.

9 O'Donovan, *Begotten or Made?*, p. 65.

10 John Stott, 1984, *Issues Facing Christians Today*, Basingstoke: Marshalls, p. 287.

11 Thomas F. Torrance, 1989, 'The Soul and Person in Theological Perspective in Religion, Reason and Self', in S. R. Sutherland and T. A. Roberts (eds), *Essays in Honour of Hywel D. Lewis*, Cardiff: University of Wales Press.

12 Rollinson, 'Incarnation and Status', p. 221.

13 Although penetration of an ovum membrane by spermatozoa can be defined precisely, the genetic contribution from the sperm and egg do not fuse until up to 24–7 hours later. Prior to this, paternal and maternal genetic contributions are still separate.

14 Helen Oppenheimer, 'Ourselves, Our Souls and Bodies', *Studies in Christian Ethics* 4 (1991), pp. 1–21 (p. 1).

15 In the same way as it is impossible to determine the precise moment of the death of an individual in the dying process, there is still a point in time, however, when it is possible to state for certain that an embryo exists or that death has occurred. It is interesting that the state of Victoria, Australia, known for its 'conservative' views, declared that the human embryo is deserving of protection in law only after the pronuclear fusion. P. Braude, 1989, 'Research on Early Embryos', in G. R. Dunstan and E. A. Shinebourne (eds), *Doctors' Decisions: Ethical Conflicts and Medical Practice*, Oxford: Oxford University Press, pp. 35–43.

16 'I believe it is ethically imperative that human dignity and integrity be rigorously safeguarded for present and future generations by banning destructive embryonic research or risky manipulation of human embryos.' Norman M. Ford, 2002, *The Prenatal Person: Ethics from Conception to Birth*, Oxford: Blackwell, pp. 64, 70.

17 John Wyatt, 1998, *Matters of Life and Death: Today's Healthcare Dilemmas in the Light of Christian Faith*, Leicester: Inter-Varsity Press, p. 152.

18 Wyatt, *Matters of Life*, p. 152.

19 Sacred Congregation for the Doctrine of the Faith, *Declaration on Procured Abortion*, 18 November 1974.

20 Congregation for the Doctrine of the Faith, Instruction on Respect for Human Life in its Origin and on the Dignity of Procreation *Donum Vitae* (22 February 1987), I, No. 1: *Acta Apostolicae Sedis* 80 (1988), pp. 78–9; John Paul II, *Evangelium Vitae* (25 March 1995), paragraph 60.

21 Jean Porter, 'Is the Embryo a Person? Arguing with the Catholic Traditions', *Commonweal* 129:3 (8 February 2002), pp. 8–10.

22 David A. Jones et al., 'A Theologian's Brief: On the Place of the Human Embryo Within the Christian Tradition and the Theological Principles for Evaluating Its Moral Status', *Ethics & Medicine* 17:3 (2001), pp. 143–53.

23 O'Donovan, *Begotten or Made?*, p. 66.

24 Robert Song, 2003, 'To Be Willing to Kill What for All One Knows Is a Person Is to Be Willing to Kill a Person', in B. Waters and R. Cole-Turner (eds), *God and the Embryo*, Washington, DC: Georgetown University Press, p. 103. Similarly Song notes: 'The substantive arguments in favor of embryo research may not be able to demonstrate embryonic non-personhood beyond reasonable doubt, and the substantive arguments against it may not be able to show that their scruples on behalf of embryos are reasonable' (p. 105).

25 Oliver O'Donovan, 1973, *The Christian and the Unborn Child*, Bramcote, Nottinghamshire: Grove Books, p. 5.

26 Michael Banner, 1999, *Christian Ethics and Contemporary Moral Problems*, Cambridge: Cambridge University Press, p. 112.

27 Neil Messer, 2011, *Respecting Life: Theology and Bioethics*, London: SCM Press, p. 117.

28 Bernhard Häring, 1963, *The Law of Christ: Moral Theology for Priests and Laity*. Cork, Ireland: Mercier Press, p. 206.

29 Germain Grisez, 1983, *The Way of the Lord Jesus*, Vol. 2. Quincy, IL: Franciscan Herald Press, p. 497. Quoted by Song, 'To Be Willing to Kill', p. 102.

30 Pope John Paul II, 'Mentally Ill Are Also Made in God's Image', *L'Osservatore Romano*, 11 December 1996.

31 John R. Ling, 2011, *When Does Human Life Begin?*, Newcastle upon Tyne: The Christian Institute, p. 8.

32 Tertullian, *On the Resurrection of the Flesh*, ch. 6.

33 Paul VI, *Gaudium et Spes* (7 December 1965), paragraph 22.

34 Pia Matthews, 'Human Dignity and the Profoundly Disabled', *Human Reproduction and Genetic Ethics* 17:2 (2011), pp. 185–203 (p. 197).

35 Brendan McCarthy, 1997, *Fertility & Faith*, Leicester: InterVarsity Press, pp. 124–5.

36 Thomas F. Torrance, 1984, *Test-tube Babies: Morals – Science – and the Law*, Edinburgh: Scottish Academic Press, p. 10.

37 Egbert Schroten, 'What Makes a Person?', *Theology* 97:776 (1994), p. 103.

38 Wyatt, *Matters of Life*, p. 173.

39 Reports to the General Assembly, 1985, p. 288.

40 Thomas F. Torrance, 1999, *The Soul and Person of the Unborn Child*, Edinburgh: Scottish Order of Christian Unity/Handsel Press, p. 19.

41 Pia Matthews, 'Discerning Persons: How the early theology can illuminate contemporary bioethical approaches to the concept of person', doctoral thesis, Saint Mary's University College, 2010, p. 9.

42 John F. Kilner, 2015, *Dignity and Destiny: Humanity in the Image of God*, Grand Rapids: Eerdmans, p. 319.

43 William E. Channing, 1841, 'Spiritual Freedom', in *The Works of William E. Channing*, Boston, MA: James Monroe, Vol. 4, p. 76, mentioned by Kilner, *Dignity and Destiny*, p. 117.

44 Andrew Hough, '1.7 million human embryos created for IVF thrown away', *Daily Telegraph*, 31 December 2012.

Appendix

The Moral Status of
New Kinds of Embryos

With the development of modern embryology, new kinds of biological entity are now being created for which it is very difficult to know, for certain, whether they can even be assimilated to living organisms and whether they can, as a result, be considered as embryos.[1] Many of these entities are severely compromised and, in some cases, divide only into a cluster of a few cells. Some have not even been created through fertilization but through other means such as cloning.

Because of this, their biological, moral and legal status remains unclear and is not likely to be resolved in any appropriate manner in the near future.[2] At present it is very difficult even to assess in many cases (1) when human life actually begins since, on a cellular level, early human life is a continuum, and (2) whether the entities obtained can even be considered as human embryos.

But when there is considerable uncertainty about whether an embryo is even present, the only appropriate and responsible way forward may be to give them the benefit of the doubt as to their moral status based on the precautionary principle. In this context, it should be noted that even with normally fertilized eggs it is difficult to know exactly when they become embryos during the first 24 hours after fertilization. Thus, it is likely that the exact moment when these new entities may become organisms will never be exactly determined since it will always be possible to reduce this moment to an ever smaller band of time.

Different Procedures for Creating New Kinds of Embryos

In the following section, a number of embryonic entities will be presented to inform a discussion about their nature and moral status. To do this, they will be classified by the number of persons who actually took part in bringing them into existence from a biological perspective. As will be seen, however, this is rather a loose form of classification and it is possible that some of these entities could be arranged in different groups or in another way based on different aspects of biology. For example, the cloning of a man could be considered the result of just one biological person who was responsible for providing the genetic material in the chromosomes. Or it could be considered the result of two biological persons if the chromosomes of a man and the empty egg of a woman are used in the cloning procedure.

Uniparental Embryos

Uniparental embryos are those in which only one person is responsible, from a biological perspective, for bringing into existence an embryo. These are quite rare in nature and usually do not take place in human beings.

The Creation of New Embryos through Parthenogenesis

Parthenogenesis, from the Greek words for 'virgin' and 'birth', is a procedure which tricks a female egg into becoming an embryo, on its own, as if it had been fertilized by sperm. This happens naturally with a number of female sap-sucking insects (aphids), some turkeys, several fish, certain forms of female reptiles[3] and other animals such as giant lizards. Different forms of parthenogenesis exist[4] and have been artificially induced in frogs and snakes although they quite often result in abnormal development.[5]

Embryonic parthenogenesis in mammals and even humans has been known to occur spontaneously in nature though no live births have ever been recorded.[6]

Using chemicals that mimic a sperm cell's fertilization properties, scientists in recent years have triggered artificial parthenogenesis in the eggs of a few mammals, including rabbits, cows, pigs and goats. But again, the resulting embryos have never developed beyond the early foetal stages.[7]

For example, researchers in the USA were reported in 2001 to have used chemical activation to trick unfertilized mouse eggs to develop into embryos with a full complement of two sets of chromosomes coming from the mother's chromosomes. Of 60 such embryos transferred into the reproductive tracts of female mice, 12 survived to the thirteenth day of gestation and were found to be developmentally normal (the full gestation period for a mouse is about 19–21 days).[8]

In the same year of 2001 other scientists from the USA were reported to have undertaken a similar experiment on 77 monkey eggs which were exposed to chemicals designed to trick them into the fertilization process. Only 28 of the eggs started dividing like embryos, with four continuing to develop up to about the 100-cell stage.[9]

Some experiments on human parthenogenesis have been undertaken with human eggs, which normally halve their genetic complement (going from 46 (diploid) to 23 chromosomes (haploid)) relatively late in their maturation cycle. This means that, if early activation is initiated by stimulating eggs that are still diploid to begin developing by forming new cells, a full set of chromosomes is retained in all the new cells. Alternatively, it is possible to stimulate a haploid egg with 23 chromosomes to replicate its genetic material, resulting in a full genetic complement of 46 chromosomes which can then develop into an embryonic entity.[10]

Scientists working with the company Advanced Cell Technology (ACT) in the USA were reported in 2001 to have used chemicals to stimulate human eggs to grow into embryo-like balls of about 100 cells. In this first creation of human parthenotes, the stimulus was applied before the eggs underwent the normal ejection of half their chromosomes, which typically occurs at the time of fertilization in order to accommodate the sperm's chromosomes.

In ACT's experiments, 22 eggs were exposed to chemical activation. After five days of growing in culture dishes, six eggs had developed into what appeared to be embryos, but none clearly contained the so-called inner cell mass.[11] But related research suggests the goal of obtaining stem cells from human parthenotes is achievable. In 2003, researchers from the biotech company Stemron in the USA reported that they had grown parthenogenetic human embryos to about the 100-cell stage.[12] A statement from ACT in December 2003 also indicated that they had managed to coax five out of eight human eggs into becoming 100-cell embryos through parthenogenesis.[13]

When parthenogenesis occurs naturally in humans the embryos may reach the stage of implantation but then do not survive early gestation.[14] Interestingly, as will be shown later, in the very rare case when a parthenogenetic human embryo fuses with a normal embryo giving rise to a chimeric individual, this new embryo can result in a living child.[15]

The above results indicate that it is impossible to come to a final conclusion as to whether parthenogenetic mammalian entities should be considered as living organisms expressing an integrated coordination of parts and be recognized, therefore, as embryos.[16] This means that, until further biological information is forthcoming, it may be appropriate to use the precautionary principle by giving them the benefit of the doubt for full moral status.

Bi-parental Unisexual Embryos

When an embryo is developed using the chromosomes of two sperm or two egg cells, respectively, originating from two different persons of the same sex, such an entity can be defined as a bi-parental unisexual embryo. If, on the other hand, two eggs are used from the same person, then they could be included in the previous section relating to uniparental embryos. Such embryos are very rare but should be mentioned in order to present a more complete picture of what is scientifically possible.

The Creation of New Embryos from the Association of Two Eggs

In order to create a female unisex embryo it is possible, in certain circumstances, for a female egg to be presented with the nucleus of another egg, which contains half the full set of chromosomes, and then left to develop.

In 2004, scientists from Japan were reported to have 'fertilized' a mouse egg with another mouse egg (which had been genetically modified) to give a mouse with two sets of chromosomes from two female mice (biparental gynogenones), rather than one from the mother and one from the father as happens in a normally fertilized embryo. This was the first time the procedure was successful in mammals.

To do this, the researchers injected the genetic material from immature mouse eggs (in which the expression of a key gene had been blocked) into mature eggs with their own set of chromosomes. They then 'activated' the combined eggs, prompting them to start growing as embryos which were then implanted into surrogate mice. As a result, just two out of 598 mice embryos were born alive.[17]

If this key gene in the immature mouse eggs is not blocked, however, the embryos formed from two eggs do not complete the normal stages of embryonic development.[18]

The Creation of New Embryos from the Association of Two Sperm Nuclei

Scientists from the company Advanced Cell Technology in the USA have speculated, in 2001, that it may be possible to transfer two sperm cell nuclei (containing half the chromosomes originating from a man), one of which should contain the X chromosome, into a donated egg stripped of its own nucleus which is then activated to give a male unisex (androgenetic) embryo.[19] However, it was recognized that a lot more research was necessary before such an embryo would be able to develop without any biological dysfunctions. Indeed, as will be discussed later, these entities are at risk of developing into hydatidiform moles.

With mice, reports show the ability of male unisex embryos (containing two sets of male chromosomes) to be produced by *in vitro* fertilization and to develop to day 9.5 of gestation.[20]

Complete Hydatidiform Moles

A complete hydatidiform mole is an embryonic entity which only contains chromosomes coming from sperm cells. They are formed by either:

1 two sperm cells fertilizing an egg which has lost its own chromosomes (or in which they are non-functional) and the chromosomes of these sperm cells fusing to from an entity with a full set of 46 chromosomes; or

2 androgenesis, whereby a single sperm cell fertilizes an egg which has lost its own chromosomes (or in which they are non-functional or have been expelled by the fertilization process) and the chromosomes of this sperm cell then duplicate to form an entity with a full set of 46 chromosomes.[21]

A complete hydatidiform mole usually results in a tumour-forming cell which is quite different from a one-cell embryo. The tumour cell develops and divides in a disorganized manner and does not result in an integrated whole which can be considered as an organism. Although it consists of human tissue, it is not a separate being and cannot be considered as a person. Hydatidiform moles actually grow relatively rapidly and, in some respects, can result in a similar experience to a pregnancy for a woman (they are often called 'molar pregnancies').[22] If this happens, they are usually evacuated as soon as possible from the woman to avoid risks of serious complications.

The Creation of New Embryos from the Association of Eggs with the Nuclei of Adult Cells

A team of reproductive biologists in Australia was reported, in 2001, to have injected adult mouse male cells (i.e. not sperm cells) into immature mouse eggs that still contained two sets of chromosomes.[23]

Unlike sperm, an adult cell has two sets of chromosomes. To overcome this problem, the team exploited the cellular machinery that is used by an unfertilized egg to eject a spare set of chromosomes when it encounters sperm. For example, during normal fertilization, two sets of chromosomes in an immature egg cell are separated, with one being ejected in a package that biologists call the polar body, leaving a single set of chromosomes to combine with another set from the sperm of the father.

But in this experiment, after 'fertilization' of the mouse egg by the adult male cell, the Australian scientists used chemicals to trick the egg to initiate the first steps of normal fertilization with the release of its spare set of chromosomes into a polar body. This time, however, the adult body cell also expelled its spare set into a second polar body. The researchers thus obtained two polar bodies and a fertilized egg, with one set of chromosomes from the mother and the second from the adult cell.

The fertilized egg went on to develop relatively normally for a few days in the laboratory (50 per cent reached the 16–32-cell stage), by which time the team considered transferring the embryos into the wombs of surrogate mice.[24] Whether the resulting embryos could have developed up to birth, however, was not demonstrated.[25]

The Creation of New Embryos from the Association of Eggs with Half the Genetic Material of Adult Cells

In a very similar experiment to the previous one, scientists from the USA in 2002 were reported to have created a procedure for any adult cell in a person's body to be used to fertilize a woman's egg. The method involves taking half the genetic material from a cell from an adult person by creating 'artificial sperm' and injecting it into a woman's egg, resulting in an embryo which contains half of the mother's chromosomes and half of the cell donor's chromosomes. After the process proved successful in experiments on mice, the method could theoretically be used with human eggs with the aim of producing functional human embryos.[26]

The Creation of New Embryos from the Association of Eggs Stripped of Their Chromosomes and the Nuclei of Adult Cells

In 1997, scientists in Scotland announced that a lamb called Dolly had been created through cloning.[27] In this procedure, the nucleus of an adult cell, which contains all the chromosomes of an adult sheep, was fused with an egg from another sheep which had been emptied of its own chromosomes. After being triggered by chemicals and an electric shock, the resulting entity was then made to develop into an embryo before being transferred into a surrogate sheep which gave birth to the lamb.

The Scottish experiment occurred after 277 nucleus fusions took place, whereby eight embryos were obtained but only one healthy lamb was born.

Since the creation of Dolly, researchers have cloned a number of large and small animals including sheep, goats, cows, mice, pigs, cats, dogs and rabbits.

Altered Nuclear Transfer

Altered Nuclear Transfer is a procedure in which the nucleus of an adult cell or the contents of an egg stripped of its chromosomes are modified so that when the two are brought together (in a similar manner to the cloning procedure) they do not produce a one-cell embryo. Instead it is suggested that they would produce a 'non-embryonic biological entity'.[28]

However, it is difficult to be certain with any confidence that only a non-embryo is created rather than just an embryo with a serious disorder,[29] and disagreement remains as to the exact nature of the entity.[30]

Bi-parental Bisexual Embryos

Bi-parental bisexual embryos are those in which two persons of different sex are responsible, from a biological perspective, for bringing them into existence. They may be formed by a number of procedures.

Normal Fertilization

When two persons of different sex are responsible for the development of an embryo, this is the usual manner in which an embryo is brought into existence. This has already been discussed at the beginning of the book in the section headed 'Early Embryonic Developments'.

Artificial Splitting of an Embryo

Another way of producing new embryos can be achieved by simply splitting an existing very early embryo in a laboratory to form new embryos. In a way, this is the artificial version of what already happens naturally in the creation of identical twins, triplets etc.

A good example of this procedure was reported in 2008 when the cells of a four-cell human embryo were isolated whereby each one then developed *in vitro* into a complete new embryo.[31]

The Creation of New Embryos by the Fertilization of a One-cell Haploid Parthenogenote by a Sperm Cell

Scientists in 2016 announced that they were able to fertilize a mouse one-cell haploid (containing half the full number of chromosomes) parthenote (an egg developing all by itself) with mouse sperm to give rise to an embryo which can later develop until birth.[32]

Partial Hydatidiform Moles

When two sperm cells both manage to fertilize the same egg, a partial hydatidiform mole may be obtained, resulting in an embryonic entity with three sets of 23 chromosomes, i.e. 69 chromosomes. Since the normal number of chromosomes in an embryo is only 46, the abnormality usually results in the death of the embryo either early in the pregnancy or, in some rare cases, as a more developed foetus. Because of the disorganization that arises in the development of the embryo or foetus, the partial hydatidiform mole usually presents itself as tumour cells to which is associated something that can be recognized as a foetus.[33] Unfortunately, in some situations, a partial hydatidiform mole could become life-threatening for the woman.

As a result of these observations, it may be appropriate to consider partial hydatidiform moles as embryonic organisms, i.e. as human embryos or foetuses. As such, they could be compared to the rare occurrence when children are born with cells containing three sets of 23 chromosomes (in which one set of chromosomes has replicated itself) but who do not, unfortunately, usually survive beyond ten months after birth.[34]

Tetraploid 'Embryos'

Tetraploid 'embryos' (with four sets of chromosomes) are sometimes created in the laboratory using mouse embryos. To create such entities, the two cells of a normal two-cell embryo created through fertilization are fused together and left to develop. Although it is unclear whether such an entity is an organism (i.e. a genuine embryo, since they usually only produce the cells forming the outer layer of an embryo, which provide nutrients, and not the body of a foetus), some have been known to develop without any additional cells to mid-gestation in mice with all the necessary organs and, in some rare cases, have even been known to be born alive. This may mean that some rare tetraploid entities are genuine embryos.[35]

Multi-parental Embryos

Multi-parental embryos are those in which more than two persons are responsible, from a biological perspective, for bringing into existence an embryo. They may be formed by a number of procedures.

Maternal Spindle and Cytoplasmic Transfer

New solutions have already been proposed to overcome some cases where women are unable to produce healthy eggs. For example, some procedures may enable a woman to have a child whom she may consider to be 'chromosomally her own' and who is free from some of the effects of mitochondrial disorders present in her eggs. Mitochondria are very small entities (containing 37 genes) found in all the cells of the human body giving them the energy to survive.[36]

The Nuffield Council on Bioethics in the UK has enumerated, in 2012, a number of procedures which could, speculatively, be considered in women unable to produce eggs with healthy mitochondria. These include:

- Maternal Spindle Transfer whereby the chromosomes of an unfertilized egg, containing dysfunctional mitochondria, from the woman wanting a child are transferred to another donated unfertilized egg, from a second woman, stripped of its own chromosomes and which contains healthy mitochondria.[37] Since the empty donated egg will be partly responsible for bringing into existence the future embryo, the woman providing the donor egg may be considered as a kind of biological 'mother' to the resulting child.
- Cytoplasmic Transfer whereby healthy cytoplasm, containing healthy mitochondria, is taken from a donated unfertilized egg and injected into the egg of a recipient woman wanting a child and who has difficulties in conceiving.[38] Since the cytoplasm from the donated egg will be partly responsible for bringing into existence the future embryo, the woman providing the donor cytoplasm may also be considered as a kind of biological 'mother' to the resulting child.

Maternal Spindle Transfer and Cytoplasmic Transfer would eventually give rise to children generated, from a biological perspective, from three different individuals (a chromosomal mother, a partial egg or cytoplasmic mother and a sperm father).

Pronuclear Transfer

Another procedure which could, speculatively, be considered in women unable to produce eggs with healthy mitochondria is called Pronuclear Transfer. In this, the 46 chromosomes of a fertilized egg, containing the dysfunctional mitochondria, from the woman wanting a child and her partner, are transferred to another donated fertilized egg, obtained from a second woman and a man's sperm, which was stripped of its own chromosomes and which contains healthy mitochondria.[39]

Pronuclear Transfer would eventually give rise to children generated, from a biological perspective, from several different individuals (a chromosomal mother, a chromosomal father, a partial egg mother and a sperm father). An example of this procedure in humans was reported in 2003 by researchers from China and the USA.[40]

The Creation of New Embryos from the Association of One-cell Embryos Stripped of Their Chromosomes and the Nuclei of Adult Cells

A very similar procedure to the previous Pronuclear Transfer method was announced in 2007 with mice when the chromosomes from an adult cell (instead of a fertilized egg) were transferred to another fertilized mouse egg which was stripped of its own chromosomes to form a new embryo.

When this procedure was replicated a number of times, the embryos obtained were shown to be able to develop into the birth of cloned mice.[41] However, this experiment did not seem to be successful when human material was used in 2011.[42]

The Creation of New Embryos from the Association of Two-cell Embryos Stripped of Their Chromosomes and the Nuclei of Adult Cells

Another very similar procedure to the previous one was announced in 2014 when the chromosomes from two adult mouse cells were transferred respectively to both the cells of a two-cell mouse embryo which had been stripped of their own chromosomes to form a new embryo. The research then showed that such embryos could develop to produce living mouse clones.[43]

The Creation of New Human–Human Hybrid Embryos

A number of procedures exist in the production of human embryonic combinations in which the genetic material would come from different sources and which may give rise to a limitless number of permutations.

The first kind of embryonic combination consists of human hybrid embryos, in which the genetic material from more than two persons would be combined inside all the cells of the embryos by transferring new chromosomes or changing the genes inside the chromosomes. For instance, it may be theoretically possible to create an embryo whose chromosomes originated from three or more persons.

The Creation of New Genetic Human–Human Chimeric Embryos[44]

The second kind of embryonic combination that may be created consists of chimeras, in which an embryo is formed through the combination of early embryonic cells originating from one or more other embryos.

The potential for cells from two different embryos to fuse and become a combination of individuals is well known in nature where genetic human–human chimeras can occur naturally when two different early embryos fuse in the womb a few days after conception.[45] The resulting babies contain genetic material from both embryos.

For example, this can take place when a woman produces two different eggs at the same time which are both fertilized by two different sperm cells into early embryos but which then combine naturally to give rise to one single (chimeric) embryo which develops into a being with two quite distinct genetic compositions.

This was noticed, for instance, when a 52-year-old woman with renal failure was being considered for a kidney transplant. During the initial process, medical tests were undertaken to examine whether any of her close relatives could be considered as a suitable kidney donor. But the results indicated that the woman could not have been the genetic mother of two of her three sons though they did all have the same father who was the husband of the woman.

This came as a very real shock to the woman who knew that she had conceived naturally with her husband and given birth to all three of her sons. After further tests, it was eventually discovered that the woman was a chimera, the result of two different embryos which had combined. She was, in fact, the result of the fusion in the womb of two non-identical embryonic twin sisters. Her body, including her ovaries which had produced her eggs, was a mixture of two genetically distinct lines of cells originating from the two embryos which had fused.[46]

If the embryos are of different sex, the babies are often noticed to resemble boys but have characteristics of both sexes.[47] For example, scientists in Scotland presented the case in 1998 of an otherwise unremarkable boy who was discovered to be a hermaphrodite. What was originally diagnosed as an un-descended testis turned out to be an ovary, a fallopian tube and part of a uterus. Further investigation revealed that some parts of his body were genetically female but the rest, which contained a different combination of his parents' genes, were male. He was believed to be the result of two eggs, fertilized by two different sperm cells, to form two embryos of different sex which then fused giving one single embryo inside his mother's womb.[48]

Another example was reported in 1995 by the same researchers in Scotland who described a boy who was partially parthenogenetic with cells from his blood and other tissues containing none of his father's chromosomes. Instead, they featured a duplicate set of one half of his mother's.[49] Although it is not unknown for an egg to start developing without being fertilized, it is believed that fully parthenogenetic human embryos cannot develop to term. The scientists suggested that the partially parthenogenetic boy owed his unusual genetic constitution to an egg that spontaneously divided, without fertilization, into two cells, one of which was fertilized. The second cell then copied its maternal chromosomes, allowing the resulting chimera to form a viable embryo.[50]

Artificial human–human embryonic chimeras were first reported in 2003. A team of scientists from the USA reported that they had made such chimeras by taking cells from three-day-old male embryos (consisting of around eight primitive cells) and combining them with female embryos at the same stage of development. The resulting embryos were part male, part female and could potentially have developed into healthy foetuses. The chimeras obtained in this way would have had four biological parents. After three days, the male cells appeared to be evenly distributed in a number of the chimeric embryos which were then destroyed.[51]

Another example of how artificial chimeras could be created is for some or all of the cells of the inner cell mass of an embryo at the blastocyst stage (containing about 100 cells) to be taken out and transferred to a second embryo from which its own inner cells had been removed. The new embryo would then be implanted and left to develop until birth.[52] In this regard, it should be noted that the cells of the inner cell mass of an embryo do not form an organism on their own. They can only do this if they are surrounded by the outer cells of the blastocyst.[53]

Human–Nonhuman Embryonic Combinations[54]

Interest in human–nonhuman embryonic combinations has recently been increasing in biomedical research. As a result, certain procedures have even been legalized in countries such as the United Kingdom.

However, defining the different kinds of human–nonhuman combination is a major challenge for both scientists and legislators, and one with direct practical consequences. Nevertheless, there have been attempts to clarify and standardize terminology, and these are surely to be welcomed.

The Creation of New Human–Nonhuman Chimeric Embryos

Human–nonhuman chimeric embryos are biological organisms that are made up of genetically distinct populations of human and nonhuman cells.

In 2003, scientists at the South Korean firm Maria Biotech were reported (without confirmation) to have injected human embryonic stem cells, labelled with a fluorescent protein, into 11 mouse blastocysts which later developed. The embryos were then carried by foster mice, whereby five offspring were born with fluorescence in tissues including the heart, bones, kidney and liver. However, the scientists terminated the project after having to address 'severe protests' from the public.[55]

Other researchers from the USA announced, in 2006, that human embryonic stem cells could engraft into mouse blastocysts where they proliferate and differentiate *in vitro* and persist in mouse–human embryonic chimeras that implant and develop in the uterus of foster mice. Interestingly, the scientists found that the human embryonic stem cells engrafted seemed to prefer occupying the inner cell mass of the mouse blastocysts which parallels that of their origin in human embryos. They did not contribute to the cells of the outer layers of the embryo. However, the researchers did indicate that the influence of these human embryonic stem cells seemed to disrupt, in most cases, the development of the human–mouse embryonic chimeras.[56]

The Creation of New Human–Nonhuman Hybrid Embryos

Human–nonhuman hybrid embryos are biological organisms in which most or all the cells have human and nonhuman origin. These include:

A *true hybrid,* whereby:

- a human ovum has been fertilized by sperm of a nonhuman life form;
- an ovum of a nonhuman life form has been fertilized by human sperm.

A combination created by the fusion of gametes from two different species represents an interspecies hybrid and sometimes the word 'hybrid' is used with this restricted use. However, because the word is often applied to a wider range of human–nonhuman combinations, the hybrid created by a fusion of gametes is sometimes referred to as a 'true hybrid'.

The 'Hamster Egg Penetration Test' (HEPT), in which human sperm is mixed with a hamster's egg, was one of the few valid tests available, in the past, to measure the viability of some patients' sperm. The hamster test was, in fact, a well established test in the UK used to examine the motility and normality of sperm.[57] Whereas the zona pellucida[58] of the ovum and the tip of the sperm are generally species specific, very closely related species such as the horse and the donkey can interbreed. The hamster is the only known exception to possess a removable zona pellucida which would otherwise repel the sperm from another species.

In the procedure, the hamster zona is removed following a specific biochemical treatment in order to undertake what is known as a zona free hamster oocyte penetration test which generally requires the mixing of 40 golden hamster eggs with a man's sperm. After being incubated for three hours or more at 37°C, the percentage of eggs that have been penetrated by the sperm is examined, on the basis of which a conclusion is made as to the fertility of this sperm. If the test is continued until 24 hours have elapsed following fusion, the embryo would normally have divided into two cells, at which stage it is destroyed.

The importance of the test is its value in studying the chromosomal constitution of human sperm, and hence the male contribution to genetic abnormalities and infertility, thought to affect one in 16 of the male population.[59]

It should be noted that the introduction of other fertility procedures has now made HEPT effectively obsolete for testing sperm prior to use in fertilization. A similar technique has sometimes been used in the UK for research into the viability of sperm. Although there are no current research projects licensed for HEPT in the UK, the case for its use is still legally valid.

A cybrid, whereby:

- the nucleus of a cell of a nonhuman life form has been introduced into a human ovum;
- the nucleus of a human cell has been introduced into an ovum of a nonhuman life form.

The company Advanced Cell Technology was reported, in 1999, to have created the first human embryo clone using human–nonhuman cybrid technology. This was achieved when the nucleus of an adult human cell was inserted into a cow's egg stripped of its chromosomes in order to create a cloned embryo. This embryo was then left to develop and divide for 12 days before being destroyed.[60]

Similarly, scientists in the USA claimed, in 2003, to have created around 200 cow–human cybrid embryos that lived for around two weeks and grew to several 100 cells in size and beyond the stage at which cells showed the first signs of development into tissue and organs. It was noted that they appeared to have normal human DNA.[61] The research team also indicated, in experiments published in 2006, that human mito-chondrial DNA was detected in almost all samples of interspecies cloned embryos, including morulae and blastocysts. This clearly indicated that mitochondria from the human donor cells were carried over to the enu-cleated bovine oocytes.[62]

In 2008, scientists in the UK claimed that they had created human–nonhuman cytoplasmic hybrids by injecting the nuclei of human skin cells into eggs taken from cow ovaries which had virtually all their genetic material removed.[63] The embryos survived for up to three days and were part of medical research into a range of illnesses. However, a team of scientists from Advanced Cell Technology in the USA reported in 2009 that human–cow hybrid embryos failed to grow beyond the 16-cell stage. They also failed to properly express genes thought to be critical for the creation of pluripotent cells.[64]

In 2003, scientists in China announced that rabbit–human cybrid embryos had been created by fusing adult human cells with rabbit eggs stripped of their chromosomes. Using donor cells from the foreskins of a five-year-old boy and two men, and facial tissue from a woman, the researchers created rabbit–human hybrid embryos which developed to the approximately 100-cell stage that forms after about four days of development. Moreover, the scientists claimed that they were able to derive human embryonic stem cells from these embryos which were simi-lar to those of conventional human embryonic stem cells, including the ability to undergo multilineage cellular differentiation.[65]

This research, nevertheless, has yet to be replicated by an independent group, though Hui Zhen Sheng's team did indicate that they were able to make new human–bovine cybrid embryos in 2008.[66] But again, a team of scientists from Advanced Cell Technology in the USA reported in 2009 that human–rabbit hybrid embryos failed to grow beyond the 16-cell stage. They also failed to properly express genes thought to be critical for the creation of pluripotent cells.[67]

Notes

1 Nancy L. Jones and William Cheshire, 'Can Artificial Techniques Supply Morally Neutral Human Embryos for Research? – Part 1. Creating Novel Categories of Human Embryos', *Ethics & Medicine* 21:1 (2005), pp. 29–40 (p. 30).

2 Maureen L. Condic, 2011, 'Preimplantation Stages of Human Development: The Biological and Moral Status of Early Embryos', in Antoine Suarez and Joachim Huarte (eds), *Is This Cell a Human Being?*, Berlin/Heidelberg: Springer, p. 25.

3 Christoph Vorburger, 'Geographic Parthenogenesis: Recurrent Patterns Down Under', *Current Biology* 16:16 (2006), R641–3; Robert G. Edwards, 'The Significance of Parthenogenetic Virgin Mothers in Bonnethead Sharks and Mice', *Reproductive Bio-Medicine Online* 15:1 (2007), pp. 12–15; T. V. Groot, E. Bruins and J. A. Breeuwer, 'Molecular Genetic Evidence for Parthenogenesis in the Burmese Python, Python Molurus Bivittatus', *Heredity* 90:2 (2003), pp. 130–5; G. Cassar, T. M. John and R. J. Etches, 'Observations on Ploidy of Cells and on Reproductive Performance in Parthenogenetic Turkeys', *Poultry Science* 77:10 (1998), pp. 1457–62.

4 The first is called heterozygous parthenogenesis in which the two sister chromatids of each maternal chromosome remain present in the egg. The second is called homozygotous parthenogenesis whereby, after the second chromatids of each chromosome have been extruded, the remaining ones duplicate themselves in the egg. See: A. Bos-Mikich et al., 'Parthenogenesis and Human Assisted Reproduction', *Stem Cells International* 2016 (2016).

5 'Scientists use "virgin birth" technique', *BBC News*, 26 November 2001, http://news.bbc.co.uk/1/hi/sci/tech/1676240.stm (accessed 2 January 2017).

6 N. J. Winston, P. R. Braude, S. J. Pickering, M. A. George, A. Cant, J. Currie and M. H. Johnson, 'The incidence of abnormal morphology and nucleocytoplasmic ratios in 2-, 3- and 5-day human pre-embryos', *Human Reproduction* 6:1 (1991), pp. 17–24.

7 Patrick Lee, 2011, 'Distinguishing Embryos from Non-embryos', in Suarez and Huarte, *Is This Cell a Human Being?*, p. 81.

8 P. Goodenough, 'Creating embryos without sperm could be ethical minefield', *CNSNews.com*, 25 October 2001, http://news.bbc.co.uk/1/hi/sci/tech/1794661.stm (accessed 2 January 2017).

9 'Unfertilised monkey eggs give stem cells', *BBC News*, 31 January 2002; Sylvia Pagan Westphal, 'Virgin birth method could found stem cells', *New Scientist* 178:2392 (26 April 2003); Kent E. Vrana et al., 'Nonhuman primate parthenogenetic stem cells', *Proceedings of the National Academy of Sciences USA* 100: suppl. 1 (2003), pp. 11911–16.

10 Jones and Cheshire, 'Can Artifical Techniques', p. 32.

11 'Scientists use "virgin birth" technique'.

12 H. Lin et al., 'Multilineage Potential of Homozygous Stem Cells Derived from Metaphase II Oocytes', *Stem Cells* 21 (2003), pp. 152–61.

13 'Human cloning experiment repeated successfully', *CNN.com*, 16 December 2003, http://edition.cnn.com/2003/HEALTH/12/16/science.clones.reut/ (accessed 5 January 2017).

14 L. I. Penkov and E. S. Platonov, 'New DA. Prolonged Development of Normal and Parthenogenetic Postimplantation Mouse Embryos *in vitro*', *International Journal of Developmental Biology* 39:6 (1995), pp. 985–91.

15 L. Strain, J. P. Warner, T. Johnston and D. T. Bonthron, 'A human parthenogenetic chimaera', *Nature Genetics* 11:2 (1995), pp. 164–9.

16 See the discussion of human parthenogenesis in Mahendra Rao and Maureen L. Condic, 'Alternative Sources of Pluripotent Stem Cells: Scientific Solutions to an Ethical Dilemma', *Stem Cells and Development* 17:1 (2008), pp. 1–10; Maureen L. Condic, 'When Does Human Life Begin? A Scientific Perspective', White Paper, *The Westchester Institute for Ethics & The Human Person* 1:1 (2008), 1–18 (p. 9).

17 H. Pearson, 'Mouse created without father', *Nature*, 22 April 2004, http://www.nature.com/news/2004/040422/news040419-8.html (accessed 2 January 2017); T. Kono et al., 'Birth of parthenogenetic mice that can develop to adulthood', *Nature* 428:6985 (2004), pp. 860–4.

18 J. McGrath and D. Solter, 'Completion of mouse embryogenesis requires both the maternal and paternal genomes', *Cell* 37:1 (1984), pp. 179–83; M. A. H. Surani, S. C. Barton and M. L. Norris, 'Development of reconstituted mouse eggs suggests imprinting of the genome during gametogenesis', *Nature* 308:5959 (1984), pp. 548–50.

19 'Cloning still to prove itself', *BBC News*, 25 November 2001, http://news.bbc.co.uk/1/hi/sci/tech/1675906.stm (accessed 2 January 2017); Jones and Cheshire, 'Can Artificial Techniques', p. 34. A similar proposal was made by Calum MacKellar in 2000 who suggested that the nucleus of a sperm cell could be transferred into an egg emptied of its own chromosomes to form a 'male egg' which could then be fertilized by another sperm cell. See M. Henderson, 'Male couples could have own babies', *The Times*, 25 September 2000.

20 Y. Obata, Y. Ono, H. Akuzawa, O. Y. Kwon, M. Yoshizawa and T. Kono, 'Post-implantation development of mouse androgenetic embryos produced by *in-vitro* fertilization of enucleated oocytes', *Human Reproduction* 15:4 (2000), pp. 874–80.

21 Lee, 'Distinguishing Embryos from Non-embryos', pp. 79–80.

22 Condic, 'When Does Human Life Begin?', p. 10.

23 C. Dennis, 'Developmental biology: Synthetic sex cells', *Nature* 424:6947 (2003), pp. 364–6.

24 R. Highfiles, 'How to make babies without a man', *Daily Telegraph*, 10 July 2001; O. Lacham-Kaplan, R. Daniels and A. Trounson, 'Fertilization of mouse oocytes using somatic cells as male germ cells', *Reproductive BioMedicine Online* 3:3 (2001), pp. 205–11.

25 Dennis, 'Developmental biology'.

26 'Lesbian couples "could have own baby"', *BBC News*, 18 January 2002, http://news.bbc.co.uk/1/hi/sci/tech/1769356.stm (accessed 2 January 2017). See also 'Process may help men and lesbians father children', *Washington Times*, 27 January 2002.

27 I. Wilmut, A. E. Schnieke, J. McWhir, A. J. Kind and K. H. Campbell, 'Viable offspring derived from fetal and adult mammalian cells', *Nature* 385:6619 (1997), pp. 810–13.

28 William B. Hurlbut, 'Alterest Nuclear Transfer', *Stem Cell Reviews* 1:4 (2005), pp. 293–300; M. L. Condic, 'Alternative sources of pluripotent stem cells: altered nuclear transfer', *Cell Proliferation* 41 (2008), pp. 7–19.

29 Condic, 'Alternative sources'.

30 Lee, 'Distinguishing Embryos', pp. 84–5.

31 H. Van de Velde et al., 'The four blastomeres of a 4-cell stage human embryo are able to develop individually into blastocysts with inner cell mass and trophectoderm', *Human Reproduction* 23:8 (2008), pp. 1742–7. See also M. Geens et al., 'Human embryonic stem cell lines derived from single blastomeres of two 4-cell stage embryos', *Human Reproduction* 24:11 (2009), pp. 2709–17.

32 T. Suzuki et al., 'Mice produced by mitotic reprogramming of sperm injected into haploid parthenogenotes', *Nature Communications* 7:12676 (2016).

33 Nicanor Pier Giorgio Austriaco, 2011, 'Complete Moles and Pathenotes Are Not Organisms', in Suarez and Huarte, *Is This Cell a Human Being?*, p. 46.

34 J. Sherard et al., 'Long survival in a 69, XXY triploid male', *American Journal of Medical Genetics* 25 (1986), pp. 307–12; Austriaco, 'Complete Moles and Pathenotes', p. 47.

35 Lee, 'Distinguishing Embryos', p. 89.

36 Mitochondria are very small entities found in all the cells of the human body and constitute 15 to 35 per cent of a cell's total mass. Depending on its function, a cell may contain a few hundred to several thousand mitochondria. They are considered to be the power source of the cells giving them the energy to survive. But for a cell to function and replicate properly, the 37 genes in every mitochondria must interact correctly with the 20,000–30,000 genes in its chromosomes.

37 Nuffield Council on Bioethics, 2012, *Novel Techniques for the Prevention of Mitochondrial DNA Disorders: An Ethical Review*, London: Nuffield Council on Bioethics, pp. 34–6.

38 Nuffield Council on Bioethics, *Novel Techniques*, pp. 36–9.

39 Nuffield Council on Bioethics, *Novel Techniques*, pp. 32–4.

40 The researchers, first of all, fertilized the eggs of five infertile women with their husbands' sperm through IVF, creating one-cell embryos and, in addition, fertilized the eggs of a fertile woman with sperm from anonymous donors.

The scientists then transferred the 'pronuclei' (the combined set of maternal and paternal chromosomes) of the fertilized eggs resulting from the infertile women into the fertilized eggs created with the eggs of the fertile woman whose own pronuclei had been removed. Finally, these fertilized eggs were implanted into the wombs of the infertile women, whereby one 30-year old woman became pregnant with triplets.

After a month of pregnancy, one of the foetuses was selectively terminated to increase the chances of survival for the other two. But after 24 weeks of pregnancy, one of the remaining foetuses was delivered prematurely because of ruptured membranes and died of 'respiratory distress'. As a result of a 'silent infection' triggered by the miscarriage, the last remaining foetus was delivered stillborn at 29 weeks' gestation. The researchers indicated that there was no evidence to suggest that the technique itself was the problem.

Rick Weiss, 'Woman Became Pregnant Through Egg Transfer Technique but Lost All Three Fetuses', *Washington Post*, 14 October 2003, p. A10.

41 D. Egli et al., 'Developmental reprogramming after chromosome transfer into mitotic mouse zygotes', *Nature* 447:7145 (2007), pp. 679–85.

42 D. Egli et al., 'Reprogramming within hours following nuclear transfer into mouse but not human zygotes', *Nature Communications* 2:488 (2011), p. 488.

43 E. Kang et al., 'Nuclear reprogramming by interphase cytoplasm of two-cell mouse embryos', *Nature* 509:7498 (2014), pp. 101–04.

44 Chimeras generally represent organisms containing cells of different genetic origins.

45 Jones and Cheshire, 'Can Artificial Techniques'.

46 Neng Yu et al., 'Disputed Maternity Leading to Identification of Tetragametic Chimerism', *New England Journal of Medicine* 346:20 (2002), pp. 1545–52. See also Jessica Richardson, 'Man fails paternity test due to passing on unborn twin's DNA', *BioNews* 826 (2 November 2015).

47 D. Derbyshire, 'Test-tube "monster" condemned by scientists', *Daily Telegraph*, 3 July 2003.

48 L. Strain, J. C. S. Dean, M. P. R. Hamilton and D. T. Bonthron, 'A true hermaphrodite chimera resulting from embryo amalgamation after *in vitro* fertilization', *New England Journal of Medicine* 338:3 (1998), pp. 166–9.

49 L. Strain, J. P. Warner, T. Johnston and D. T. Bonthron, 'A human parthenogenetic chimaera', *Nature Genetics* 11 (1995), pp. 164–9.

50 H. Pearson, 'Human genetics: Dual identities', *Nature* 417:6884 (2002), pp. 10–11.

51 Derbyshire, 'Test-tube "monster"'; 'Mixed-sex human embryo created', *BBC News*, 3 July 2003, http://news.bbc.co.uk/1/hi/health/3036458.stm (accessed 2 January 2017).

52 Antoine Suarez, 2011, 'Is This Cell Entity a Human Being? Neural Activity, Spiritual Soul, and the Status of the Inner Cell Mass and Pluripotent Stem Cell', in Suarez and Huarte, *Is This Cell a Human Being?*, p. 181; Y. Nakamura et al., 'A tetraploid liveborn neonate: cytogenetic and autopsy findings', *Archives of Pathology Laboratory Medicine*, 127 (2003), pp. 1612–14; Condic, 'Preimplantation Stages', p. 36.

53 Austriaco, 'Complete Moles and Pathenotes', p. 52.

54 This section was based on Calum MacKellar and David Albert Jones (eds), 2012, *Chimera's Children: Ethical, Philosophical and Religious Perspectives on Human–Nonhuman Experimentation*, London: Continuum.

55 N. Boyce, 'Mixing species – and crossing a line?', *usnews.com*, 27 October 2003.

56 D. James, S. A. Noggle, T. Swigut and A. H. Brivanlou, 'Contribution of human embryonic stem cells to mouse blastocysts', *Developmental Biology* 295:1 (2006), pp. 90–102.

57 This is variously known as 'Hamster Egg Penetration Test' (HEPT), the 'Hamster Zona-Free Ovum test' (HZFO test), or the 'Sperm Penetration Assay' (SPA). It is a test of the ability of a man's sperm to penetrate a hamster egg that has been stripped of its outer layer, the 'zona pellucida'. The test focuses on the ability of the sperm to begin the process of fertilization by progressing through the membrane of the egg – in scientific terminology it tests the sperm's ability to 'undergo capacitation and the acrosome reaction'.

58 The zona pellucida is a membrane surrounding an ovum and is vital for its survival and enabling fertilization. In humans, five days after fertilization the membrane degenerates and decomposes to be replaced by the underlying layer of trophoblastic cells.

59 R. G. Lee and D. Morgan, 2001, *Human Fertilisation & Embryology: Regulating the Reproductive Revolution*, London: Blackstone Press, pp. 89–90.

60 'Company "cloned human cells"', *BBC News*, 13 November 1998, http://news.bbc.co.uk/1/hi/sci/tech/213663.stm (accessed 2 January 2017); 'Details of hybrid clone revealed', *BBC News*, 18 June 1999, http://news.bbc.co.uk/1/hi/sci/tech/371378.stm (accessed 2 January 2017).

61 A. Coghlan, 'First human clone embryo ready for implantation', *NewScientist.com*, 15 September 2003; J. Leake, 'Cloning expert claims to have created "human-cow" embryo', *Times Online*, 14 September 2003.

62 K. Illmensee, M. Levanduski and P. M. Zavos, 'Evaluation of the embryonic pre-implantation potential of human adult somatic cells via an embryo interspecies bioassay using bovine oocytes', *Fertility and Sterility*, 85: suppl. 1 (2006), pp. 1248–60.

63 'UK's first hybrid embryos created', *BBC News*, 1 April 2008, http://news.bbc.co.uk/1/hi/health/7323298.stm (accessed 2 January 2017).

64 Y. Chung et al., 'Reprogramming of Human Somatic Cells Using Human and Animal Oocytes', *Cloning and Stem Cells* 11:2 (2009), pp. 213–23.

65 A. Abbott and D. Cyranoski, 'China plans "hybrid" embryonic stem cells', *Nature* 413:6854 (2001), p. 339; H.-Z. Sheng et al., 'Embryonic stem cells generated by nuclear transfer of human somatic nuclei into rabbit oocytes', *Cell Research* 13:4 (2003), pp. 251–64.

66 H.-Z. Sheng et al., 'Activation of human embryonic gene expression in cytoplasmic hybrid embryos constructed between bovine oocytes and human fibroblasts', *Cloning and Stem Cells* 10:3 (2008), pp. 297–305.

67 Y. Chung et al., 'Reprogramming of Human Somatic Cells'.

Glossary

Aneuploidy: a condition in which the number of chromosomes in the cell differs from the normal number.

Assisted Reproductive Technologies (ARTs): the collective name for all artificial procedures used to assist women to bear children.

Blastocyst: a hollow ball of 50 to 120 cells obtained after about four to five days of human embryonic development just before implantation in the uterus. It includes the inner cell mass (a group of cells in the blastocyst which would eventually develop into the foetus and some of the surrounding membranes) and trophoblast cells (which form the outer layer of a blastocyst).

Blastomere: a single cell in an embryo just after fertilization.

Cell line: cells of common descent and type cultured in the laboratory.

Cell nuclear replacement (also called somatic cell nuclear transfer): the procedure of replacing the cell nucleus of an egg with the nucleus from another cell.

Cell type: one of over 200 different types of cell in the human body such as blood cells, liver cells and neuronal cells. Each of these cell types has a different subset of genes switched on ('expressed') and therefore specific characteristics which allow these cells to serve a specific function in the body.

Chimera: an organism composed of cells derived from at least two genetically different cell types. The cells could be from the same or separate species.

Chromosome: a feature of all plant and animal cells composed of DNA and protein. Chromosomes carry the information necessary for the development and functioning of the body. Humans normally have 46 chromosomes in the nucleus of their body's cells (22 pairs plus two sex chromosomes, denoted X or Y) which contain the 20,000 to 25,000 human genes.

Clone: a cell or organism derived from, and genetically identical to, another cell or organism.

Congenital: refers to a characteristic present at birth, though not necessarily evident at birth. Often used in the context of negative traits, i.e., 'congenital malformations', deformities, diseases, etc. but perceived positive conditions may also be congenital.

Cytoplasm: a gel-like substance surrounding the nucleus inside the cell.

Dedifferentiation: the process of inducing a specialized cell to revert towards pluripotency.

Differentiation: the process by which less specialized cells develop into more specialized cell types.

Diploid: having the normal two sets of chromosomes, usually one paternal and one maternal.

DNA: deoxyribonucleic acid – the cell's and the body's genetic material.

Ectoderm: the outermost of the three primitive germ layers of the embryo. It gives rise to skin, nerves and brain, and appears about 16 days after fertilization for the human embryo.

Egg: the gamete produced by a woman during her monthly cycle. The nucleus of an egg contains an X chromosome, having 23 chromosomes in all.

Embryo (human): a human being during the first 56 days (eight weeks) of his or her development following his or her creation, excluding any time during which the development has been suspended.

Embryo biopsy: removal and examination of one or more cells from a developing embryo for diagnostic purposes.

Embryonic stem cells (ES cells): cells originating from an embryo which can proliferate indefinitely and differentiate into many different tissues. These are pluripotent cells.

Endoderm: the innermost of the three primitive germ layers of the embryo. It later gives rise to the lungs, liver and digestive organs and appears about 16 days after fertilization for the human embryo.

Enhypostasis: describes the reality that the humanity of Jesus had real personal being in the person of the Son as a result of the incarnation.

Enucleated: describes a cell (usually an egg cell) from which the nucleus, containing all the chromosomes, has been removed.

Epistemology: describes the philosophy of knowledge, its nature, methods, sources and limits.

Fertilization: the joining of a sperm cell and an egg to produce an embryo. Naturally, fertilization occurs in the woman's body (*in vivo*) but it can also occur in the laboratory (*in vitro*).

Foetus: the developed embryo at eight–nine weeks of gestation. By this time, different tissues have begun to differentiate.

Gametes: the general term for eggs and sperm cells. A gamete usually has half the number of chromosomes of any other cell.

Gastrulation: the procedure by which an animal embryo at an early stage of development produces the three primary germ layers, ectoderm, mesoderm and endoderm. This takes place about 16 days after fertilization for the human embryo.

Gene: the genetic information required to form a protein.

Genome: the complete genetic material or make-up of an individual.

Germ line: the cells of an organism which, during the usual course of reproduction, may pass on their genetic material to progeny.

Haploid: having one set of chromosomes as normally carried by a sperm cell or egg.

Hydatidiform mole: a mass of cells in the uterus growing in clusters resembling grapes. Such an entity often results from dysfunctional fertilization.

Hypostasis: describes the unique reality or 'personal subsistence' of the three persons in the one essential being of God. The formula 'three hypostasis in one ousia', or 'three persons in one being', became the orthodox doctrine of the Trinity in Christianity since the Council of Constantinople in 381.

Hypostatic union: describes the two distinct natures, divine and human, in the one person of Jesus.

Implantation: a process which lasts about one week, beginning when the blastocyst attaches to the wall of the uterus of the woman and ending when the embryo is fully embedded in the wall of the uterus, or exceptionally in an extra-uterine place.

Inner cell mass (ICM): a group of cells in the blastocyst which eventually develop into the foetus and some of the surrounding membranes. The cells of the inner cell mass are pluripotent. They are not totipotent because they cannot develop into a foetus on their own.

Insemination: the introduction of sperm into a woman's body to create a pregnancy. Artificial insemination can be done using either freshly ejaculated sperm or sperm that has been frozen. Where the sperm of a donor is used (donor insemination or DI) this will usually have been frozen, to allow time for the donor to be screened for transmissible diseases, before insemination takes place.

In vitro **fertilization (IVF):** a common technique for overcoming infertility whereby eggs are collected from the woman and fertilized with sperm in the laboratory. Up to two resulting embryos are then generally transferred to the woman's uterus to begin a pregnancy.

Kenotic theory: the theory that, when Christ became man, he emptied himself in some sense of his divinity or of some of his divine characteristics in order to become human with limited knowledge and power.

Meiosis: the process by which germ cells (i.e. reproductive cells from the ovary or the testes) divide to produce haploid gametes (those which contain only one set of chromosomes resulting from the recombination between the maternal and paternal chromosome sets of an organism).

Mitosis: the process that takes place in the nucleus of a dividing adult cell which results in the formation of two new nuclei each having the same number of chromosomes as the original parent nucleus.

Monogenic disorders: disorders arising from defects in a single gene.

Monozygotic: derived from one zygote (a fertilized egg).

Mesoderm: the middle layer of the embryonic disc, which consists of a group of cells derived from the inner cell mass of the blastocyst. It is formed at gastrulation and is the precursor to bone, muscle and connective tissue; it appears about 16 days after fertilization for the human embryo.

Mitochondria: present in all cells, they are sometimes described as 'cellular power plants' because they convert organic materials into energy. They do not form part of the nucleus (containing the chromosomes) of a cell but contain 37 genes.

Morula: a solid mass of 16–32 cells resulting from the cell division of a zygote (a fertilized egg).

Multipotent: having the capacity to develop into multiple (but not all) cell types.

Nucleus: a cellular organelle enclosed in a membrane which contains the chromosomes of a cell.

GLOSSARY

Ontological: describes the very nature of things in their being or inner reality.

Onto-relations: the idea that a person is intrinsically defined by relationships with other persons.

Oocyte: immature female egg.

Ovum (pl. ova): mature female egg (mature oocyte) possessing a genome reduced by half (haploid genome), i.e. normally 23 chromosomes in humans.

Parthenote: a living entity usually formed by the development of an unfertilized egg by itself.

Pelagianism: the belief in a human capacity and freedom to cooperate with divine grace for salvation (originating from Pelagius, *c.* 354–415).

Perichoresis: the mutual indwelling and communion of the persons of the Father, Son and Holy Spirit, who share the same nature, will and acts in the one God.

Personhood: the status of being a person (often in the context of having rights).

Pluripotent: having the capacity to develop into every cell type in the human body, but not the extra-embryonic tissues such as the placenta and the umbilical cord.

Pre-implantation genetic diagnosis: the use of genetic testing on a live embryo to determine the presence, absence or change in a particular gene or chromosome prior to implantation of the embryo in the uterus of a woman.

Pre-natal diagnosis: a procedure that aims to provide a diagnosis of a particular condition that the foetus might have. There are two primary types:

1 Amniocentesis – This method involves examining foetal cells taken between 15 and 16 weeks of pregnancy from the amniotic fluid which surrounds the foetus. The foetal cells are cultured and the genetic make-up of the foetus determined. This allows testing for chromosomal abnormalities such as Down's syndrome and other birth defects.
2 Chorionic Villus Sampling (CVS) – This method involves the removal of a small sample of placental tissue between 9 and 11 weeks of pregnancy which is tested for genetic abnormalities.

Pre-natal screening: a public health service that offers pregnant women a test to see if the baby is at an increased risk of having a particular disorder such as Down's syndrome. If a screening test reveals an increased risk, it is followed by the offer of a diagnostic test to clarify the cause of the screening test results and any implications for the health of the baby.

Primates: the group of mammals which includes monkeys, apes and humans.

Primitive streak: appears around the fourteenth day after creation of the embryo in humans. This is the latest stage at which identical twins can occur. The streak includes precursor cells to the spinal cord.

Pronucleus (pl. pronuclei): the haploid nucleus (containing only half the chromosomes) of the egg and the sperm cell after fertilization but before the dissolution of their membranes and the first division of the fertilized egg.

Providence: that activity by which God holds in being the order of creation including the human and nonhuman realms.

Redifferentiation: the process of inducing a dedifferentiated cell to differentiate into a specialized cell type (usually different from the original).

Replication: the production of two identical DNA molecules from an original DNA molecule.

RNA: ribonucleic acid – a molecule essential for the functioning of genes.

Somatic cells: all body cells that are not part of the germ line.

Sperm cell: the gamete produced by the male, usually through ejaculation. Millions of sperm cells are present in each ejaculate and roughly half of these will carry X chromosomes, the other half carrying Y chromosomes.

Spermatid: immature spermatozoon. Haploid (having one set of chromosomes) germ cell resulting from the second meiotic division of spermatogenesis which will then differentiate into spermatozoa.

Spermatocyte: diploid (having two sets of chromosomes) germ cell which will undergo two meiotic divisions to give haploid spermatids.

Spermatozoon (pl. spermatozoa): male germ cell (cells).

Stem cell: a cell that has the ability to divide for an indefinite period *in vivo* or in culture and to give rise to specialized cells.

Syngamy: the mingling of the male and female haploid chromosome following the breakdown of the pronuclear membranes approximately 24 hours after the fusion between the sperm cell and egg. This results in the formation of the zygote.

Teleology: the doctrine of the end of history or the interpretation of history with respect to its ends, purpose or goals.

Teratoma: an uncontrolled growth of cells that are the result of an abnormal fertilization without any potential to develop into an embryo proper.

Totipotent: demonstrates the ability of a cell to develop into every cell type required for human development, including extra-embryonic tissues, and to produce a fertile, adult individual. An individual cell that is totipotent and on its own is also a one-cell embryo; i.e. a cell that is capable of generating a globally coordinated developmental sequence.

Transcription: the synthesis of RNA under the direction of DNA.

Trophectoderm: the extra-embryonic part of the ectoderm of mammalian embryos at the blastocyst stage before the mesoderm becomes associated with the ectoderm. It is the cell layer from which the trophoblast differentiates (i.e. the trophectoderm is formed from trophoblasts). The trophectoderm is responsible for the nutritional supply and for implanting the embryo into the uterus.

Trophoblasts (from Greek *threphein*, to feed, and *blastos*, germinator): cells forming the outer layer of a blastocyst, which provide nutrients to the embryo and develop into a large part of the placenta. They are formed during the first stage of pregnancy and are the first cells to differentiate from the fertilized egg. Trophoblasts mediate the implantation of the embryo into the endometrium, but they are never incorporated into the mother's body or the foetus. They are not foetal cells. Trophoblasts become inert during pregnancy and are completely rejected by the foetus and mother at delivery.

Zona pellucida: a thick, transparent layer surrounding the oocyte, zygote and early embryo. It degenerates after several days allowing the embryo to emerge and bind to the uterus.

Zygote: the final stage of fertilization, the single cell formed when the two sets of chromosomes, one from the male sperm cell, the other from the female egg, have joined.

Index

Printed in the USA
CPSIA information can be obtained
at www.ICGtesting.com
LVHW042052121023
760842LV00004B/391

9 780334 055217